Symptom Management in Advanced Cancer

Fourth edition

Robert Twycross DM Oxon, FRCP London
Emeritus Clinical Reader in Palliative Medicine,
Oxford University

Andrew Wilcock DM Nottm, FRCP London
Macmillan Clinical Reader in Palliative Medicine and Medical
Oncology, Nottingham University
Consultant Physician, Hayward House, Nottingham University
Hospitals NHS Trust, City Campus

Claire Stark Toller BM, BCh MA MRCP
Specialist Registrar in Palliative Medicine,
Oxford Postgraduate Deanery

Published by palliativedrugs.com Ltd.

Palliativedrugs.com Ltd
Hayward House Study Centre
Nottingham University Hospitals NHS Trust, City Campus
Nottingham NG5 1PB
United Kingdom

www.palliativedrugs.com

First edition 1995
Second edition 1997
Third edition 2001
Revised and reprinted 2002

British Library Cataloguing in Publication Data

A catalogue record for this book is available from the British Library.

ISBN 978-0-9552547-3-4

Typeset by Alden Prepress Services Private Limited, Chennai, India
Printed by Halstan Printing Group, Amersham, UK.

DISCLAIMER

Every effort has been made to ensure the accuracy of this text, and that the best information available has been used. However, palliativedrugs.com Ltd. neither represents nor guarantees that the practices described herein will, if followed, ensure safe and effective patient care. The recommendations contained in this book reflect the authors' judgement regarding the state of general knowledge and practice in the field as of the date of publication. Recommendations such as those contained in this book can never be all-inclusive, and therefore will not be appropriate in all and every circumstance. Those who use this book should make their own determinations regarding specific safe and appropriate patient-care practices, taking into account the personnel, equipment, and practices available at the hospital or other facility at which they are located. Neither palliativedrugs.com Ltd. nor the authors can be held responsible for any liability incurred as a consequence of the use or application of any of the contents of this book. Mention of specific drug product brands does not imply endorsement. As always, doctors are advised to make themselves familiar with the manufacturer's recommendations and precautions before prescribing any drug or using any device.

CONTENTS

Contents

PREFACE

Symptom Management in Advanced Cancer is the companion volume to the *Palliative Care Formulary (PCF)*. More information about the drugs (or classes of drug) referred to in *Symptom Management in Advanced Cancer* can be found in the *Palliative Care Formulary, 3rd edition (PCF3)*, and on the website www.palliativedrugs.com.

Symptom Management in Advanced Cancer is written primarily for doctors, but will also be of value to nurses working with cancer patients, particularly in palliative care. It provides a framework of knowledge which will enable both doctors and nurses to develop a scientific and systematic approach to the management of symptoms in advanced cancer.

In palliative care, many drugs are used 'beyond the licence' or 'off label'. For example, few drugs are licensed (labelled) for use by continuous subcutaneous infusion (CSCI) but many are given this way. Because of the costs involved, it is unlikely that this situation will ever be rectified. Unlicensed use is not routinely indicated in *Symptom Management in Advanced Cancer*. However, details of licensed and unlicensed indications are given in *PCF3* (and the *Hospice and Palliative Care Formulary USA, 2nd edition*), and on www.palliativedrugs.com.

Physicians have a duty in common law to act with reasonable care and skill in a manner consistent with the practice of professional colleagues of similar standing. Thus, when prescribing outside the terms of a licence, doctors must be fully informed about the actions and uses of the drug and be assured of the quality of the particular product.

For this fourth edition of *Symptom Management in Advanced Cancer*, the authorship has been extended to ensure continuity for the future. All the chapters have been updated, and some extensively revised. Chapter 12, Emergencies, has been much expanded to encompass the list of emergencies in the UK Palliative Medicine Specialty Training Curriculum. Chapter 13, Last days, is entirely new. *Inter alia*, it discusses the implications for clinicians in England and Wales of the Mental Capacity Act 2005 (and reflected in common law in Scotland and Northern Ireland), as well as consideration of other important end-of-life issues such as palliative sedation.

Scattered throughout the book is a series of Guidelines. These provide practitioner-friendly clinical advice, purposely restricted to 1–2 pages to facilitate their use in patient care. For the justification of the opinions expressed in the Guidelines, the reader should refer to the main text and to the articles referenced there.

We thank Susan Wright and Karen Isaac for preparing the typescript for publication, and Susan Brown for her painstaking copy-editing.

Robert Twycross
Andrew Wilcock
Claire Stark Toller
March 2009

ACKNOWLEDGEMENTS

The contents of a textbook can never be wholly original. Over many years, much information and help has been received from our clinical colleagues, the Editorial Team of the *Palliative Care Formulary* (notably Julie Mortimer, Sarah Charlesworth, and Paul Howard), and many others. With this fourth edition, we are particularly grateful to the following for their advice in relation to part or all of a chapter:

Pain relief, Lee Jays (orthopaedics), Zbigniew Zylicz (opioid-induced hyperalgesia);

Alimentary symptoms, Claud Regnard (dysphagia), Paul Howard (anti-emetics), Simon Parsons (bowel obstruction and paracentesis), Robert MacDonald, Kate Pointen, Kathy Teahon (paracentesis);

Respiratory symptoms, David Baldwin, Anne Tattersfield;

Biochemical syndromes, Josie Drew and Renee Page (diabetes mellitus);

Haematological symptoms, David Keeling (for providing the content of figures 7.2 and 7.4), Nikki Curry, Miriam Johnson, Tim Littlewood, David Morgan, Simon Noble, Peter Prinsloo;

Neurological symptoms, Paul Maddison (paraneoplastic syndromes), Jenifer Jeba, Pradeep Poonnoose and Reena George (spinal cord compression), Paul Howard (epilepsy);

Oedema, Tim Dale, Vaughan Keeley;

Skin care, Jenny Millward (for permission to reproduce Plate 1), ConvaTec (for permission to reproduce Plates 2 and 4), George Cherry (for permission to reproduce Plate 3), Zbigniew Zylicz (pruritus), Julia Williams (stomas), Vanessa Halliday (diet and stomas), Patricia Grocott (decubitus ulcers), Suresh Kumar, MR Rajagopal and Tim Boswell (fungating cancer).

DRUG NAMES

All drugs marketed in Europe are now officially known by their recommended International Non-proprietary Names (rINNs). Previously, in the UK, drugs were known by their British Approved Names (BANs). Differences between BANs and rINNs are listed in Table 1. In the USA, most official drug names (United States Adopted Names; USANs) are the same as their respective rINNs. However, there are important differences; these are also listed in Table 1.

With combination products such as codeine and paracetamol (USAN acetaminophen) or diphenoxylate and atropine, the UK conventional name is shown in Table 2, e.g. co-codamol or co-phenotrope.

Table 1 Drug names relevant to palliative care for which the rINN, BAN and/or USAN differ

rINN	BAN	USAN
Alimemazine	Trimeprazine	Trimeprazine
Aluminium		Aluminum
Amfetamine		Amphetamine
Amobarbital	Amylobarbitone	
Beclometasone	Beclomethasone	Beclomethasone
Bendroflumethiazide	Bendrofluazide	Bendroflumethiazide
Benorilate	Benorylate	
Benzathine benzylpenicillin	Benzathine penicillin	Benzathine penicillin
Benzatropine	Benztropine	Benztropine
Benzylpenicillin		Penicillin G
Calcitonin (salmon)	Salcatonin	Calcitonin
Carmellose		Carboxymethylcellulose
Cefalexin (etc.)	Cephalexin (etc.)	Cephalexin (etc.)
Chlorphenamine	Chlorpheniramine	Chlorpheniramine
Ciclosporin	Cyclosporin	Cyclosporine
Clomethiazole	Chlormethiazole	
Colestyramine	Cholestyramine	Cholestyramine
Dantron	Danthron	
Dexamfetamine	Dexamphetamine	Dextroamphetamine
Dextropropoxyphene		Propoxyphene
Dicycloverine	Dicyclomine	Dicyclomine
Dienestrol	Dienoestrol	
Diethylstilbestrol	Stilboestrol	Diethylstilbestrol
Dimeticone	Dimethicone	Dimethicone

continued

Table I Continued

rINN	BAN	USAN
Dosulepin	Dothiepin	Dothiepin
Estradiol	Oestradiol	
Etamsylate	Ethamsylate	
Furosemide	Frusemide	
Glibenclamide		Glyburide
Glyceryl trinitrate		Nitroglycerin
Glycopyrronium		Glycopyrrolate
Guaifenesin	Guaiphenesin	
Hyoscine		Scopolamine
Indometacin	Indomethacin	Indomethacin
Isoprenaline		Isoproterenol
	Ispaghula	Psyllium
Levomepromazine	Methotrimeprazine	
Levothyroxine	Thyroxine	
Lidocaine	Lignocaine	
Liquid paraffin		Mineral oil
Meclozine		Meclizine
Methenamine hippurate	Hexamine hippurate	
Mitoxantrone	Mitozantrone	
Oxetacaine	Oxethazine	Oxethazine
Paracetamol		Acetaminophen
Pethidine		Meperidine
Phenobarbital	Phenobarbitone	
Phenoxymethylpenicillin		Penicillin V
Phytomenadione		Phytonadione
Procaine benzylpenicillin	Procaine penicillin	Procaine penicillin
Retinol	Vitamin A	Vitamin A
Rifampicin		Rifampin
Salbutamol		Albuterol
Simeticone[a]	Simethicone	Simethicone
Sodium cromoglicate	Sodium cromoglycate	Cromolyn sodium
Sulfasalazine	Sulphasalazine	
Sulfathiazole	Sulphathiazole	
Sulfonamides	Sulphonamides	
Tetracaine	Amethocaine	
Trihexyphenidyl	Benzhexol	Trihexyphenidyl

a. silica-activated dimeticone; known in some countries as activated dimethylpolysiloxane.

Table 2 UK names for combination products

Contents	UK name
Amoxicillin-clavulanate	Co-amoxiclav
Diphenoxylate-atropine	Co-phenotrope
Magnesium hydroxide-aluminium[a] hydroxide	Co-magaldrox
Paracetamol[b]-codeine phosphate	Co-codamol
Paracetamol-dextropropoxyphene[c]	Co-proxamol
Paracetamol-dihydrocodeine	Co-dydramol
Sulfamethoxazole-trimethoprim	Co-trimoxazole

a. aluminum (USAN)
b. acetaminophen (USAN)
c. propoxyphene (USAN).

LIST OF ABBREVIATIONS

Drug administration

In 2007, in the interests of greater patient safety, the Joint Commission on Accreditation of Healthcare Organizations (JCAHO, USA) published a series of recommendations about the use of abbreviations when writing prescriptions (http://www.jointcommission.org/PatientSafety/NationalPatientSafetyGoals/npsg_rfr.htm). Thus, several time-honoured abbreviations (e.g. o.n. for 'at bedtime') are no longer used in SMAC. Instead, the following times of administration are written in full:

- at bedtime
- once daily
- each morning
- every other day.

However, other traditional UK abbreviations are still used (Table 3).

Table 3 Drug administration

Times	UK	Latin	USA	Latin
Twice daily	b.d.	*bis die*	b.i.d.	*bis in die*
Three times daily	t.d.s.	*ter die sumendus*	t.i.d.	*ter in die*
Four times daily	q.d.s.	*quarta die sumendus*	q.i.d.	*quarta in die*
Every 4 hours, etc.	q4h	*quaque quarta hora*	q4h	*quaque quarta hora*
Rescue medication (as needed, as required)	p.r.n.	*pro re nata*	p.r.n.	*pro re nata*
Give immediately	stat		stat	

a.c.	ante cibum (before food)
amp	ampoule containing a single dose (cf. vial)
CD	preparation subject to prescription requirements under the Misuse of Drugs Act (UK); for regulations see BNF
CIVI	continuous intravenous infusion
CSCI	continuous subcutaneous infusion
e/c	enteric-coated
ED	epidural
IM	intramuscular
IT	intrathecal
IV	intravenous
IVI	intravenous infusion

m/r	modified-release; alternatives, slow-release, sustained-release, controlled-release, extended-release
N̶H̶S̶	not prescribable on NHS prescriptions
OTC	over the counter (i.e. can be obtained without a prescription)
p.c.	post cibum (after food)
PO	per os, by mouth
POM	prescription-only medicine
PR	per rectum
PV	per vaginum
SC	subcutaneous
SL	sublingual
TD	transdermal
vial	sterile container with a rubber bung containing either a single or multiple doses (cf. amp)
WFI	water for injections

General

BMA	British Medical Association
BNF	British National Formulary
BP	British Pharmacopoeia
CHM	Commission on Human Medicines
CSM	Committee on Safety of Medicines (now part of CHM)
EMEA	European Medicines Agency
EORTC	European Organisation for Research and Treatment of Cancer
FDA	Food and Drug Administration (USA)
GMC	General Medical Council (UK)
IASP	International Association for the Study of Pain
IDIS	International Drug Information Service
MCA	Medicines Control Agency (now MHRA)
MHRA	Medicines and Healthcare products Regulatory Agency (formerly MCA)
NICE	National Institute for Health and Clinical Excellence
NPF	Nurse Prescribers' Formulary
PCS/PCU	Palliative care service/unit
PIL	Patient Information Leaflet
rINN	recommended International Non-proprietary Name
SPC	Summary of Product Characteristics
UK	United Kingdom
USA	United States of America
VAS	visual analogue scale, 0–100mm
WHO	World Health Organization

Medical

ACD	anaemia of chronic disease
ACE	angiotensin-converting enzyme
ADH	antidiuretic hormone (vasopressin)
AED	automated external defibrillator
ALS	amyotrophic lateral sclerosis (motor neurone disease)
APPT	activated partial thromboplastin time

AUC	area under the plasma concentration-time curve
β_2	beta 2 adrenergic (receptor)
BUN	blood urea nitrogen
CBT	Cognitive behavioural therapy
CHF	congestive heart failure
CNS	central nervous system
COPD	chronic obstructive pulmonary disease
COX	cyclo-oxygenase; alternative, prostaglandin synthase
CPR	Cardiopulmonary resuscitation
CRP	C-reactive protein
CSF	cerebrospinal fluid
CT	computed tomography
δ	delta-opioid (receptor)
D_2	dopamine type 2 (receptor)
DIC	disseminated intravascular coagulation
DVT	deep vein thrombosis
ECG	electrocardiogram
ECT	electroconvulsive therapy
EEG	electro-encephalograph
FBC	full blood count
FEV_1	forced expiratory volume in 1 second
FRC	functional residual capacity
FSH	follicle-stimulating hormone
FVC	forced vital capacity of lungs
GABA	gamma-aminobutyric acid
GI	gastro-intestinal
H_1, H_2	histamine type 1, type 2 (receptor)
Hb	haemoglobin
HIV	human immunodeficiency virus
HT	hydroxytriptamine
Ig	immunoglobulin
IL	interleukin
INR	international normalized ratio
ITU	intensive therapy unit
IVC	inferior vena cava
JVP	jugular venous pressure
κ	kappa-opioid (receptor)
LABA	long-acting β_2-adrenergic receptor agonist
LDH	lactate dehydrogenase
LFTs	liver function tests
LH	luteinising hormone
LMWH	low molecular weight heparin
MAOI	mono-amine oxidase inhibitor
MARI	mono-amine re-uptake inhibitor
MND	motor neurone disease (amyotrophic lateral sclerosis)
MRI	magnetic resonance imaging
MSU	mid-stream specimen of urine
μ	mu-opioid (receptor)
NaSSA	noradrenergic and specific serotoninergic antidepressant
NDRI	noradrenaline (norepinephrine) and dopamine re-uptake inhibitor

NG	nasogastric
NJ	nasojejunal
NMDA	N-methyl D-aspartate
NNH	number needed to harm, i.e. the number of patients needed to be treated in order to harm one patient sufficiently to cause withdrawal from a drug trial
NNT	number needed to treat, i.e. the number of patients needed to be treated in order to achieve 50% improvement in one patient compared with placebo
NRI	noradrenaline (norepinephrine) re-uptake inhibitor
NSAID	non-steroidal anti-inflammatory drug
NSCLC	non-small-cell lung cancer
$PaCO_2$	arterial partial pressure of carbon dioxide
PaO_2	arterial partial pressure of oxygen
PCA	patient-controlled analgesia
PCC	prothrombin complex concentrates
PE	pulmonary embolism/emboli
PEF	peak expiratory flow
PG	prostaglandin
PPI	proton pump inhibitor
PT	prothrombin time
PUB	gastro-intestinal perforation, ulceration or bleeding (in relation to serious GI events caused by NSAIDs)
RBC	red blood cell
RCT	randomized controlled trial
RIMA	reversible inhibitor of mono-amine oxidase type A
RTI	respiratory tract infection
SaO_2	oxygen saturation
SCLC	small-cell lung cancer
SNRI	serotonin and noradrenaline (norepinephrine) re-uptake inhibitor
SSRI	selective serotonin re-uptake inhibitor
SVC	superior vena cava
TCA	tricyclic antidepressant
TIBC	total iron-binding capacity; alternative, plasma transferrin concentration
Tl_{CO}	transfer factor of the lung for carbon monoxide
TNF	tumour necrosis factor
UTI	urinary tract infection
VEGF	vascular endothelial growth factor
VIP	vaso-active intestinal polypeptide
WBC	white blood cell

Units

cm	centimetre(s)
cps	cycles per sec
dL	decilitre(s)
g	gram(s)
Gy	Gray(s), a measure of radiation
h	hour(s)

Hg	mercury
kg	kilogram(s)
L	litre(s)
mg	milligram(s)
microL	microlitre(s)
micromol	micromole(s)
min	minute(s)
mL	millilitre(s)
mm	millimetre(s)
mmol	millimole(s)
mosmol	milli-osmole(s)
msec	millisecond
nm	nanometre(s)
nmol	nanomole(s); alternative, nM
sec	second(s)

1: GENERAL PRINCIPLES

BIOPSYCHOSOCIAL CARE

Symptom management must always be provided within a holistic framework. Symptoms are never purely physical or purely psychological. The discomforts of the body always and inevitably impact on the mood and morale of the individual (and thence to the bystanders – family, friends, work colleagues). Likewise, the mind always impacts on the body. An understanding of this fundamental body–mind interaction is one of the basic principles underlying palliative care with its commitment to 'the active total care of patients with advanced progressive disease'.

Because it is focused on end-stage disease, palliative care is more patient-centred than disease-focused. It includes supporting:
- patients as they adjust to decreasing physical ability, and as they mourn in anticipation the loss of family, friends and all that is familiar
- families as they adjust to the fact that one of them is dying.

Palliative care neither intentionally hastens nor intentionally postpones death. The goal is the best possible quality of life for patients and their families. Many aspects of palliative care are also applicable early in the course of the illness together with disease-specific treatments.

Although psychologically demanding for doctors, nurses and other carers, caring for patients at the end of life is potentially one of the most rewarding of their responsibilities. Good communication is the key to success, together with an attitude of partnership between the caring team and the patient and family (Table 1.1). Palliative care is a partnership between experts. The health professionals are experts in relation to their knowledge of the disease and its management, whereas patients (and their families) are experts in relation to the personal impact of the illness and the disruption it causes.

Table 1.1 Partnership with the patient

Attitudes	Actions
Show respect	Explain and discuss treatment options
Do not be condescending	Take the patient's priorities into account
Be honest	Share decision-making
Listen	Accept treatment refusal

For a professional to be maximally supportive, it is necessary to show genuine concern about the patient as a person, not just about the physical symptoms. Starting consultations with an open question helps with this. For example:

'Where would you like to begin?'

'How are you feeling today?'

'How have you been coping since we last met?'

An enquiry from time to time about how the family is coping is also interpreted by the patient as an indication of your general interest and concern. Finally, at the end of each consultation, check whether the patient has any more questions they would like to ask.

ETHICAL CONSIDERATIONS

Society's commission to health professionals is succinctly summarized in the aphorism 'to cure sometimes, to relieve often, to comfort always'. The same mandate applies in palliative care, even though the possibility of cure is limited to intercurrent events or complications such as infection. Given that the primary disease is incurable, the emphasis in end-stage disease shifts decisively to relief and to comfort.

Cardinal principles
Because there is an imbalance of power in the relationship between any professional and any client, professional behaviour is governed by ethical codes of practice. In this way, it is hoped that abuses of professional power can be avoided.

In relation to medical care, the same cardinal principles apply 'across the board', from obstetrics to geriatrics, and from acute care to palliative care, namely:
- respect for patient autonomy (patient choice)
- beneficence (do good)
- non-maleficence (minimize harm)
- justice (fair use of available resources).[1]

These four principles are applied against the background of respect for life and an acceptance of the ultimate inevitability of death.[2] Thus, in practice, there are three dichotomies which need to be held in balance:
- the potential benefits of treatment versus the potential risks and burdens
- striving to preserve life but, when the burdens of life-sustaining treatments outweigh the potential benefits, withdrawing or withholding such treatments and providing comfort in dying
- individual needs versus the needs of society.

A sense of urgency is also needed, just as much in palliative care as in acute care. This aspect of applied ethics is encapsulated in what has been called the emancipation principle of palliative care:

'No efforts should be spared to free dying persons from intoleable suffering which invades and dominates their consciousness, and leaves no space for other things.'[3]

Patient autonomy
Doctors often act as if patients have an obligation to accept medically recommended treatment. However, legally a person is not obliged to accept medical treatment, even

if refusal may result in an earlier death.[4,5] Thus, doctors have an obligation to discuss treatment options and their implications with patients, and to obtain their informed consent before proceeding with treatment.

Without consent, a doctor risks being found liable in battery.[6] If a patient lacks capacity to give or withhold consent, a doctor's legal obligation is to treat in what he perceives as the patient's best interests.[7] Severe depression, delirium (acute confusional state) or dementia are common causes of lack of capacity to give consent.

Principle of double effect

The principle of double effect has been described in various ways.[8–11] In essence, the principle states that:

'A single act having two possible foreseen effects, one good and one harmful, is not always morally prohibited if the harmful effect is not intended and there is no other way of achieving the same result.'

The principle is generally ascribed to Thomas Aquinas, a 13th century theologian and philosopher.[12] It was originally enunciated in relation to self-defence. If I defend myself when attacked and my attacker is severely injured or killed, I can invoke this principle in my defence against a charge of grievous bodily harm or homicide. The principle of double effect is thus a universal principle which is invoked to exculpate someone when a good action results in unintended harm. The practice of medicine would be impossible without such a principle. It is essential because all treatment has an inherent risk and, inevitably, things go wrong occasionally.

Discussion of the principle of double effect often focuses on the use of morphine or similar drugs to relieve pain in terminally ill patients. This gives the false impression that the use of morphine in this circumstance is a high-risk strategy.[13] When correctly used, morphine (and other strong opioids) are very safe drugs, almost certainly safer than non-steroidal anti-inflammatory drugs (NSAIDs). The use of both classes of analgesic is justified on the basis that the benefits of pain relief far outweigh the risk of serious undesirable effects. Indeed, clinical experience suggests that those whose pain is relieved live longer than would have been the case if they had continued to be exhausted and demoralized by severe unremitting pain.

The situation in the UK is encapsulated in a classic legal judgement:

'A doctor who is aiding the sick and the dying does not have to calculate in minutes or even in hours, and perhaps not in days or weeks, the effect upon a patient's life of the medicines which he administers or else be in peril of a charge of murder. If the first purpose of medicine, the restoration of health, can no longer be achieved, there is still much for a doctor to do, and he is entitled to do all that is proper and necessary to relieve pain and suffering, even if the measures he takes may incidentally shorten life.'[14]

Similar sentiments have been expressed in other countries, and reflect a broad international consensus.

However, the intended aim of treatment must be the relief of suffering and not the patient's death. Although a greater risk is acceptable in more extreme circumstances, it remains axiomatic that effective measures which carry less risk to life should normally be used. Thus, in an extreme situation, it is widely regarded to be ethically acceptable to use drugs to heavily sedate a patient into unconsciousness (because less extreme measures have failed to bring relief; see p.430). On the other hand, it is still generally considered unacceptable to precipitate death deliberately (euthanasia) and, in all but 2–3 countries, it remains illegal.

Appropriate treatment

'Treatment that does not provide net benefit to the patient may, ethically and legally, be withheld or withdrawn and the goal of medicine should shift to the palliation of symptoms.'[15]

Doctors must keep in mind the self-evident fact that all patients must die eventually. Thus, part of the skill of medicine is to decide when to allow death to occur without further impediment. A doctor is not obliged legally or ethically to preserve life 'at all costs'. Priorities change when a patient is clearly dying. There is no obligation to employ treatments if their use can best be described as prolonging the process of dying.[16,17] A doctor has neither a duty nor the right to prescribe a lingering death. In palliative care, the primary aim of treatment is not to prolong life but to make the life which remains as comfortable and as meaningful as possible.

Further, because there is an ethical imperative incumbent upon health professionals collectively to ensure continuity of care, it should never be a question of to treat or not to treat. Rather, the question should be reformulated as 'what is the most appropriate treatment given the patient's biological prospects and his personal and social circumstances?'. Appropriate treatment for an acutely ill patient may be inappropriate in the dying (Figure 1.1 and Figure 1.2). Nasogastric tubes, IV infusions, antibiotics, cardiac resuscitation, and artificial respiration are all primarily support measures for use in acute or acute-on-chronic illnesses to assist a patient through the initial crisis towards recovery of health. The use of these measures in patients who are irreversibly close to death is generally inappropriate (and thus bad practice) because the burdens of such treatments exceed their potential benefits.

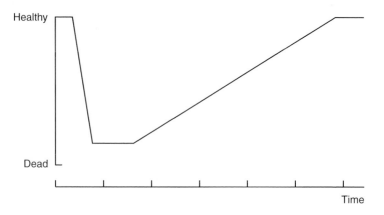

Figure 1.1 A graphical representation of acute illness. Biological prospects are generally good. Acute resuscitative measures are important and enable the patient to survive the initial crisis. Recovery is aided by the natural forces of healing: rehabilitation is completed by the patient on his own, without continued medical support.

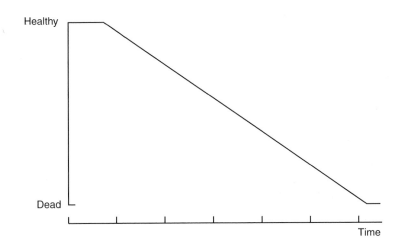

Figure 1.2 A graphical representation of terminal illness. Biological prospects progressively worsen. Acute and terminal illnesses are thus distinct pathophysiological entities. Therapeutic interventions which can best be described as prolonging the distress of dying are futile and inappropriate.

Thus, therapeutic recommendations are based on a consideration of the possible advantages (benefits) and disadvantages (risks and burdens) which might accrue for the patient. A doctor is not a technician and, in practice, there are generally several courses of action which might legitimately be adopted. Arguments in favour of a certain treatment revolve around the question of the anticipated effectiveness of intervention. Linked with this are considerations of the consequences and implications for the patient, the family and society as a whole. In other words, the doctor seeks, on the basis of the biological and social facts at his disposal, to offer the patient the most appropriate form of care, heavily influenced by what is perceived to be the patient's likely prognosis. Because death is inevitable for everyone, doctors ultimately have no choice but to 'let nature take its course'.

Medical care is a continuum, ranging from complete cure at one end to symptom relief at the other. Many types of treatment span the entire spectrum, notably radiotherapy and, to a lesser extent, chemotherapy and surgery. It is important to keep the therapeutic aim clearly in mind when employing any form of treatment. In deciding what is appropriate, the key points to bear in mind are:
• the patient's biological prospects
• the therapeutic aim and benefits of each treatment
• the undesirable effects of treatment
• the need not to prescribe a lingering death.

Although the possibility of unexpected improvement or recovery should not be totally ignored, there are many occasions when it is appropriate to 'give death a chance'. As death draws near, interest in hydration and nutrition often becomes minimal, and it is inappropriate to force someone to accept food and fluid. The patient's disinterest or positive disinclination is part of the process of letting go.

SYMPTOM MANAGEMENT

The scientific approach to symptom management can be encapsulated in the acronym *EEMMA*:
- *Evaluation*: diagnosis of each symptom before treatment
- *Explanation*: explanation to the patient before treatment
- *Management*: individualized treatment
- *Monitoring*: continuing review of the impact of treatment
- *Attention to detail*: no unwarranted assumptions.

Evaluation

A wide range of symptoms is experienced by patients with advanced cancer, but no symptom occurs invariably.[18] Evaluation must always precede treatment, and is based on *probability* and *pattern recognition*. For example, hiccup in advanced cancer is mostly associated with gastric stasis or distension, and the most common cause of pruritus is dry skin. Except for confirming or excluding a biochemical cause (e.g. hypercalcaemia), few patients need additional tests at this stage in their illness.

What is the impact of the symptom on the patient's life?

The severity of a symptom is measured by determining the impact the symptom is having on a patient's life. Questions to ask include:

'How much does the pain [or other symptom] affect your life?'

'Does anything make it worse, or make it better?'

'Is it worse at any particular time of the day or night?'

'Does it disturb your sleep?'.

What is the cause of the symptom?

The cancer itself is not always the cause of a symptom. Causal factors include:
- the cancer itself
- anticancer or other treatment
- cancer-related debility
- a concurrent disorder.

Some symptoms are caused by several factors. All symptoms are made worse by insomnia, exhaustion, anxiety and depression.

What is the underlying pathological mechanism?

Even when the cancer is responsible, a symptom may be caused by different mechanisms, e.g. vomiting may be caused by hypercalcaemia or raised intracranial pressure. Treatment varies accordingly.

What treatment has been tried?

Knowing this helps in planning the most appropriate management strategy by excluding certain treatment options, provided they were used optimally. If not, a further trial of treatment may be indicated.

Explanation

Explain the underlying mechanism(s) in simple terms

Treatment begins with an explanation by the doctor of the reason(s) for the symptom. This knowledge does much to reduce the psychological impact of the symptom on the sufferer. Thus, for example, 'The shortness of breath is caused partly by cancer itself and partly by the fluid at the base of the right lung ... and, in addition, you are anaemic'.

If explanation is omitted, patients may think that their condition is shrouded in mystery. This can be frightening if they conclude, 'This is terrible: even the doctors don't know what's going on'.

Discuss treatment options with the patient
Generally, doctors should discuss treatment options with the patient and give reasons for their recommendations. This allows the patient to ask for clarification and to express an alternative view. Few things are more damaging to a person's self-esteem than to be excluded from such discussions.

Explain the treatment to the family
Discussion with close relatives generally enlists their co-operation and helps to re-inforce symptom management strategies. This is particularly important when the patient is at home. If actively involved in supporting the patient, the family have a right to be informed, subject to the patient's approval. However, it is important not to let the family take over. Generally speaking, the patient's wishes must prevail.

Management
Management falls into three categories:
- correct the correctable
- non-drug treatment
- drug treatment.

Although the underlying disease cannot be cured, it is often possible to obtain significant (and sometimes complete) relief by adopting an appropriate multimodal approach. Achievable goals should be set. For example, with inoperable chronic partial (subacute) intestinal obstruction, it is not always possible to relieve vomiting completely. It is better to aim initially to reduce it to once or twice a day.

It may also be necessary to compromise in order to reduce undesirable effects. For example, drug-induced dry mouth or visual disturbance may limit the dose escalation of a drug with antimuscarinic effects, e.g. amitriptyline. With some symptoms, such as anorexia, weakness and fatigue, helping the patient (and family) accept the irreversible physical limitations of end-stage disease is often the focus of management.

Correct the correctable
Palliative care often includes disorder-specific treatment when it is practical and not disproportionately burdensome. For example, patients with breathlessness and bronchospasm benefit from bronchodilators. Likewise, an emollient will relieve pruritus associated with dry skin.

Non-drug treatment
This includes palliative radiotherapy for metastatic bone pain, dietary modification in patients with taste changes, and advice about breathing technique and relaxation in patients with breathlessness. Other examples of non-drug treatment are given in the sections dealing with individual symptoms.

Drug treatment
Prescribe drugs prophylactically for persistent symptoms
When treating a persistent symptom with a drug, it should be administered regularly on a prophylactic basis, and also 'as needed' (p.r.n.). The latter alone is the cause of much unrelieved distress.

Keep drug treatment as straightforward as possible
When an additional drug is considered, the following questions should be asked:

'What is the treatment goal?'

'How can it be monitored?'

'What is the risk of undesirable effects?'

'What is the risk of a drug–drug interaction?'

'Is it possible to stop any of the current medications?'.

Written advice is essential
Precise guidelines are necessary to achieve maximum patient co-operation. 'Take as much as you like, as often as you like' is a recipe for anxiety, poor symptom relief and maximum undesirable effects. The drug regimen should be written out in full for the patient and family to work from (Figure 1.3 and Figure 1.4). Times to be taken, names of drugs, reason for use ('for pain', 'for bowels', etc.) and dose (x mL, y tablets) should all be stated. The patient should be advised how to obtain further supplies, e.g., from his general practitioner.

Seek a colleague's advice in seemingly intractable situations
No one can be an expert in all aspects of patient care. For example, the management of an uncommon genito-urinary problem is likely to be enhanced by advice from a urologist or gynaecologist.

Never say 'I have tried everything' or 'There's nothing more I can do'
It is generally possible to develop a repertoire of alternative measures. Although it is sensible not to promise too much, it is important to assure the patient that you are going to stand by him and do all you can to help, e.g. 'No promises but we'll do our best'. However, instead of expecting immediate complete relief, be prepared to chip away at symptoms a bit at a time. When tackled in this way it is often surprising how much can be achieved with determination and persistence.

Monitoring
Review! review! review!
Patients vary and it is not always possible to predict the optimum dose of opioids, laxatives and psychotropics. Undesirable effects put drug adherence in jeopardy. Dose adjustments will be necessary, particularly initially. This should be anticipated and arrangements made for ongoing supervision. Cancer is a progressive disease, and new symptoms occur. These must be dealt with promptly.

Attention to detail
Attention to detail makes all the difference to palliative care; without it success may be forfeited and patients suffer needlessly. It is important not to make unwarranted assumptions. Remember: to *ass-u-me* means to make an *ass* of *u* and *me*.[19]

Attention to detail requires an inquisitive mind, one which repeatedly asks 'Why?':

'Why is this patient with breast cancer vomiting? She's not taking morphine; she's not hypercalcaemic. Why is she vomiting?'

'This patient with cancer of the pancreas has pain in the neck. It does not fit with the typical pattern of metastatic spread. Why does he have pain there?'.

St Elsewhere's Hospice

Name Mary Brown   **Age** 58   **Date** June 15, 2009

TABLETS/MEDICINES	2 am	On waking	10 am	2 pm	6 pm	Bedtime	PURPOSE
MORPHINE (Oramorph 2mg in 1ml)		5ml	5ml	5ml	5ml	10ml	pain relief
METOCLOPRAMIDE (10mg tablet)		1		1		1	anti-sickness
IBUPROFEN (400mg tablet)		2		2		2	pain relief
CO-DANTHRUSATE (capsules)			2			2	for bowels
AMITRIPTYLINE (50mg tablet)						1	for sleep and to help mood

If troublesome pain: take an extra 5ml of MORPHINE (Oramorph) between regular doses.
If bowels remain constipated: increase CO-DANTHRUSATE to 3 capsules twice a day.

- Keep this chart with you so you can show your doctor or nurse this list of what you are taking.
- Ask for a fresh supply of your medication 2–3 days before you need it.
- Sometimes your medication may be supplied in different strengths or presentations. If you have any concerns about this, check with your pharmacist.
- In an emergency, phone_____ and ask to speak to _____

Figure 1.3 Example of a patient's home medication chart (q4h).

St Elsewhere's Hospice

Name Mary Brown   **Age** 58   **Date** June 15, 2009

TABLETS/MEDICINES	Breakfast	Midday meal	Evening meal	Bedtime	PURPOSE
ASILONE (suspension)	10ml	10ml	10ml	10ml	for hiccup
MORPHINE m/r (MST 100mg tablet)	1			1	pain relief
NAPROXEN (500mg tablet)	1			1	pain relief
HALOPERIDOL (1.5mg tablet)				1	anti-sickness
CO-DANTHRUSATE (capsules)	2			2	for bowels
TEMAZEPAM (20mg tablet)				1	for sleeping

If troublesome pain: take MORPHINE SOLUTION (Oramorph 20mg in 1ml) 1.5ml, up to every 2h.
If troublesome hiccup: take extra 10ml of ASILONE, up to every 2h.

- Keep this chart with you so you can show your doctor or nurse this list of what you are taking.
- Ask for a fresh supply of your medication *2–3 days* before you need it.
- Sometimes your medication may be supplied in different strengths or presentations. If you have any concerns about this, check with your pharmacist.
- In an emergency, phone _____ and ask to speak to _____

Figure 1.4 Example of a patient's home medication chart (q.d.s.).

Attention to detail is important at every stage; in evaluation, explanation (e.g. avoid jargon, use simple language), when deciding management (e.g. drug regimens which are easy to follow, providing written advice) and when monitoring the impact of the treatment. Attention to detail is equally important in relation to the non-physical aspects of care; all symptoms are exacerbated by anxiety and fear.

1 Beauchamp T and Childress J (1994) *Principles of Biomedical Ethics*. Oxford University Press, New York, pp. 206–211.
2 Gillon R (1994) Medical ethics: four principles plus attention to scope. *British Medical Journal*. **309**: 184–188.
3 Roy DJ (1990) Need they sleep before they die? *Journal of Palliative Care*. **6**: 3–4.
4 Re T (adult: refusal of treatment) (1992). 4 *All England Reports*.
5 Re MB (an adult: medical treatment) (1997). 2 *Family Court Reports*, 541.
6 Fleming JG (1998) *Law of Torts* (9e). LBC Information Services, p. 29.
7 Anonymous (2005) Mental Capacity Act 2005: Elizabeth II. Chapter 9 Reprinted May and December 2006; May 2007. Available from: www.opsi.gov.uk/acts/acts2005/20050009.htm
8 Dunphy K (1998) Sedation and the smoking gun: double effect on trial. *Progress in Palliative Care*. **6**: 209–212.
9 Thorns A (1998) A review of the doctrine of double effect. *European Journal of Palliative Care*. **5**: 117–120.
10 Randall F and Downie R (1999) *Palliative Care Ethics. A companion for all specialties* (2e). Oxford University Press, Oxford, pp. 119–121.
11 Beauchamp TL and Childress JF (2001) *Principles of Biomedical Ethics* (5e). Oxford University Press, Oxford, pp. 128–132 and p.161.
12 Beauchamp TL and Childress JF (2001) *Principles of Biomedical Ethics* (5e). Oxford University Press, Oxford, p. 160.
13 Gilbert J and Kirkham S (1999) Double effect, double bind or double speak? *Palliative Medicine*. **13**: 365–366.
14 Devlin P (1985) *Easing the Passing. The trial of Dr John Bodkin Adams*. The Bodley Head, London, pp. 171–182.
15 BMA (1999) *Withholding or Withdrawing Life-prolonging Medical Treatment. Guidance for decision making*. BMA, London.
16 Gillon R (1999) End-of-life decisions. *Journal of Medical Ethics*. **25**: 435–436.
17 London D (2000) Withdrawing and withholding life-prolonging medical treatment from adult patients. *Journal of the Royal College of Physicians of London*. **34**: 122–124.
18 Walsh D et al. (2000) The symptoms of advanced cancer: relationship to age, gender, and performance status in 1000 patients. *Supportive Care in Cancer*. **8**: 175–179.
19 Gordon L (1997) *If You Really Loved Me*. Science and Behaviour Books, Palo Alto.

2: PAIN RELIEF

PAIN

'Pain is what the patient says hurts.'

Pain is an unpleasant *sensory* and *emotional* experience associated with actual or potential tissue damage or described in terms of such damage (see Appendix 1, p.56).[1] Thus, pain is a *somatopsychic* phenomenon modulated by:

- the patient's mood and morale
- the meaning of the pain for the patient.

The meaning of persistent pain in advanced cancer is 'I am incurable; I am going to die'. Common factors affecting pain threshold are shown in Table 2.1. Because pain is multidimensional, it helps to think in terms of total pain, encompassing physical, psychological, social and spiritual aspects of suffering (Figure 2.1).

People with chronic pain generally do not look in pain because of the absence of autonomic concomitants (Table 2.2). In cancer, acute pain concomitants may be evident, particularly, if the pain is severe and of recent onset, or is paroxysmal.

Table 2.1 Factors affecting pain sensation

Pain increased	Pain decreased
Anger	Acceptance
Anxiety	Reduction in anxiety, relaxation
Boredom	Creative activity
Depression	Elevation of mood
Discomfort	Relief of other symptoms
Grieving	Vent feelings, empathic support
Insomnia → fatigue	Sleep
Lack of understanding about condition	Explanation
Mental isolation, social abandonment	Companionship

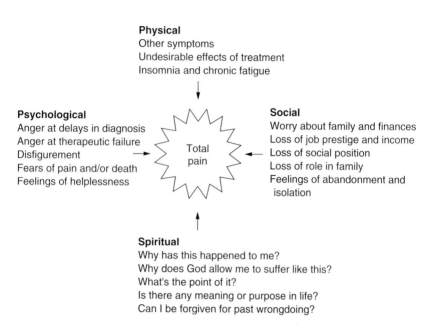

Physical
Other symptoms
Undesirable effects of treatment
Insomnia and chronic fatigue

Psychological
Anger at delays in diagnosis
Anger at therapeutic failure
Disfigurement
Fears of pain and/or death
Feelings of helplessness

Total pain

Social
Worry about family and finances
Loss of job prestige and income
Loss of social position
Loss of role in family
Feelings of abandonment and
    isolation

Spiritual
Why has this happened to me?
Why does God allow me to suffer like this?
What's the point of it?
Is there any meaning or purpose in life?
Can I be forgiven for past wrongdoing?

Figure 2.1 The four dimensions of pain.

Table 2.2 Temporal classification of pain

	Acute	Chronic	
Time course	Transient	Persistent	
Meaning to patient	Positive draws attention to injury or illness	Negative serves no useful purpose	Positive patient obtains secondary gain
Concomitants	Fight or flight pupillary dilation increased sweating tachypnoea tachycardia shunting of blood from viscera to muscles	Vegetative sleep disturbance anorexia decreased libido no pleasure in life constipation somatic pre-occupation personality change lethargy	

About 1/2 of all cancer patients receiving anticancer treatment report pain.[2] Even with advanced cancer, pain is not universal:
• 3/4 of patients experience pain
• 1/4 of patients do not.[2–4]

Multiple concurrent pains are common in those who have pain. Approximately:

- 1/3 have a single pain
- 1/3 have two pains
- 1/3 have three or more pains.[5]

Break-through (episodic) pain

Break-through (episodic) pain is a term used to describe a transient exacerbation of pain which occurs either spontaneously or in relation to a specific trigger despite adequately relieved background pain.[6] Patients with poorly relieved background pain are excluded because this suggests overall poor management, and is an indication for an increase in regular analgesia. Similarly, pain recurring shortly before the next dose of regular analgesic ('end-of-dose-interval pain') is not a true break-through pain. There are two main types of break-through pain:

- predictable (incident) pain, an exacerbation of pain caused by weight-bearing and/or activity (including swallowing, defaecation, coughing, nursing/medical procedures) which may or may not be at the same location as the underlying pain[7]
- unpredictable (spontaneous) pain, unrelated to movement or activity, e.g. colic, stabbing pain associated with nerve injury.

In patients receiving opioid medication for persistent pain, break-through pain is common in both cancer (up to 90%) and non-cancer (up to 75%).[8,9] It may be functional (e.g. tension headache) or pathological, either nociceptive (associated with tissue distortion or injury) or neuropathic (associated with nerve compression or injury). Patients may experience more than one type of break-through pain, and these may have different causes.

Pathogenesis of cancer pain

Also see Appendix 1: IASP pain definitions (p.56), and Appendix 2: Supplementary pain definitions (p.59).

The peripheral nerve endings of C and Aδ primary afferent fibres detect noxious stimuli (i.e. actual or potentially tissue-damaging mechanical, thermal and/or chemical stimuli). They are stimulated and/or sensitized by substances produced by:

- cancer cells
- immune cells, e.g. macrophages, neutrophils, lymphocytes, as part of an inflammatory response to the cancer ± associated tissue damage
- other cells, e.g. osteoclasts
- sympathetic nerve fibres, which sprout at sites of nerve injury and the dorsal root ganglion.

These substances include:

- prostaglandins, produced by cancer cells and macrophages which express high levels of COX-2
- kinins, released in response to tissue injury
- endothelin-1, produced by cancer cells
- growth factors, e.g. nerve growth factor, produced by cancer and immune cells
- H^+/acid metabolites, produced by inflammation, cell death and osteoclasts
- catecholamines, e.g. noradrenaline (norepinephrine).

The C and Aδ fibres can also be directly compressed or injured by the cancer.

Ongoing stimulation leads to lowering of activation thresholds, the recruitment of otherwise 'silent' nociceptors and sensitization of the dorsal horn via activation of the NMDA-receptor-channel complex. These changes result in:
- mild noxious stimuli becoming more intensely noxious (hyperalgesia)
- non-noxious stimuli becoming noxious (allodynia)
- ongoing generation, amplification, and maintenance of pain.

The prolonged and amplified pain signals are relayed to higher cortical and midbrain centres important in sensation (e.g. thalamus, cortex), emotion (e.g. limbic system) and level of arousal. Excitatory and inhibitory pathways descend from the higher centres to modulate pain signal transmission in the dorsal horn.

Other contributing factors vary with the underlying nature of the pain, e.g.:
- cancer-related bone pain
  ▷ an increase in osteoclast number and activity → increased acidity, direct injury of sensory nerves, loss of bone mineral
  ▷ cancer cell necrosis → further increased acidity
  ▷ mechanical stresses arise as a result of bone distension (cancer expansion) or bone instability (loss of bone mineral), triggering mechanoreceptors in the periosteum and pain on movement
- neuropathic pain
  ▷ loss of opioid receptors in sensory afferents and an increased release of glutamate (a neuro-excitatory amino acid) in the dorsal horn
  ▷ other changes which facilitate pain transmission and result in sensitization of the dorsal horn and higher centres, e.g. activation of glial cells (microglia, astrocytes), neuroma formation, increase in sodium channels, calcium-channel activation
  ▷ the resultant hyperexcitability causes spontaneous pain, hyperalgesia and allodynia in the areas adjacent to the nerve damage
  ▷ abnormal or absent sensation in the area served by the compressed or injured sensory nerve.

Thus, the pattern of neurotransmitter release and the response in the spinal cord vary according to the type of pain.[10] The changes which accompany nerve injury help to explain the variable response to opioids seen with neuropathic pain.[11]

EVALUATION

Evaluation is a multidimensional process (Figure 2.2). It is partly sequential and partly synchronous. It begins by asking the patient to identify the location of the pain ('Where exactly is your pain?') and its duration ('When did it start?'). Then, while the patient describes the pain (Box 2.A), the practitioner reflects on:
- the cause of the pain (cancer vs. non-cancer)
- the underlying mechanism (functional vs. pathological; nociceptive vs. neuropathic)
- the contribution of non-physical factors.

Causes of pain
Pain in advanced cancer can be grouped into four causal categories:
- the cancer itself, e.g. soft tissue, visceral, bone, neuropathic
- anticancer or other treatment, e.g. chemotherapy-related mucositis

- cancer-related debility, e.g. constipation, muscle tension/spasm
- a concurrent disorder, e.g. spondylosis, osteo-arthritis.

In 15% of patients with advanced cancer and pain, none of their pain is caused by the cancer itself.[5]

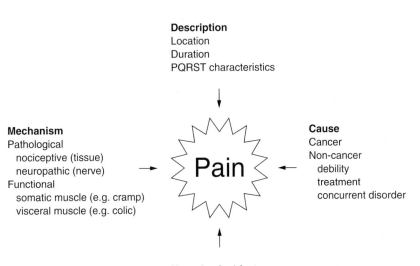

Description
Location
Duration
PQRST characteristics

Mechanism
Pathological
  nociceptive (tissue)
  neuropathic (nerve)
Functional
  somatic muscle (e.g. cramp)
  visceral muscle (e.g. colic)

Pain

Cause
Cancer
Non-cancer
  debility
  treatment
  concurrent disorder

Non-physical factors
Psychological
Social
Spiritual

Figure 2.2 The four dimensions of pain evaluation.

Box 2.A The *PQRST* characteristics of pain

*P*alliative factors	'What makes it better?'
*P*rovocative factors	'What makes it worse?'
*Q*uality	'What exactly is it like?'
*R*adiation	'Does it spread anywhere?'
*S*everity	'How severe is it?'
	'How much does it affect your life?'
*T*emporal factors	'Is it there all the time or does it come and go?'
	'Is it worse at any particular time of the day or night?'

In practice it may be better to begin with T and end with P, i.e. TSRQP!

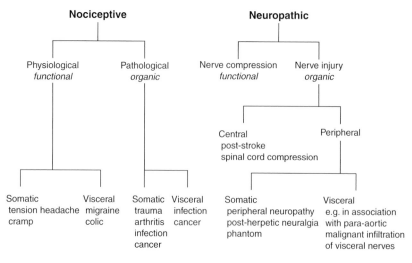

Figure 2.3 Classification of pain.

Mechanisms of pain

It is important to distinguish between functional and pathological pains (Figure 2.3). Functional muscle pains are part of everybody's general life experience:

- somatic muscle-tension pains, e.g. tension headache, cramp, myofascial
- visceral muscle-tension pains, e.g. distension and colic.

Myofascial pain is a specific form of cramp related to myofascial trigger points.[12] These occur most commonly in the muscles of the pectoral girdle and neck, and are likely to be more troublesome in physically debilitated and anxious people (Figure 2.4).[13] Functional muscle pains are common in patients with advanced cancer, in whom they may become persistent.

Pathological pains can be divided into:

- nociceptive (pain associated with tissue distortion or injury)
- neuropathic (pain arising as a direct consequence of a lesion or disease affecting the somatosensory system, e.g. that associated with nerve compression or injury; Figure 2.3).

Pain in an area of abnormal or absent sensation is always neuropathic.

There are many potential causes of neuropathic pain in cancer (Box 2.B). Note:

- when directly caused by the cancer, nerve compression generally precedes nerve injury
- pain associated with compression of a single peripheral nerve or plexus is typically a deep ache of variable intensity, neurodermatomal in distribution
- pain associated with peripheral nerve injury pain is often superficial and burning ± a spontaneous stabbing/lancinating component (± a deep aching component as well), but with a similar neurodermatomal distribution
- the distribution (and associated pain) of paraneoplastic, diabetic, and drug-induced peripheral polyneuropathy is typically 'glove and stocking' (Box 2.B).

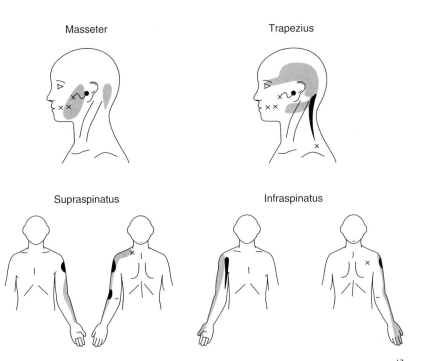

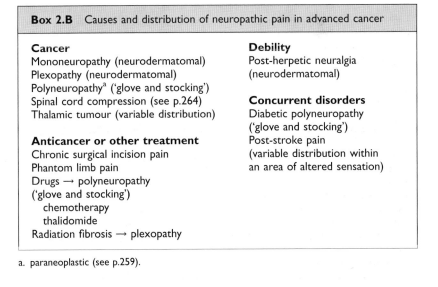

Figure 2.4 Selected trigger points and associated patterns of myofascial pain.[13]
Site of pain ■■; trigger area ×.

Box 2.B Causes and distribution of neuropathic pain in advanced cancer

Cancer
Mononeuropathy (neurodermatomal)
Plexopathy (neurodermatomal)
Polyneuropathy[a] ('glove and stocking')
Spinal cord compression (see p.264)
Thalamic tumour (variable distribution)

Anticancer or other treatment
Chronic surgical incision pain
Phantom limb pain
Drugs → polyneuropathy
('glove and stocking')
 chemotherapy
 thalidomide
Radiation fibrosis → plexopathy

Debility
Post-herpetic neuralgia
(neurodermatomal)

Concurrent disorders
Diabetic polyneuropathy
('glove and stocking')
Post-stroke pain
(variable distribution within
an area of altered sensation)

---

a. paraneoplastic (see p.259).

The characteristics of nerve injury pain stem from pathological changes in the nervous system:
- neuronal hyperexcitability and spontaneous activity at the site of injury
- a cascade of neurochemical and physiological changes in the CNS, particularly in the dorsal horn of the spinal cord ('central sensitization').[14]

The relative importance of the various mechanisms differs between patients, and probably contributes towards the variation seen in the clinical presentation and responses to drug treatment (Box 2.C).[15]

Box 2.C   Clinical features of nerve injury pain

Quality
One or more of the following:
- superficial burning/stinging pain, particularly if a peripheral lesion
- spontaneous stabbing/lancinating pain
- a deep ache.

Concomitants
Often there is:
- allodynia (light touch exacerbates pain), e.g. unable to bear clothing on the affected area
- a sensory deficit, generally numbness.

Occasionally there is a sympathetic component manifesting as:
- cutaneous vasodilation → increased skin temperature
- sweating.

Patients also become exhausted and demoralized, particularly if there is insomnia.

Relief from analgesics
About 1/2 of nerve injury pains caused by cancer respond to the combined use of an NSAID and a strong opioid; the rest need adjuvant analgesics.[16]

Non-physical factors
Because non-physical factors influence pain intensity, psychosocial evaluation is essential. Most patients benefit if they are enabled to express their fears and anxieties. Sometimes specific intervention is needed, e.g. treatment of depression (see p.194).

The help of a clinical psychologist or psycho-oncologist may be necessary if the patient seems to be using pain to express otherwise inexpressible negative emotions ('somatization'). The aim is to encourage the patient to discover and utilize coping strategies which help them:
- control pain or continue to function despite the pain
- accept and adapt to their situation, e.g. switching their focus to activities and goals less affected by pain
- to pursue a meaningful and valued life.[17]

EXPLANATION

Given that many patients have pain which is not caused by the cancer, the positive value of an explanation of the causes and mechanisms of their pains is self-evident. In relation to neuropathic pain which is not responding to standard analgesics, it is important to tell the patient that:
- nerve compression pain 'often needs a corticosteroid as well as painkillers'
- nerve injury pain 'does not always respond to painkillers like naproxen and morphine ... Because of this we need to start a different type of painkiller ... And an important step is to get you a good night's sleep'.

MANAGEMENT

With cancer pain, multiple mechanisms may co-exist, and optimal relief may require a combination of treatments.

Different types of pain may well need different types of treatment (Table 2.3). A broad-spectrum multimodal approach is often necessary (Box 2.D). For pain caused by the cancer itself, drugs may well give adequate relief (provided the right drugs are administered in the right doses at the right time intervals) but, with bone metastases in particular, palliative radiotherapy is often crucially important.

If anticancer treatment is recommended, analgesics should be given until the treatment ameliorates the pain; this may take several weeks. It is important to avoid various forms of bad practice (Box 2.E).

It is often best to aim at progressive pain relief:
- relief at night
- relief at rest during the day
- relief on movement (not always completely possible).

Correct the correctable
When possible and appropriate, modification of the pathological process can improve and sometimes eliminate the pain. Treatments include radiotherapy, hormone therapy (e.g. in breast, endometrial and prostate cancer), chemotherapy and surgery.

Non-drug treatment
The perception of pain requires both consciousness and attention. Pain is worse when it occupies a person's whole attention. Activity, particularly when creative, does much more than pass the time; it aids coping and diminishes pain. Further, professional time spent exploring a patient's worries and fears is time well spent, and relates directly to pain management (see p.13).

Radiotherapy
This should be considered when pain is caused by bone metastases, nerve compression or soft tissue infiltration (Box 2.F). Radiotherapy is generally inappropriate in patients with a very short prognosis, i.e. <2 weeks.[18]

In bone pain, a single-dose treatment with 8–10Gy is often possible, particularly in peripheral sites.[20] One month after radiation, pain is reduced by >50% in 40%

Table 2.3 Mechanisms of pain in cancer and implications for treatment

Type of pain	Mechanism	Example	Response to opioid	Typical first-line treatment
Nociceptive				
Muscle spasm	Stimulation of nerve endings	Cramp	–	Skeletal muscle relaxant
Somatic		Soft tissue, bone pain	±	NSAID ± opioid
Visceral		Liver pain	±	NSAID ± opioid
Neuropathic				
Compression				
Peripheral nerve	Stimulation of nervi nervorum	Brachial plexus compression by apical lung cancer	±	Corticosteroid + opioid
CNS (central)	Neural ischaemia (→ irreversible injury if prolonged)	Spinal cord compression	±	Corticosteroid + opioid
Injury				
Peripheral nerve	Neural injury	Neuroma or nerve infiltration, e.g. brachial or lumbosacral plexus	±	NSAID + opioid and/or TCA ± anti-epileptic
CNS (central)	Neural injury	Thalamic metastasis	±	TCA ± anti-epileptic

Box 2.D Examples of treatment modalities for cancer pain management

Explanation
Tends to reduce the negative
psychological impact of
unexplained pain

Modification of the pathological process
Radiotherapy
Hormone therapy
Chemotherapy
Percutaneous interventions
  vertebroplasty
  kyphoplasty
Surgery
  orthopaedic
  other

Analgesics
Non-opioid
Opioid
Adjuvant
  corticosteroids
  antidepressants
  anti-epileptics
  NMDA-receptor-channel blockers
  muscle relaxants
  bisphosphonates

Non-drug methods
Physical
  massage
  heat pads
  TENS

Psychological
Identify and address psychological issues
Relaxation
CBT

Neural blockade and neurosurgery
Local anaesthesia
  lidocaine
  bupivacaine
Neurolysis
  chemical, e.g. alcohol, phenol
  cryotherapy
  thermocoagulation
Neurosurgery, e.g.
  cervical cordotomy

Modification of way of life and environment
Avoid pain-precipitating activities
Immobilization of the painful part
  cervical collar
  surgical corset
  slings
  orthopaedic surgery
Walking aid
Wheelchair
Hoist

of patients and completely relieved in 25% with benefit often maintained for the remainder of the patient's life. Median duration of complete pain relief is 3 months.[21] Recalcification occurs in most cases. Response is more likely in breast, prostate and myeloma (about 80%) than lung, kidney or colorectal cancer (about 60–65%).[22]

There is no difference in overall pain response between single-dose treatment and fractionated (multiple doses) radiotherapy for bone pain. However, patients treated with single rather than fractionated treatment are more likely to need retreatment, and have a small increased risk of pathological fracture. The risk of these must be balanced against the inconvenience and possible discomfort of multi-dose treatment.[23] There is a 50–90% response to retreatment.[22]

If there are widespread bone metastases causing pain at several different sites, wide field or hemibody radiotherapy may be appropriate. IV radio-isotope therapy is an

Box 2.E Common reasons for unrelieved pain in advanced cancer

Associated with patient or family
A belief that pain in cancer is inevitable and untreatable.
Failure to contact a doctor.
Patient misleads the doctor by 'putting on a brave face'.
Patient fails to take prescribed medication because they do not 'believe' in tablets.
Belief that analgesics should be taken only 'if absolutely necessary'.
Not adhering to the prescribed regimen because of fears of addiction or that tolerance could mean that there will be nothing left 'for when things get really bad'.
Patient stops medication because of undesirable effects, and does not notify doctor.

Associated with doctor or nurse
Doctor ignores the patient's pain, believing it to be inevitable and untreatable.

Poor communication with patient and family
Failure to listen to the patient.
Failure to appreciate the severity of the patient's pain, often because of a failure to get behind the patient's 'brave face'.
Failure to distinguish between pain caused by cancer and pain related to other causes.
Failure to evaluate each pain individually and to plan treatment accordingly.
Lack of attention to psychosocial issues; failure to give psychological support to the patient and family.

Poor drug management
Failure to use non-drug treatments, particularly for muscle spasm pain.
Failure to give the patient adequate instructions about how best to take the prescribed analgesics.
Prescription of an analgesic to be taken only 'as needed'.
Prescription of an analgesic which is too weak to relieve the pain; reluctance to prescribe morphine.
Fear that the patient will become addicted if morphine (or an alternative) is prescribed.
Belief that morphine should be reserved until patients are 'really terminal' (moribund), and continuing to prescribe inadequate doses of less effective analgesics.
Failure to use an NSAID and an opioid in combination.
Failure to appreciate that the necessary dose of morphine varies between patients.
Changing to an alternative analgesic before optimizing the dose and timing of the previous analgesic.
Changing from another strong opioid, e.g. buprenorphine or oxycodone, to an inadequate dose of morphine.
Ignorance about adjuvant analgesics, notably antidepressants and anti-epileptics.
Failure to monitor the patient's response to the prescribed analgesics.
Failure to anticipate, monitor and control undesirable effects, particularly constipation.

Box 2.F   Indications for radiotherapy in symptom management (*BUMP*)[19]

Bleeding
Haemoptysis
Haematuria
Vaginal

Ulceration
Superficial
Mucosa
 oronasopharyngeal
 rectal

Mass effect
SVC obstruction
Oesophagus (dysphagia)

Pain
Bone metastases
Soft tissue infiltration
 headache from brain metastases
 liver pain
 splenic pain
 para-aortic lymphadenopathy
Plexopathy
 brachial plexus
 lumbosacral plexus
Spinal cord compression (see p.264)

---

alternative, e.g. strontium for bone metastases from prostate cancer, but response takes up to 3 months.[24]

Whole-brain radiotherapy can be given to relieve headache caused by cerebral metastases, e.g. 20Gy in five fractions. Relief is obtained in >70% of patients.[25,26] Patients with primary brain tumours and significant neurological deficit with poor performance status respond less well.

Orthopaedic surgery
Bone metastases are common in cancer and can lead to pain, pathological fracture and spinal cord compression. Orthopaedic intervention has a role for each of these, helping to relieve pain and maintain function (Box 2.G). Orthopaedic interventions are more likely to be used because improved survival increases the likelihood of bony complications. Appropriate patient selection is important, taking into account factors such as symptom and disease burden, performance status, prognosis and cancer type.

Neural blockade and neurosurgery
Neural blockade ('nerve blocks') and neurosurgery for pain management in advanced cancer are important for a small number of patients. In a recent survey of patients receiving specialist palliative care, overall <5% received such interventions, and <2% if under the care of a service whose lead physician was not an anaesthetist.[29] Half of the interventions comprised spinal analgesia with local anaesthetics ± opioids. Other interventions included blocks of:
• various peripheral nerves with local anaesthetic
• sympathetic nerve plexuses with a neurolytic (nerve-destructive) agent
• various nerve roots with intrathecal phenol.

Since the advent of spinal analgesia and the increased use of local anaesthetic and corticosteroid injections (for more information, see *PCF3*), neurolytic procedures are rarely done in palliative care services in the UK. At many centres, a coeliac plexus block with alcohol for epigastric visceral pain is the only neurolytic block still used, and only infrequently (Box 2.H).

In addition to the use of analgesics and the non-drug measures detailed above, pain on movement may be helped by suggesting modifications to the patient's way of life and

---

Box 2.G Orthopaedic interventions for the complications of bone metastases[22,27,28]

General

Requires specialist orthopaedic expertise:

- about 30–50% of the bone has to be destroyed before there are radiographic changes; thus damage is generally more extensive than the radiograph suggests
- in pathological fracture, bone union occurs in only about 1/3 and standard fracture implants may fail
- the intervention must be appropriate for the survival of the patient, i.e. recovery time must be shorter than the prognosis
- the method of fixation must allow immediate weight-bearing, outlive the patient, and avoid bone grafts if postoperative radiotherapy is planned.

An optimal approach requires the additional input of radiology, oncology, rehabilitation and palliative care.

Percutaneous therapies

- cement augmentation, increasingly used:
  - ▷ vertebroplasty, eases pain and helps prevent further collapse
  - ▷ kyphoplasty, a balloon is used to restore height to a collapsed vertebra before injection of cement
  - ▷ pediculoplasty
  - ▷ sacroplasty
  - ▷ acetabuloplasty
- radiofrequency ablation, provides a well-demarcated focal thermal injury; used to destroy painful solitary lesions when radiotherapy not possible
- embolization, selective arterial embolization of vascular cancers, e.g. renal cell, thyroid, generally undertaken pre-operatively to reduce risk of serious bleeding.

Prevention of pathological fracture

Prophylactic surgical fixation when there is risk of fracture.
Various risk factors have been suggested:

Risk factor	Score		
	1	*2*	*3*
Site	Upper limb	Lower limb	Peritrochanteric
Lesion	Osteoblastic	Mixed	Osteolytic
Width of cortex involved	< 1/3	1/3–2/3	> 2/3
Pain	Mild	Moderate	Severe

Risk of fracture
Total score from above
  ≤7 Low risk
   8 15% risk
  ≥9 ≥33% risk; consider prophylactic fixation

continued

Box 2.G Continued

However, a consistent relationship between size and risk of fracture has not been found, probably because the degree of bone destruction can be difficult to measure, particularly when diffuse and with osteoblastic metastases. Further, these criteria are less applicable where the cortex cannot be easily measured, e.g. vertebrae. A pragmatic rule is to stabilize bony metastases in the weight-bearing skeleton if they cause pain on movement.

Treatment of pathological fracture
Generally, the optimal approach is to excise and replace any destroyed bone and stabilize any weakened bone. If fracture union is unlikely, an implant must outlive the patient. Approaches include:
- plaster of Paris + radiotherapy; when surgery not appropriate, non-weight-bearing bones, radiosensitive cancer, long time to unite
- percutaneous fixation; e.g. intramedullary nails, good for diaphyseal lesions, recovery time 3–6 weeks
- curettage and cementation ± fixation; e.g. large lytic lesions with minimal structural bone remaining, radio-insensitive cancers such as renal cell, recovery time 4–6 weeks
- arthroplasty/endoprosthetic reconstruction; e.g. proximal femur and humerus, good prognosis (>6 months), recovery time several months
- pelvic reconstruction.

Spinal surgery
Indications include, particularly in radio-insensitive cancers:
- intractable pain; sustained improvement in the majority, about 1/4 obtain complete relief
- spinal instability ± collapse
- imminent cord compression ('threatened cord')
- progressive neurological deficit.

environment. This is where the help of a physiotherapist and an occupational therapist is invaluable.

Relief should be evaluated in relation to each pain. If there is severe anxiety and/or depression, it may take 3–4 weeks to achieve maximum benefit. Re-evaluation is a continuing necessity; old pains may get worse and new ones develop.

Drug treatment
For more information, see *PCF3*.

For convenience, analgesics can be divided into three classes:
- non-opioid
- opioid
- adjuvant.

Paracetamol (acetaminophen), NSAIDs and opioids all have peripheral and central effects, although to a different extent.[34,35] Adjuvant analgesics act in various ways (see p.45).

The principles governing analgesic use have been summarized by the WHO as:[36,37]
- *by the mouth*: the oral route is the standard route for analgesics, including morphine and other strong opioids

---

Box 2.H Coeliac plexus block[30–33]

The coeliac plexus consists of several ganglia lying anterior to the aorta, generally at the level of the T12–L1 disc space, surrounding the origin of the superior mesenteric artery. It conveys visceral sensory afferents from all the abdominal viscera except the left half of the colon, the rectum and the pelvic organs. The afferents run alongside the sympathetic and parasympathetic efferent nerves to respectively reach the spinal cord (via the sympathetic chain) or the brain stem (via the vagal nerve).

The main indication for neurolytic coeliac plexus block with 50–100% alcohol is intractable pain from cancer of the upper GI tract. It is generally undertaken using radiological guidance via a posterior or anterior approach. It is sometimes carried out during elective surgery.

Robust efficacy data are limited:
- about 50–75% of patients get complete pain relief, the remainder partial or none
- most continue to require other analgesics, although a reduction in dose may be possible
- benefit can last up to 1 year, but in 1/4 of patients pain recurs within 1 month.

Because the block only removes the visceral component, complete pain relief may only be possible when the cancer is confined to the viscera. If the cancer has already extended beyond the viscera, e.g. into surrounding tissues or local lymph nodes, the likelihood of benefit is much reduced. Thus, some recommend that the procedure should not be performed in patients with locally advanced pancreatic cancer.

Common complications include:
- hypotension, results from a loss of sympathetic tone, is generally postural and improves within 3–5 days; however, when severe may require IV fluids, vasopressors, and compression stockings
- pain:
  - ▷ in response to the alcohol injection; there may be immediate epigastric, chest or mid-back pain lasting about 30min or more prolonged mid-back pain lasting <48h. Both may require additional analgesia; the former may be reduced by an initial injection of bupivacaine
  - ▷ colic can occur because of the removal of the sympathetic 'brake' on GI motility
- diarrhoea, generally improves within a few days.

Rare complications include weakness and/or numbness in the distribution of the T10–L2 nerve roots, impotence, loss of sphincter control, paraplegia, pneumothorax and retroperitoneal haematoma.

- *by the clock*: persistent pain requires preventive therapy. Analgesics should be given regularly and prophylactically, and also as needed (p.r.n.); the latter alone is irrational and inhumane (Figure 2.5)
- *by the ladder*: use the 3-step analgesic ladder (Figure 2.6). If after optimizing the dose a drug fails to give adequate relief, move up the ladder; do not move sideways in the same efficacy group
- *individualized treatment*: the right dose is the one which relieves the pain; if necessary doses should be titrated upwards until the pain is relieved or undesirable effects prevent further escalation

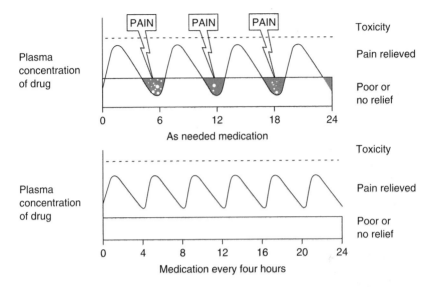

Figure 2.5 A comparison of 'as needed' (p.r.n.) dosing and regular q4h morphine.

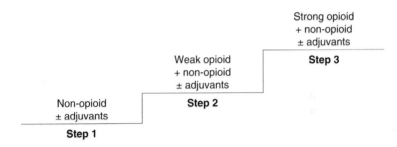

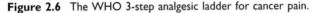

Figure 2.6 The WHO 3-step analgesic ladder for cancer pain.

- *use adjuvants*: in the context of the analgesic ladder these include:
  ▷ other drugs which relieve pain in specific situations
  ▷ drugs to control the undesirable effects of analgesics, e.g. laxatives, anti-emetics
  ▷ concurrently prescribed psychotropic medication, e.g. anxiolytics.

Comparable recommendations are available from other sources.[38,39]

A key concept underlying the analgesic ladder is 'broad-spectrum analgesia', i.e. drugs from each of the three classes of analgesic are used appropriately, either singly or in combination, to maximize their impact (Figure 2.7). Relief with morphine and other opioids is often limited when there is neural sensitization (Figure 2.8). Because peripheral sensitization occurs in association with both inflammation and nerve injury, it is important to use an NSAID and an opioid in combination for most pains caused by cancer; not only for bone and soft tissue pain but also for nerve injury pain.

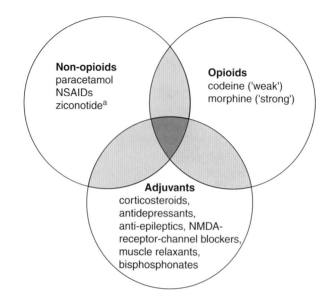

Figure 2.7 Broad-spectrum analgesia; drugs from different categories are used singly or in combination according to the type of pain and response to treatment.

a. an N-type calcium-channel blocker, the first of a new type of non-opioid. Its place in palliative care has still to be determined.

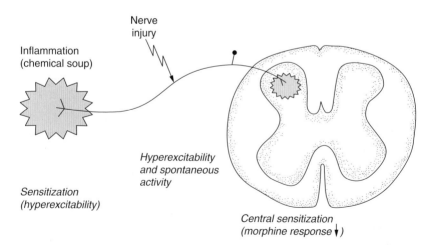

Figure 2.8 Peripheral sensitization leads to central sensitization and a reduced response to opioids.

Break-through pain

Various strategies reduce the impact of break-through (episodic) pain (Figure 2.9).[40]

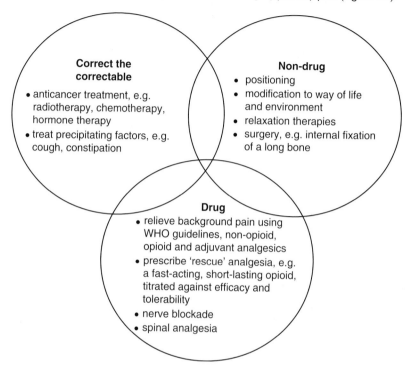

Figure 2.9 A multimodal approach to managing break-through pain.

A widespread drug treatment is to give an extra dose of the regular analgesic, e.g. a p.r.n. dose of normal-release morphine for patients taking morphine regularly round the clock. A traditional practice, dating from before m/r opioid products were available, was to give an extra dose of the regular q4h dose of oral morphine (i.e. 1/6 of the total daily dose). However, many break-through pains are short-lived and this approach effectively doubles the patient's opioid intake for the next 4h.

Increasingly, a more measured approach has been adopted, i.e. many centres recommend that the patient initially takes, as a normal-release formulation, 10% of the total daily regular dose as the p.r.n. dose.[41,42] However, a standard fixed dose is unlikely to suit all patients and all pains, particularly because the intensity and the impact of break-through pain vary considerably. Thus, when patients are encouraged to optimize their rescue dose, the chosen dose varies from 5–20% of the total daily dose.[43,44]

Generally, break-through pain has a relatively rapid onset and short duration (e.g. 20–30min, ranging from <1min to >3h), whereas oral morphine has a relatively slow onset of action (30min) and long duration of effect (3–6h).[45] This helps to explain why many patients choose *not* to take a rescue dose of PO opioid with every episode of break-through pain, particularly when predictable, mild in intensity, and of relatively short duration.[46,47]

Strategies to circumvent the mismatch between break-through pain duration and drug effect latency include:

- timing a predictable painful activity or procedure to coincide with the peak plasma concentration after a regular or rescue PO dose of morphine (1–2h) or other strong opioid
- using routes of administration, e.g. buccal, intranasal, SL, which permit more rapid absorption of some (lipophilic) opioids, e.g. fentanyl.[48]

Transmucosal fentanyl products include Abstral®, Actiq® and Effentora®. Experience with such products to date indicates:[49]

- there is little or no correlation between the dose of the regularly administered strong opioid and the satisfactory rescue dose
- that the rescue dose needs to be individually titrated
- that different products will not be bio-equivalent and cannot be substituted for one another (the formulation and route of administration differ)
- that the cost will be substantially more than PO opioids
- serious adverse events and deaths can occur with inappropriate:
  ▷ patient selection, e.g. opioid non-tolerant, transient pain (postoperative, migraine)
  ▷ product use, e.g. exceeding recommended frequency of administration, dose-for-dose substitution of one product with another, i.e. Actiq® for Effentora®.

NON-OPIOID ANALGESICS

For more information, see *PCF3*.

The main non-opioid analgesics are:
- paracetamol (acetaminophen)
- non-steroidal anti-inflammatory drugs (NSAIDs).

Paracetamol

Paracetamol is a synthetic centrally-acting non-opioid analgesic. Although some studies have suggested a peripheral action,[50,51] most evidence points to a purely central effect.[52] Like NSAIDs, paracetamol is antipyretic; unlike NSAIDs, it has no peripheral anti-inflammatory effect.

Paracetamol reduces the production of prostanoids in the CNS by inhibiting cyclo-oxygenase (COX).[53] It is possible that paracetamol reduces the active oxidized form of COX to an inactive form. Thus, the mechanism by which paracetamol inhibits COX activity could be different from that of NSAIDs. Paracetamol also interacts with the L-arginine-nitric oxide, serotonin and opioid systems.[54,55]

The following features distinguish paracetamol from NSAIDs:
- undesirable effects are uncommon
- does not injure the gastric mucosa, although it may cause non-specific dyspepsia
- is well tolerated by patients with peptic ulcers
- does not affect plasma uric acid concentration.

Paracetamol also has no effect on platelet function. It can be taken by 2/3 of patients who are hypersensitive to aspirin.[56] NSAIDs and paracetamol can be used together with an additive effect. Recent animal studies suggest that this effect may be synergistic.[57] The main drawback with paracetamol is the frequency of administration, generally q6h, and its potential for hepatotoxicity.[52]

Non-steroidal anti-inflammatory drugs
Non-steroidal anti-inflammatory drugs (NSAIDs) inhibit cyclo-oxygenase (COX), an important enzyme in the arachidonic acid cascade which results in the production of tissue and inflammatory PGs.[53] NSAIDs are essential drugs for cancer pain management.[58,59] They prevent or reverse inflammation-induced hyperalgesia by both peripheral and central effects.[60]

Unfortunately, NSAIDs cause a range of serious undesirable effects, notably in relation to the GI tract,[61] kidneys, and cardiovascular system. The relevance and importance of these effects varies according to the patient population. In those with advanced disease, the benefit associated with greater physical comfort is likely to outweigh the potential harm from serious GI or thrombotic complications, even if this leads to an earlier death. In some patients, NSAIDs cause bronchospasm.

Gastro-intestinal effects
Data derived from cohort studies in patients taking an NSAID for >2 months indicate that the risk of a bleeding ulcer or perforation is about 1 in 500.[62] On average, 1 in 1,200 patients taking NSAIDs for at least 2 months will die from gastroduodenal complications.[62]

Cardiovascular
Recent data show an increased risk of thrombotic events with many NSAIDs.[63] The risk is established with the coxibs (selective COX-2 inhibitors), and this has led to two drugs being withdrawn.[64] Although celecoxib was not implicated initially, more recent data suggest an increased risk.[65–67]

Of the non-selective COX inhibitors, evidence suggests an increased risk with diclofenac (particularly at 150mg/day) and high-dose ibuprofen (2,400mg/day), but no increased risk with naproxen or low-dose ibuprofen (≤1,200mg/day).[63,68] Thus, thrombosis should not be regarded as a class effect.

However, the increased risk must be kept in perspective. Even for coxibs, the number of additional thrombotic events (mainly myocardial infarctions) is only 3 per 1,000 patients per year of use.[63] It is not clear how many of these are fatal. If 1/6–1/3, this would give a death rate from thrombosis of about 1 in 1,000–2,000 patients per year of use.

Bronchospasm
Most NSAIDs, and sometimes paracetamol, induce bronchospasm in certain patients. However, benzydamine (oral rinse) does not. Meloxicam (preferential COX-2 inhibitor) and celecoxib also seem to be safe in this respect.[69]

Renal effects
All NSAIDs cause salt and water retention which may result in ankle oedema, antagonizing the effect of diuretics. Also, <1% of patients prescribed an NSAID will develop renal impairment sufficient to necessitate its discontinuation.[70] The risk is associated with hypovolaemia and is similar with different NSAIDs, including coxibs.[71] Thus, except in patients expected to die in a few days, dehydrated patients should be rehydrated when starting treatment with an NSAID.

Choice of NSAID
Pain relief is a priority in palliative care, and even high-risk patients should not be denied the benefit of an NSAID if its use provides definitely better relief than, say, paracetamol and morphine (Box 2.I). Even so, it is important to heed the official warnings and, as a general rule, to use the lowest effective dose for the shortest possible length of time,[68,72] although this is likely to be indefinite in advanced cancer.

Box 2.I   Choice of NSAID: PO route

As first-line NSAID, consider:
• nabumetone and no gastroprotection *or*
• ibuprofen or naproxen plus a PPI or misoprostol as gastroprotection.
Reserve celecoxib for patients with particularly high GI risk but with low cardiovascular risk.

In patients undergoing chemotherapy or with thrombocytopenia from other causes, use an NSAID which has no effect on bleeding time, e.g. a non-acetylated salicylate, nabumetone, diclofenac, meloxicam, a coxib.

It is unclear if some cancer patients obtain more benefit from one particular NSAID as is anecdotally reported in rheumatoid arthritis, or if apparent differences simply relate to a relative increase in inhibition of PG synthesis. Patients with hypertension[73] and with cardiac, hepatic or renal impairment may deteriorate, and should be monitored appropriately.

Except for biliary and renal colic,[74] NSAIDs should generally be given PO or PR because, except in the case of ketorolac,[75,76] there is no evidence of greater efficacy by injection (Box 2.J).[77]

Box 2.J   Choice of NSAID: alternatives to PO route

Orodispersible tablet
Piroxicam[a] 20mg once daily, given as an orodispersible tablet (Feldene Melt®), dissolves rapidly and completely if placed on the tongue or in the mouth. However, absorption is from the GI tract, which means that Feldene Melt® tablets can be used only in patients who can swallow their saliva.

Injection
Generally use SC diclofenac 150mg/24h CSCI.
Reserve ketorolac[a] 30–90mg/24h CSCI for patients with nociceptive pain who fail to obtain good relief with other (less gastrotoxic) NSAIDs.[75,76]

---

a. because of the higher risk of serious adverse GI events (piroxicam and ketorolac) and serious skin reactions (piroxicam), neither should be used first-line, and both should be used at the lowest effective dose for as short a period of time as possible.

WEAK OPIOIDS

For more information, see *PCF3*.

There is no pharmacological need for Step 2 of the WHO analgesic ladder. Low doses of morphine, or an alternative strong opioid, can be used instead of a weak opioid.[78,79] Moving directly from Step 1 to Step 3 is the preferred option at some centres. However, from an international perspective, Step 2 remains a practical necessity because of the highly restricted availability (or even non-availability) of oral morphine and other strong opioids in many countries.

Codeine is the archetypal weak opioid (and morphine the archetypal strong opioid).[80] However, the division of opioids into 'weak' and 'strong' is to a certain extent arbitrary. In reality, opioids manifest a range of strengths which is not fully reflected in two discrete categories. High-dose codeine (or alternative) is comparable to low-dose morphine (or alternative), and vice versa. By IM injection, weak opioids can provide analgesia equivalent, or almost equivalent, to IM morphine 10mg. However, not all weak opioids are marketed as injections.

Weak opioids are said to have a 'ceiling' effect for analgesia. This is an oversimplification; whereas mixed agonist-antagonists such as pentazocine have a true ceiling effect, the maximum effective dose of weak opioid agonists is arbitrary. At higher doses there are progressively more undesirable effects, notably nausea and vomiting, which outweigh any additional analgesic effect. Further, the upper dose limit is determined in practice by the number of tablets a patient will accept, which may only be 2–3 of any one product.

There is little to choose between weak opioids in terms of efficacy. Available products are not Controlled Drugs, which makes prescribing more straightforward compared with morphine and other strong opioids. Several combination products are available (Table 2.4). The following should be noted:

- there is good evidence for additional benefit from the combination of paracetamol 1g with codeine 30–60mg;[81–84] lower doses of codeine have not been examined to the same extent
- codeine is more constipating than dextropropoxyphene and tramadol.[85] Further, it has little or no analgesic effect unless metabolized to morphine mainly via CYP2D6; it is thus essentially ineffective in poor metabolizers (5–10% of the Caucasian population)
- dextropropoxyphene has effectively been withdrawn in the UK; this is because of its relatively common use in intentional overdose, and its potential fatal toxicity in accidental overdose[86]
- dihydrocodeine is widely used either alone or as a combination product; it is analgesic in its own right and, like codeine, has an active metabolite, dihydromorphine[87]
- pentazocine should not be used; it often causes psychotomimetic effects (dysphoria, depersonalization, frightening dreams, hallucinations)[88]
- tramadol, if used with another drug which affects serotonin metabolism/availability, can cause serotonin toxicity, particularly in the elderly (see p.392); it also lowers seizure threshold. Further, it has little or no analgesic effect unless metabolized to O-desmethyltramadol (M1) via CYP2D6; it is thus essentially ineffective in poor metabolizers (5–10% of the Caucasian population).

Table 2.4 Commonly used weak opioid combination products (UK)

Generic name		Drug content	
		Weak opioid	Non-opioid
Co-codaprin	8/400	Codeine 8mg	Aspirin 400mg
Co-codamol	8/500	Codeine 8mg	Paracetamol 500mg
Co-codamol	30/500	Codeine 30mg	Paracetamol 500mg
Co-dydramol	10/500	Dihydrocodeine 10mg	Paracetamol 500mg

The following general rules should be observed:
• a weak opioid should be added to, not substituted for, a non-opioid
• generally it is inappropriate to switch from one weak opioid to another weak opioid
• if a weak opioid is inadequate when given regularly, change to morphine (or an alternative strong opioid).

As with all opioids, patients must be monitored for undesirable effects, particularly nausea and vomiting, and constipation. Depending on individual circumstances, an anti-emetic should be prescribed for regular or p.r.n. use (Guidelines: Management of nausea and vomiting, p.106) and, routinely, a laxative prescribed (Guidelines: Opioid-induced constipation, p.117).

STRONG OPIOIDS

For more information, see *PCF3*.

'*Strong opioids exist to be given, not merely to be withheld; their use is dictated by therapeutic need and response, not by brevity of prognosis.*'

'*Pain is a physiological antagonist to the central depressant effects of opioids.*'

Strong opioids are indicated when weak opioids ($\pm$ non-opioids) are no longer adequate. Contrary to popular belief, strong opioids, rightly used, do not cause clinically important respiratory depression in patients in pain.[89] Naloxone, a specific opioid antagonist, is rarely needed in palliative care. In contrast to postoperative patients, cancer patients with pain:
• have generally been receiving a weak opioid for some time, i.e. are not opioid naïve
• take medication by mouth (slower absorption, lower peak concentration)
• titrate the dose upwards step by step (less likelihood of an excessive dose being given).

The relationship of the therapeutic dose to the lethal dose of a strong opioid (the therapeutic ratio) is greater than commonly supposed. For example, patients who take a double dose of morphine at bedtime are no more likely to die during the night than those who do not.[90]

Tolerance to strong opioids is not a practical problem.[91] Psychological dependence (addiction) to morphine is rare in patients.[92,93] Physical dependence does not prevent a reduction in the dose of morphine if the patient's pain ameliorates, e.g. as a result of radiotherapy or a nerve block.[94]

Strong opioids are not the panacea for cancer pain; generally they are best administered with a non-opioid. Further, even combined use does not guarantee success, particularly with neuropathic pain and if the psychosocial dimension of suffering is ignored. Other reasons for poor relief include:
• underdosing (failure to titrate the dose upwards)
• poor patient compliance (patient not taking medication)
• poor alimentary absorption because of vomiting
• genetic variation in the μ-opioid receptor reducing the response to morphine, e.g.:
  ▷ single-nucleotide polymorphisms
  ▷ splice variants leading to multiple receptor subtypes.

Oral morphine
Morphine by mouth is the global strong opioid of choice for cancer pain.[37,95] It is available in normal-release and m/r formulations. Normal-release morphine is

administered as tablets, e.g. 10mg, 20mg, or in aqueous solutions, e.g. 2mg in 1mL. An increasing range of m/r formulations is available, i.e. tablets, capsules, suspensions. Most are administered b.d., some once daily. The pharmacokinetic profiles of different proprietary products of m/r morphine are broadly similar (Box 2.K).[96]

Traditionally, to make things easier for patients, morphine q4h has been given on waking, 1000h, 1400h, 1800h, with a double dose at bedtime. When adjusting the dose of morphine, generally increase by 33–50%. Two-thirds of patients never need >30mg q4h (or m/r morphine 100mg q12h); the rest need up to 200mg q4h (or m/r morphine 600mg q12h), and occasionally more.[97]

Instructions must be clear: extra p.r.n. morphine does not mean that the next regular dose is omitted (see Figure 1.3, p.9 and Figure 1.4, p.10). *As a general rule, the p.r.n. dose must be increased when the regular dose is increased.*

A laxative should be prescribed routinely unless there is a definite reason for not doing so, e.g. the patient has an ileostomy (Guidelines: Opioid-induced constipation, p.117). Suppositories and enemas continue to be necessary in about 1/3 of patients.[98] *Constipation may be more difficult to manage than the pain.*

An anti-emetic, e.g. haloperidol 1.5mg stat & at bedtime, should be supplied for p.r.n. use during the first week or prescribed regularly if the patient has had nausea with a weak opioid. Warn patients about the possibility of initial drowsiness.

If changing from PO to IV/SC, give 1/3–1/2 of the PO dose.[99] Alternatively, morphine may be given PR (same dose as PO).

The main metabolites of morphine are morphine-3-glucuronide (M3G) and morphine-6-glucuronide (M6G). M3G is not analgesic but M6G is *more potent* than morphine. Both glucuronides accumulate in renal failure. This results in a prolonged duration of action, with a danger of severe sedation and respiratory depression if the dose or frequency of administration is not reduced (see *PCF3*, p.271).

Initial dose titration with IV morphine
For more information, see *PCF3*.

Initial dose titration with small boluses of IV morphine provides a method of rapidly determining morphine responsiveness, e.g. in 30–40min. This approach is ideal in countries where patients travel long distances and cannot readily return for monitoring.

Diamorphine
Diamorphine hydrochloride (di-acetylmorphine, heroin) is available for medicinal use only in the UK, where it is often used as an alternative to morphine when injections are necessary. Diamorphine hydrochloride is much more soluble than morphine sulphate or hydrochloride and large amounts can be given in a very small volume. Although a protracted supply problem has been resolved, because diamorphine ampoules cost about 3 times more than morphine ampoules, many palliative care units in the UK are continuing to use morphine as their standard parenteral strong opioid, unless the need for high doses means that solubility is an issue.

IV diamorphine is twice as potent as IV morphine.[100,101] By this route, its initial effects are mediated by the primary metabolite, mono-acetylmorphine.[102] However, by mouth, diamorphine is virtually a pro-drug for morphine because of its rapid de-acetylation.[103] When changing to SC diamorphine, give 1/3 of the PO dose of morphine, and adjust as necessary.[99]

Box 2.K Starting a patient on PO morphine

Oral morphine is indicated in patients with pain which does not respond to the optimized combined use of a non-opioid and a weak opioid.

The starting dose of morphine is calculated to give a greater analgesic effect than the medication already in use:

- if the patient was previously receiving a weak opioid regularly (e.g. codeine 240mg/24h or equivalent), give 10mg q4h or m/r 20–30mg q12h
- if changing from an alternative strong opioid (e.g. fentanyl, methadone) a much higher dose of morphine may be needed
- if the patient is frail and elderly, a lower dose helps to reduce initial drowsiness, confusion and unsteadiness, e.g. 5mg q4h
- because of accumulation of an active metabolite, a lower and/or less frequent regular dose may be preferable in renal failure, e.g. 5–10mg q6h.

If the patient takes two or more p.r.n. doses in 24h, the regular dose should be increased by 30–50% every 2–3 days.

As with all opioids, patients must be monitored for undesirable effects, particularly nausea and vomiting, and constipation. Depending on individual circumstances, an anti-emetic should be prescribed for regular or p.r.n. use (Guidelines: Management of nausea and vomiting, p.106) and, routinely, a laxative prescribed (Guidelines: Opioid-induced constipation, p.107).

Upward titration of the dose of morphine stops when either the pain is relieved or intolerable undesirable effects supervene. In the latter case, it is generally necessary to consider alternative measures. The aim is to have the patient free of pain and mentally alert.

Because of poor absorption, m/r morphine may not be satisfactory in patients troubled by frequent vomiting or those with diarrhoea or an ileostomy. All morphine products, particularly if given regularly, should be used with caution if there is renal impairment.

Scheme 1: ordinary (normal-release) morphine tablets or solution
- morphine given q4h by the clock with p.r.n. doses of equal amount
- after 1–2 days, recalculate q4h dose based on total used in previous 24h (regular + p.r.n. use)
- continue q4h and p.r.n. doses
- increase the regular dose until there is adequate relief throughout each 4h period, taking p.r.n. use into account
- a double dose at bedtime obviates the need to wake the patient for a dose during the night.

Scheme 2: ordinary (normal-release) morphine and modified-release (m/r) morphine
- begin as for Scheme 1
- when the q4h dose is stable, replace with m/r morphine q12h, or once daily if a 24h product is prescribed
- the q12h dose will be three times the previous q4h dose; a once daily dose will be six times the previous q4h dose, rounded to a convenient number of tablets or capsules
- continue to provide ordinary morphine tablets or solution for p.r.n. use; give the equivalent of a q4h dose, i.e. 1/6–1/10 of the total daily dose (practice varies).

Scheme 3: m/r morphine and ordinary (normal-release) morphine
- generally start with m/r morphine 20–30mg b.d.
- use ordinary morphine tablets or solution for p.r.n. medication; give about 1/6–1/10 of the total daily dose (practice varies)
- if necessary, increase the dose of m/r morphine every 2–3 days until there is adequate relief throughout each 12h period, guided by p.r.n. use.

Alternative strong opioids

There are four opioid receptor subtypes (μ, κ, δ and ORL-1) distributed in varying densities throughout the body, particularly in nerve tissue. All are involved in analgesia. Opioids differ from each other in terms of intrinsic activity, receptor site affinity, and non-opioid effects. These properties can be utilized in patients who are intolerant of morphine by switching to an alternative opioid (Table 2.5).[104]

Other reasons for prescribing an alternative strong opioid include:

- little or no benefit from morphine (in a pain anticipated to be opioid-responsive); genetic mutations of the μ-opioid receptor can result in reduced analgesia from morphine
- morphine not readily available
- transdermal route is preferable because of:
  - ▷ difficulty in swallowing
  - ▷ dislike of oral medication
  - ▷ lack of adherence to oral regimen
  - ▷ convenience
- fashion
- psychological 'allergy' to morphine
- cost (although morphine preparations are generally cheaper than the alternatives).

Globally, there is a range of strong opioids available for pain management (Table 2.6).[105] However, in many countries, not all are available.

Buprenorphine and fentanyl are both available as transdermal (TD) patches in a range of strengths which provide pain relief for several days (for more information, see PCF3). Patients who have not previously taken morphine or another strong opioid should always be started on the lowest dose. After removal of a patch, there is a reservoir of the opioid sequestered in body fat; this will be released slowly over the next few days. Although convenient, TD formulations are more expensive than standard morphine preparations and they are not generally considered for first-line use except in specific circumstances, e.g. patients with dysphagia.

Hydromorphone and oxycodone have a place in patients who are intolerant of morphine. Methadone is harder to use safely because of its long and variable halflife, and generally should be prescribed only by palliative care and pain relief specialists.

Pethidine (meperidine) is *not* a recommended alternative to morphine. By mouth it is best regarded as a weak opioid; it is relatively short-acting (2–3h) and has a neuro-excitatory metabolite, norpethidine (normeperidine).

The starting dose of the alternative opioid can be calculated approximately from the dose of the patient's current opioid (for more information, see PCF3, Chapter 15, Opioid dose conversion ratios).

Spinal morphine

If given epidurally (ED) or intrathecally (IT), a much lower dose of morphine has a much greater analgesic effect because of the proximity to the opioid receptors in the dorsal horn of the spinal cord. The ED dose is about 1/10 and the IT dose 1/100 of the dose of PO morphine. Undesirable effects are correspondingly reduced. In the UK, <5% of cancer patients needing morphine receive it spinally.

The main indications for spinal morphine are:

- intractable pain despite the appropriate combined use of standard and adjuvant analgesics
- intolerable undesirable effects with systemic opioids.

Table 2.5 Potential intolerable effects of systemic morphine

Type	Effect	Initial action	Comment
Gastric stasis	Epigastric fullness, flatulence, anorexia, hiccup, persistent nausea	Metoclopramide 10–20mg q4h	If the problem persists, change to an alternative opioid
Sedation	Intolerable persistent sedation	Reduce dose of morphine; consider methylphenidate 5–10mg once daily–b.d.	Sedation may be caused by other factors; stimulant rarely appropriate
Cognitive impairment	Agitated delirium ± hallucinations	Prescribe haloperidol 3–5mg stat & p.r.n.; reduce dose of morphine and, if no improvement, switch to an alternative opioid	Some patients develop intractable delirium with one opioid but not with an alternative opioid
Myoclonus	Multifocal twitching ± jerking of limbs	Prescribe diazepam/midazolam 5mg stat & p.r.n.; reduce dose of morphine	Uncommon with typical oral and SC doses; more common with high dose IV and spinal morphine; may be associated with opioid-induced hyperalgesia (see below)
Opioid-induced hyperalgesia (see p.43)	Hyperalgesia (increasing pain despite increasing morphine) ± whole-body allodynia	Progressively and rapidly reduce the dose of the causal opioid to about 25% of the peak dose; optimize the use of non-opioids and adjuvant analgesics; consider the use of an alternative opioid and/or ketamine	Occasionally seen with typical oral and SC doses; more common with high dose IV and spinal morphine

continued

Table 2.5 Continued

Type	Effect	Initial action	Comment
Vestibular stimulation	Movement-induced nausea and vomiting	Prescribe cyclizine 25–50mg q8h–q6h	If intractable, try levomepromazine or switch to an alternative opioid
Pruritus	Tends to affect the whole body	Stat dose of an H_1-antihistamine, e.g. chlorphenamine 4–12mg PO; if after 2–3h there is definite benefit, prescribe 4mg t.d.s.; if not, switch to an alternative opioid, e.g. oxycodone	Uncommon after systemic morphine (see p.322); does not always respond to H_1-antihistamines
Histamine release	Bronchoconstriction → breathlessness	Prescribe IV/IM antihistamine (e.g. chlorphenamine 5–10mg) and a bronchodilator; change to a chemically distinct opioid immediately, e.g. methadone	Rare

Table 2.6 Alternative strong opioids (for more details, see individual drug monographs in PCF3)

	Opioid receptor affinity			Non-opioid properties	Bio-availability[a]	Plasma halflife (h)	PO:PO potency ratio with morphine[b]
	Mu	Kappa	Delta				
Buprenorphine	pA	Ant	Ant	None	50–60% SL 100% IV[c,d]	24–69 SL 3–16 IV 13–36 TD[e] (formulation dependent)	80 SL 100 (75–115) TD
Fentanyl	A	–	–	None	100% IV[c,d]	3 IV 24 TD[e]	100 (150) TD
Hydromorphone	A	–	–	None	37–62%	2.5	4–5 (7.5)
Morphine	A	–	–	None	15–64%	2–2.5	1
Methadone	A	–	A(?)	Blocks pre-synaptic re-uptake of serotonin; NMDA-receptor-channel blocker	40–100%	8–75	5–10[f]
Oxycodone	A	A	–	None	60–87%	3.5	1.5 (2)

Key: A = strong agonist; pA = partial agonist; Ant = antagonist; – = no activity; IV = intravenous; SC = subcutaneous; SL = sublingual; TD = transdermal.
a. PO unless stated otherwise
b. numbers in parenthesis are the manufacturer's preferred ratios
c. IV and SC bio-availability are essentially the same
d. bio-availability irrelevant for TD patches; all patches have stated mean delivery rates (e.g. microgram/h), although inevitably there will be interindividual variation in the amounts delivered
e. the halflife after a patch has been removed and not replaced
f. variable long halflife leads to accumulation and a variable potency ratio, occasionally as high as 30:1.

To increase the effect of spinal analgesia in neuropathic pain, morphine is often combined with bupivacaine, and sometimes clonidine.

Topical morphine
The peripheral endings of nociceptive afferent nerve fibres contain opioid receptors which, in the presence of local inflammation, become active and increase in number, responding to opioids produced by neutrophils.[105–108] This property is exploited in joint surgery where morphine is given intra-articularly at the end of the operation.[109] Topical morphine has also been used successfully to relieve otherwise intractable pain associated with cutaneous ulceration, often sacral decubitus.[110–112] Generally, it is given as a 0.1% (1mg/mL) gel (in Intrasite®). A higher dose may be necessary, e.g. 0.3–0.5%, in other situations:
- oral mucositis
- vaginal inflammation associated with a fistula
- rectal ulceration.[111]

The amount of gel applied varies according to the size and the site of the ulcer but is typically 5–10mL applied b.d.–t.d.s. The topical morphine is kept in place with:
- a non-absorbable pad or dressing, e.g. Opsite®
- gauze coated with petroleum jelly.

OPIOID-INDUCED HYPERALGESIA

Opioid-induced hyperalgesia (OIH) appears important in both acute and chronic pain. Although poorly understood, it appears to result from sustained sensitization of the nervous system in which the excitatory amino acid neurotransmitter system and the NMDA-receptor-channel complex play important roles.[113] Possible causes include:
- opioid-induced activation of glial cells, which play a role in inflammation, pain signal transmission, pain hypersensitivity and opioid tolerance[11,114]
- alteration in the G protein coupling of opioid receptors, with G_s rather than G_i or G_o; the variant G protein complex possibly has an excitatory rather than an inhibitory effect[115]
- in the case of morphine, accumulation of M3G.[116]

Genetic make-up probably plays an important part in its development.

Clinical features
In surgical pain, OIH may contribute to exaggerated levels of pain in the immediate postoperative period and the development of a chronic pain state. In patients with cancer, OIH may manifest in various ways:
- rapidly developing tolerance to opioids
- short-lived benefit from increased doses
- a change of pain pattern (Table 2.7).

The extreme upper end of the spectrum may be those patients who manifest evidence of severe neural hyperexcitability (myoclonus, allodynia, and/or hyperalgesia), particularly when taking high doses of morphine or an alternative strong opioid. This may

Table 2.7   Opioid-induced hyperalgesia[117]

What the patient says	What the doctor finds
Increased sensitivity to pain stimulus (hyperalgesia)	Any dose of any opioid, but particularly with high-dose morphine or hydromorphone, and in renal failure
Worsening pain despite increasing doses of opioids	Pain elicited from ordinary non-painful stimuli, e.g. stroking skin with cotton (allodynia)
Pain which becomes more diffuse, extending beyond the distribution of the pre-existing pain	Presence of other manifestations of opioid-induced neural hyperexcitability: myoclonus, seizures, delirium

be accompanied by sedation and delirium (when it is often described as opioid neurotoxicity). However, OIH:
- is *not* limited to very high doses, or to any one opioid
- is probably under-diagnosed
- is more common than generally thought.

Severe pain which does not respond to increasing doses of opioids, or is complicated by severe undesirable effects, should raise the *possibility* of OIH.[117]

Evaluation
A diagnosis of OIH is generally made on the basis of a high level of clinical suspicion, probability, and pattern recognition. OIH must be differentiated from increased pain caused by disease progression or the development of opioid tolerance, both of which may be managed by increasing the opioid dose.

Management
Management is based largely on theoretical grounds and clinical observation.

Prophylaxis
Use a multimodal approach to analgesia, e.g.:
- an NSAID may help to reduce the production of excitatory amino acid neurotransmitters which activate the pronociceptive and anti-opioid systems
- gabapentin may block calcium channels which may contribute to hyperalgesia in nerve pain.

Treatment
- progressively and rapidly reduce the dose of the causal opioid to about 25% of the peak dose
- switch to an opioid with less risk of OIH, i.e. fentanyl (highest) → morphine → methadone → buprenorphine (lowest)[118]
- (rarely) if occurring at very low doses (< 10mg/24h), discontinue the opioid completely
- use a multimodal approach to analgesia, i.e. use non-opioids, e.g. paracetamol or an NSAID, and adjuvant analgesics, e.g. gabapentin
- start oral or parenteral ketamine (an NMDA-receptor-channel blocker).[119]

Note that when switching from morphine because of severe neural hyperexcitability, a lower than expected dose of the alternative opioid is likely to be needed unless the dose of morphine has been much reduced (as suggested above).[120,121] If these steps do not lead to a resolution of the OIH:

- consider spinal, regional or local analgesia (with local anaesthetics), and tail off systemic opioids completely
- check for hypomagnesaemia as this can aggravate OIH[122,123]
- consider treatment with ultralow doses of an opioid antagonist.[124-126]

ADJUVANT ANALGESICS

In the past, adjuvant analgesics were drugs primarily marketed for indications other than pain but which, in certain limited circumstances, were used beyond their licence to relieve pain. More recently, some adjuvant analgesics, e.g. duloxetine, gabapentin, pregabalin, are now licensed for the relief of various neuropathic pains. Even so, adjuvants are *not* primarily classified as analgesics even though they may relieve pain which has proved to be resistant to 'primary' analgesics such as NSAIDs and/or strong opioids. Adjuvant analgesics include:

- corticosteroids
- antidepressants
- anti-epileptics
- NMDA-receptor-channel blockers
- smooth muscle relaxants (antispasmodics)
- skeletal muscle relaxants
- bisphosphonates.

Unfortunately, the term 'adjuvant analgesic' is misleading if interpreted to mean that such drugs work only when used together with a primary analgesic. In many situations, adjuvant analgesics *alone* provide pain relief ± a reduction in undesirable drug effects. For example, although opioids have been shown in RCTs to at least partly relieve neuropathic pain,[127,128] an antidepressant and/or an anti-epileptic may be preferable in patients with a normal life expectancy, i.e. in those who do not have progressive cancer.

Systemic corticosteroids
For more information, see *PCF3*.

Systemic corticosteroids are helpful for pain and weakness associated with:
- nerve root/nerve trunk compression, e.g. dexamethasone 4–8mg once daily
- spinal cord compression, e.g. dexamethasone 12–16mg daily.[129,130]

A reduction in compression is likely to improve both function and pain (Figure 2.10). Improved pain may also relate to the anti-inflammatory effect reducing mediators such as prostaglandins which lead to peripheral and central sensitization. In a limited number of cancers, e.g. breast, lymphoma, multiple myeloma and prostate, corticosteroids can also have an anticancer effect.

In cancer-related nerve injury pain, a trial of dexamethasone for 7–10 days may be beneficial. However, systemic corticosteroids do not help in pure non-cancer nerve injury pain, e.g. chronic postoperative scar pain and post-herpetic neuralgia.

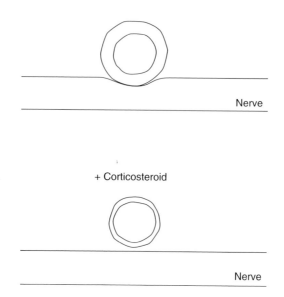

Figure 2.10 Possible mechanism of action of corticosteroids in relief of nerve compression pain. Total tumour mass = cancer + surrounding inflammation. The general anti-inflammatory effect of corticosteroids reduces the total tumour mass resulting in reduction of pain.

Antidepressants and anti-epileptics

For more information, see *PCF3*.

Antidepressants and anti-epileptics are often of benefit when used as single agents in 'pure' nerve injury pain, e.g. chronic surgical incision pain, painful diabetic neuropathy, and post-herpetic neuralgia.[131–134] However, if the nerve injury pain is associated with an infiltrating cancer, morphine and an NSAID should be tried first before *adding* an antidepressant or an anti-epileptic.[135–137]

About 90% of patients with nerve injury pain respond to the use of non-opioids, opioids and adjuvant analgesics.[16] The remainder require spinal analgesia (e.g. morphine + bupivacaine ± clonidine) or a neurolytic procedure to obtain adequate relief. Some patients derive benefit from other non-drug measures, e.g. TENS.

Antidepressants are not equally effective in relieving peripheral neuropathic pain. TCAs are the most effective followed by venlafaxine, then SSRIs, e.g. paroxetine and citalopram. TCAs have an opioid-sparing effect when used in cancer pain generally. Central pain is generally harder to relieve than peripheral neuropathic pain. Again, TCAs are the most effective antidepressant for treatment of this.

The analgesic effect of TCAs probably depends on several pharmacological mechanisms, possibly including:

- inhibition of pre-synaptic re-uptake of serotonin and noradrenaline/norepinephrine (Figure 2.11)

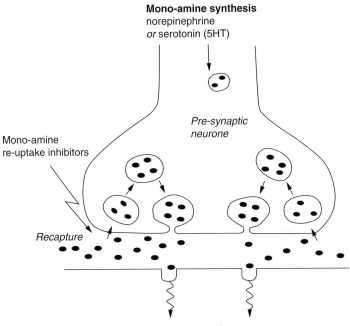

Mono-amine synthesis
norepinephrine
or serotonin (5HT)

Pre-synaptic neurone

Mono-amine
re-uptake inhibitors

Recapture

Post-synaptic neurone

Figure 2.11 Mono-amine re-uptake inhibitors, e.g. TCAs and SSRIs, facilitate one or both of the two descending spinal inhibitory pathways by blocking pre-synaptic re-uptake (one serotoninergic and the other noradrenergic). SNRIs and SSRIs also potentiate opioid analgesia by a serotoninergic mechanism in the brain stem.

- post-synaptic receptor antagonism:
  ▷ α-adrenergic
  ▷ histamine type 1 (H_1)
  ▷ μ-opioid (low affinity)
- channel blockade:
  ▷ NMDA-receptor
  ▷ sodium
  ▷ calcium.[134]

The mechanisms by which anti-epileptics relieve pain differ from the antidepressants. Some anti-epileptics act as peripheral sodium-channel blockers. Others impact mainly on the dorsal horn by inhibiting the glutamate (excitatory) system or activating the GABA (inhibitory) system, or both. Gabapentin and pregabalin, although structural analogues of GABA, act principally as $\alpha_2\delta$-type calcium-channel blockers.[138] Thus, it makes sense to combine an antidepressant with an anti-epileptic in those patients who fail to achieve satisfactory relief with either class of drug individually.

It is important to establish a straightforward practical scheme for neuropathic pain management, selecting only one or two drugs from each category of agents

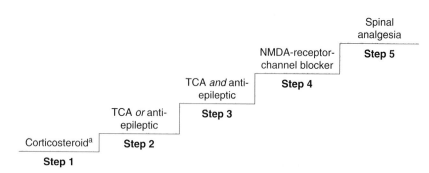

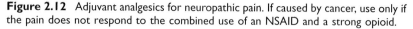

Figure 2.12 Adjuvant analgesics for neuropathic pain. If caused by cancer, use only if the pain does not respond to the combined use of an NSAID and a strong opioid.

a. a trial of a corticosteroid is important when neuropathic pain is associated with limb weakness.

(Figure 2.12).[139,140] For example, in Steps 2 and 3, although now less often used to treat depression, amitriptyline 25–75mg at bedtime is still widely used as an adjuvant analgesic.[141] For an anti-epileptic, some centres still use valproate 400mg–1g at bedtime. However, gabapentin and pregabalin are increasingly used, partly because they are licensed for treating neuropathic pain.[141,142]

When considering combining adjuvant analgesics, the following combinations should be avoided:

• two different antidepressants
• an antidepressant with tramadol (see p.392).

RCT evidence for combinations is still sparse but:

• adding venlafaxine to gabapentin in painful diabetic neuropathy results in significant additional benefit[143]
• in both diabetic neuropathy and post-herpetic neuralgia, combining morphine and gabapentin results in better pain relief at lower doses than either drug when used as a single agent.[144]

When treating nerve injury pain, the patient should be warned that major benefit often takes a week or more to manifest, although improvement in sleep may well occur immediately.

Particularly with nerve injury pain, relief is not an 'all-or-none' phenomenon. The crucial first step in many cases is to help the patient obtain a good night's sleep. The second is to reduce pain intensity and allodynia to a bearable level during the day. Initially, there may be marked diurnal variation in relief, with more prolonged periods with less or no pain rather than a decrease in worst pain intensity round the clock.

Undesirable drug effects are often a limiting therapeutic factor. To avoid excessive drowsiness with psychotropics, dose escalation generally should be relatively slow, e.g. a dose increase no more than twice per week. On the other hand, with a corticosteroid, it is generally best to start with a high dose and then reduce to a satisfactory maintenance level.

NMDA-receptor-channel blockers

For more information, see *PCF3*.

The archetypal NMDA-receptor-channel blocker is ketamine.[145–147] It is generally used when neuropathic pain does not respond well to standard analgesics together with an antidepressant and an anti-epileptic or to methadone. It has also been used in inflammatory pain, e.g. severe mucositis.[148] Undesirable effects can limit its use.

Smooth muscle relaxants (antispasmodics)

For more information, see *PCF3*.

This is a heterogeneous group of drugs encompassing antimuscarinics, glyceryl trinitrate, and calcium-channel blockers (e.g. nifedipine). Antimuscarinics are used to relieve visceral distension pain and colic. In advanced cancer, there is little place for 'weak' antispasmodics such as dicycloverine and mebeverine. In the UK, hyoscine *butylbromide* and glycopyrronium, quaternary drugs which do not cross the blood–brain barrier, are widely used. Atropine and hyoscine *hydrobromide* have comparable peripheral effects but also have central effects, either stimulation or sedation, and may precipitate delirium.

Glyceryl trinitrate and calcium-channel blockers can be used for the same range of indications, but tend to be reserved for painful spasm of the oesophagus, rectum and anus.

Skeletal muscle relaxants

For more information, see *PCF3*.

These include baclofen, diazepam, and tizanidine. However, for painful skeletal muscle spasm (cramp) and myofascial pain, non-drug treatments are generally preferable, e.g. physical therapy (massage, local heat, acupuncture). Some patients also benefit from relaxation therapy ± diazepam. Myofascial trigger points often benefit from direct injection of local anaesthetic.[149] *However severe, morphine is ineffective for the relief of cramp and trigger point pains.*

Bisphosphonates

For more information, see *PCF3*.

Bisphosphonates are osteoclast inhibitors and are used to relieve metastatic bone pain which persists despite analgesics and radiotherapy ± orthopaedic surgery. Published data relate mainly to breast cancer and myeloma; benefit is also seen with other cancers. About 50% of patients benefit, typically in 1–2 weeks, and this may last for 2–3 months. Benefit may be seen only after a second treatment but, if there is no response after two treatments, an analgesic effect is unlikely.[150] In those who respond, continue to treat p.r.n. for as long as there is benefit. However, particularly for patients with breast cancer or multiple myeloma and a prognosis of ⩾6 months, maintenance treatment with a bisphosphonate may be indicated in those who do not obtain an analgesic response to reduce the risk of additional complications from metastatic bone disease.

ALTERNATIVE ROUTES OF ADMINISTRATION

Not all patients are able to swallow tablets or capsules, and those experiencing nausea and vomiting may not be able to retain them. A range of alternative routes is available. In practice, choice is largely determined by local availability (Figure 2.13).

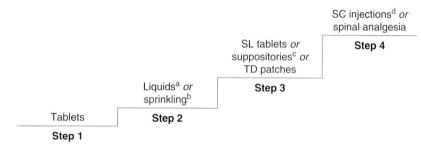

Figure 2.13 Alternative routes of administration.

a. solutions or suspensions
b. on semi-solid food
c. can use m/r tablets in an emergency
d. in the UK, CSCI generally used in preference to intermittent SC injections.

'Sprinkling' refers to the practice of emptying the contents of an m/r morphine capsule onto a teaspoon of semi-solid food immediately before swallowing, e.g. apple sauce, puree, jam, yoghurt, ice cream. Although sachets of m/r morphine granules are available for use as a suspension, they are much more expensive.

Available buccal and SL tablets include piroxicam and buprenorphine. Orodispersible piroxicam (Feldene Melt®, see Box 2.J, p.34) is a soluble oral formulation, i.e. the dissolved tablet still has to be swallowed. On the other hand, SL buprenorphine is absorbed locally, and swallowing it results in a major loss of efficacy because of first-pass hepatic metabolism.

For break-through pain, oral transmucosal fentanyl citrate (e.g. OTFC, Actiq®) or SL alfentanil are used at some centres (for more information, see *PCF3*). These will soon be joined by various tablet, spray and powder formulations of fentanyl specifically developed for delivery via the buccal/SL, pulmonary or nasal routes. Other drugs examined for nasal delivery include morphine and ketamine.

Morphine administered SL is poorly absorbed through the buccal mucosa, with most absorption resulting from it being swallowed.[151] However, it has been successfully used by this route in moribund patients cared for at home.

Buprenorphine and fentanyl TD patches are an alternative in selected patients. Lidocaine patches are also available. These are used mainly for chest wall pain caused by mesothelioma, but could probably be used successfully in other situations.

Morphine suppositories are available for PR administration, but are not always feasible. Although not licensed for this route, m/r morphine tablets have been used PR to provide emergency analgesia in moribund patients.

Battery-driven portable syringe drivers are a convenient method for administering many drugs by CSCI to patients with severe nausea and vomiting, or who cannot swallow medication for various reasons. The advantages of CSCI infusion include:

- better control of nausea and vomiting (guarantees drug absorption)
- constant analgesia (no peaks or troughs)
- generally reloaded once in 24h (saves nurses' time)
- comfort and confidence (minimal number of injections)
- does not limit mobility (lightweight and compact).

Detailed information about CSCI is available in *PCF3*, Chapter 18, Continuous subcutaneous infusions, and at www.palliativedrugs.com. In patients with venous access, e.g. a Hickman line, the IV route is an obvious alternative but CSCI is generally preferable.

1 IASP Task Force on Taxonomy (2007) Part III: Pain Terms, A Current List with Definitions and Notes on Usage. In: *Classification of Chronic Pain*. IASP Press, Seattle. Available from: http://www.iasp-pain.org/AM/Template.cfm?Section=Home&template=/CM/HTMLDisplay.cfm&ContentID=6648

2 van den Beuken-van Everdingen MH et al. (2007) High prevalence of pain in patients with cancer in a large population-based study in The Netherlands. *Pain*. **132**: 312–320.

3 Kane R et al. (1984) A randomized controlled trial of hospice care. *Lancet*. **1**: 890–894.

4 Bonica J (1990) Cancer pain: current status and future needs. In: J Bonica (ed) *The Management of Pain* (2e). Lea and Febiger, Philadelphia, pp. 400–455.

5 Grond S et al. (1996) Assessment of cancer pain: a prospective evaluation in 2266 cancer patients referred to a pain service. *Pain*. **64**: 107–114.

6 Davies AN et al. (2009) The management of cancer-related breakthrough pain: Recommendations of a task group of the Science Committee of the Association for Palliative Medicine of Great Britain and Ireland. *European Journal of Pain*. **13**: 330–337.

7 Douglas I et al. (2000) Central issues in the management of temporal variation in cancer pain. In: R Hillier et al. (eds) *The Effective Management of Cancer Pain*. Aesculapius Medical Press, London, pp. 93–106.

8 Davies A (ed) (2006) *Cancer-related Breakthrough Pain*. Oxford University Press, Oxford, UK.

9 Portenoy RK et al. (2006) Prevalence and characteristics of breakthrough pain in opioid-treated patients with chronic noncancer pain. *The Journal of Pain*. **7**: 583–591.

10 Colvin L and Fallon M (2008) Challenges in cancer pain management–bone pain. *European Journal of Cancer*. **44**: 1083–1090.

11 Romero-Sandoval EA et al. (2008) Neuroimmune interactions and pain: focus on glial-modulating targets. *Current Opinion in Investigational Drugs*. **9**: 726–734.

12 Bonica J (1990) Definitions and taxonomy of pain. In: Bonica J (ed) *The Management of Pain* (2e). Lea and Febiger, Philadelphia, pp. 18–27.

13 Travell J and Rinzler S (1952) The myofascial genesis of pain. *Postgraduate Medicine (Minneapolis)*. **11**: 425–434.

14 Baron R (2000) Peripheral neuropathic pain: from mechanisms to symptoms. *Clinical Journal of Pain*. **16**: S12–S20.

15 Sindrup S and Jensen T (1999) Efficacy of pharmacological treatments of neuropathic pain: an update and effect related to mechanism of drug action. *Pain*. **83**: 389–400.

16 Grond S et al. (1999) Assessment and treatment of neuropathic cancer pain following WHO guidelines. *Pain*. **79**: 15–20.

17 Van Damme S et al. (2008) Coping with pain: a motivational perspective. *Pain*. **139**: 1–4.

18 Hoskin PJ (1995) Radiotherapy in the management of bone pain. *Clinical Orthopaedics*. **312**: 105–119.

19 George R (1999) Unpublished work.

20 Bone Pain Trial Working Party (1999) 8Gy single fraction radiotherapy for the treatment of metastatic skeletal pain: randomized comparison with a multifraction schedule over 12 months of patient follow-up. *Radiotherapy and Oncology*. **52**: 111–121.

21 McQuay HJ et al. (2000) Radiotherapy for the palliation of painful bone metastases. *Cochrane Database Systematic Review*. CD001793.

22 Ashford RU et al. (2006) Management of metastatic disease of the appendicular skeleton. *Current Orthopaedics*. **20**: 299–315.

23 Sze WM et al. (2004) Palliation of metastatic bone pain: single fraction versus multifraction radiotherapy – a systematic review of the randomised trials. *Cochrane Database Systematic Review*. CD004721.

24 Roque M et al. (2003) Radioisotopes for metastatic bone pain. *Cochrane Database Systematic Review*. CD003347.

25 Borgelt B et al. (1980) The palliation of brain metastases: final results of the first two studies by the Radiation Therapy Oncology Group. *International Journal of Radiation Oncology, Biology, Physics*. **6**: 1–9.

26 Tsao MN et al. (2006) Whole brain radiotherapy for the treatment of multiple brain metastases. *Cochrane Database Systematic Review.* **3**: CD003869.

27 Selvaggi G and Scagliotti GV (2005) Management of bone metastases in cancer: a review. *Critical Reviews in Oncology/Hematology.* **56**: 365–378.

28 Mirels H (1989) Metastatic disease in long bones. A proposed scoring system for diagnosing impending pathologic fractures. *Clinical Orthopaedics and Related Research.* **249**: 256–264.

29 Tei Y et al. (2008) Treatment efficacy of neural blockade in specialized palliative care services in Japan: a multicenter audit survey. *Journal of Pain and Symptom Management.* **36**: 461–467.

30 Polati E et al. (2008) The role of neurolytic celiac plexus block in the treatment of pancreatic cancer pain. *Transplantation Proceedings.* **40**: 1200–1204.

31 de Leon-Casasola OA (2000) Neurolysis of the sympathetic axis for cancer pain management. *Techniques in Regional Anaesthesia and Pain Management.* **9**: 161–166.

32 Fugere F and Lewis G (1993) Coeliac plexus block for chronic pain syndromes. *Canadian Journal of Anaesthesia.* **40**: 954–963.

33 Puli SR et al. (2009) EUS-guided celiac plexus neurolysis for pain due to chronic pancreatitis or pancreatic cancer pain: a meta-analysis and systematic review. *Digestive Diseases and Sciences* [published on line 10.01.09]

34 Stein C (1993) Peripheral mechanisms of opioid analgesia. *Anesthesia and Analgesia.* **76**: 182–191.

35 Geisslinger G and Yaksh T (2000) Spinal actions of cyclooxygenase isozyme inhibitors. In: D M et al. (eds) *Proceedings of the 9th World Congress on Pain Progress in Pain Research and Management Volume 16.* IASP Press, Seattle, pp. 771–785.

36 World Health Organization (1986) *Cancer Pain Relief.* WHO, Geneva.

37 WHO (1996) *Cancer Pain Relief: with a Guide to Opioid Availability* (2e). World Health Organisation, Geneva.

38 Cormie PJ et al. (2008) Control of pain in adults with cancer: summary of SIGN guidelines. *British Medical Journal.* **337**: a2154.

39 SIGN (2008) Control of pain in adults with cancer. (Guideline No. 106.). Scottish Intercollegiate Guidelines Network, Edinburgh. Available from: www.sign.ac.uk

40 Zeppetella G and Ribeiro MD (2002) Episodic pain in patients with advanced cancer. *The American Journal of Hospice & Palliative Care.* **19**: 267–276.

41 Davis MP (2003) Guidelines for breakthrough pain dosing. *The American Journal of Hospice & Palliative Care.* **20**: 334.

42 Davis MP et al. (2005) Controversies in pharmacotherapy of pain management. *The Lancet Oncology.* **6**: 696–704.

43 Portenoy K and Hagen N (1990) Breakthrough pain: definition, prevalence and characteristics. *Pain.* **41**: 273–281.

44 Mercadante S et al. (2002) Episodic (breakthrough) pain: consensus conference of an expert working group of the EAPC. *Cancer.* **94**: 832–839.

45 Zeppetella G (2008) Opioids for cancer breakthrough pain: a pilot study reporting patient assessment of time to meaningful pain relief. *Journal of Pain and Symptom Management.* **35**: 563–567.

46 Gomez-Batiste X et al. (2002) Breakthrough cancer pain: prevalence and characteristics in Catalonia. *Journal of Pain and Symptom Management.* **24**: 45–52.

47 Davies AN et al. (2008) An observational study of oncology patients' utilization of breakthrough pain medication. *Journal of Pain and Symptom Management.* **35**: 406–411.

48 Zeppetella G and Ribeiro MD (2006) Opioids for the management of breakthrough (episodic) pain in cancer patients. *Cochrane Database Systematic Review.* CD004311.

49 Christie J et al. (1998) Dose-titration, multicenter study of oral transmucosal fentanyl citrate for the treatment of breakthrough pain in cancer patients using transdermal fentanyl for persistent pain. *Journal of Clinical Oncology.* **16**: 3238–3248.

50 Lim R et al. (1964) Site of action of narcotic and non-narcotic analgesics determined by blocking bradykinin-evoked visceral pain. *Archives Internationales de Pharmacodynamie et de Therapie.* **152**: 25–58.

51 Moore U et al. (1992) The efficacy of locally applied aspirin and acetaminophen in postoperative pain after third molar surgery. *Clinical Pharmacology and Therapeutics.* **52**: 292–296.

52 Twycross RG et al. (2000) Paracetamol. *Progress in Palliative Care.* **8**: 198–202.

53 Flower RJ and Vane JR (1972) Inhibition of prostaglandin synthetase in brain explains the anti-pyretic activity of paracetamol. *Nature.* **240**: 410–411.

54 Bjorkman R et al. (1994) Acetaminophen (paracetamol) blocks spinal hyperalgesia induced by NMDA and substance P. *Pain.* **57**: 259–264.

55 Pini L et al. (1997) Naloxone-reversible antinociception by paracetamol in the rat. *Journal of Pharmacology and Experimental Therapeutics.* **280**: 934–940.

56 Settipane R et al. (1995) Prevalence of cross-sensitivity with acetaminophen in aspirin-sensitive asthmatic subjects. *Journal of Allergy and Clinical Immunology.* **96**: 480–485.

57 Miranda HF et al. (2006) Synergism between paracetamol and nonsteroidal anti-inflammatory drugs in experimental acute pain. *Pain.* **121**: 22–28.

58 Mercadante S (2001) The use of anti-inflammatory drugs in cancer pain. *Cancer Treatment Reviews.* **27**: 51–61.

59 McNicol E et al. (2004) Nonsteroidal anti-inflammatory drugs, alone or combined with opioids, for cancer pain: a systematic review. *Journal of Clinical Oncology.* **22**: 1975–1992.

60 Koppert W et al. (2004) The cyclooxygenase isozyme inhibitors parecoxib and paracetamol reduce central hyperalgesia in humans. *Pain.* **108**: 148–153.

61 Hawkins C and Hanks G (2000) The gastroduodenal toxicity of nonsteroidal anti-inflammatory drugs. A review of the literature. *Journal of Pain and Symptom Management.* **20**: 140–151.

62 Tramer M et al. (2000) Quantitative estimation of rare adverse events which follow a biological progression: a new model applied to chronic NSAID use. *Pain.* **85**: 169–182.

63 Kearney PM et al. (2006) Do selective cyclo-oxygenase-2 inhibitors and traditional non-steroidal anti-inflammatory drugs increase the risk of atherothrombosis? Meta-analysis of randomised trials. *British Medical Journal.* **332**: 1302–1308.

64 CHM (2004) Cardiovascular safety of COX-2 inhibitors and non-selective NSAIDs. Commission on Human Medicines. Available from: www.mhra.gov.uk/home/idcplg?IdcService=SS_GET_PAGE&nodeId=227

65 Solomon SD et al. (2005) Cardiovascular risk associated with celecoxib in a clinical trial for colorectal adenoma prevention. *The New England Journal of Medicine.* **352**: 1071–1080.

66 Singh G et al. (2006) Celecoxib versus naproxen and diclofenac in osteoarthritis patients: SUCCESS-I Study. *The American Journal of Medicine.* **119**: 255–266.

67 Caldwell B et al. (2006) Risk of cardiovascular events and celecoxib: a systematic review and meta-analysis. *Journal of the Royal Society of Medicine.* **99**: 132–140.

68 Duff G (2006) Safety of selective and non-selective NSAIDs. In: *Letter to health professionals from the Chairman of the Commission on Human Medicines, 24th October 2006.* Available from: http://www.mhra.gov.uk/Safetyinformation/Safetywarningsalertsandrecalls/Safetywarningsandmessagesformedicines/CON2025040

69 Bennett A (2000) The importance of COX-2 inhibition for aspirin induced asthma. *Thorax.* **55 (suppl 2)**: s54–s56.

70 Venturini C et al. (1998) Nonsteroidal anti-inflammatory drug-induced renal failure: a brief review of the role of cyclooxygenase isoforms. *Current Opinion in Nephrology and Hypertension.* **7**: 79–82.

71 Schneider V et al. (2006) Association of selective and conventional nonsteroidal antiinflammatory drugs with acute renal failure: A population-based, nested case–control analysis. *American Journal of Epidemiology.* **164**: 881–889.

72 EMEA (2006) Questions and answers on the review of non-selective NSAIDs. European Agency for the Evaluation of Medicinal Products. Available from: www.emea.europa.eu/pdfs/human/opiniongen/nsaidsq&a.pdf

73 Whelton A et al. (2002) Effects of celecoxib and rofecoxib on blood pressure and edema in patients >65 years of age with systemic hypertension and osteoarthritis. *American Journal of Cardiology.* **90**: 959–963.

74 Lundstam SOA et al. (1982) Prostaglandin-synthetase inhibition with diclofenac sodium in treatment of renal colic: comparison with use of a narcotic analgesic. *Lancet.* **1**: 1096–1097.

75 Middleton RK et al. (1996) Ketorolac continuous infusion: a case report and review of the literature. *Journal of Pain and Symptom Management.* **12**: 190–194.

76 Hughes A et al. (1997) Ketorolac: continuous subcutaneous infusion for cancer pain. *Journal of Pain and Symptom Management.* **13**: 315–317.

77 Tramer M et al. (1998) Comparing analgesic efficacy of non-steroidal anti-inflammatory drugs given by different routes in acute and chronic pain: a qualitative systematic review. *Acta Anaesthesiologica Scandinavica.* **42**: 71–79.

78 Marinangeli F et al. (2004) Use of strong opioids in advanced cancer pain: a randomized trial. *Journal of Pain and Symptom Management.* **27**: 409–416.

79 Maltoni M et al. (2005) A validation study of the WHO analgesic ladder: a two-step vs three-step strategy. *Support Care Cancer.* **13**: 888–894.

80 WHO (1986) *Cancer Pain Relief.* World Health Organisation, Geneva.

81 Moore A et al. (2000) Single dose paracetamol (acetaminophen), with and without codeine, for postoperative pain. *Cochrane Database Systematic Review.* CD001547.

82 Smith LA et al. (2001) Using evidence from different sources: an example using paracetamol 1000mg plus codeine 60mg. *BMC Medical Research Methodology.* **1**: 1.

83 Macleod AG et al. (2002) Paracetamol versus paracetamol-codeine in the treatment of post-operative dental pain: a randomized, double-blind, prospective trial. *Australian Dental Journal.* **47**: 147–151.

84 Rodriguez RF et al. (2007) Codeine/acetaminophen and hydrocodone/acetaminophen combination tablets for the management of chronic cancer pain in adults: a 23-day, prospective, double-blind, randomized, parallel-group study. *Clinical Therapeutics.* **29**: 581–587.

85 Wilder-Smith C et al. (2001) Treatment of severe pain from osteoarthritis with slow-release tramadol or dihydrocodeine in combination with NSAID's: a randomised study comparing analgesia, antinociception and gastrointestinal effects. *Pain.* **91**: 23–31.

86 Hawton K et al. (2003) Co-proxamol and suicide: a study of national mortality statistics and local non-fatal self poisonings. British Medical Journal. 326: 1006–1008.

87 Ammon S et al. (1999) Pharmacokinetics of dihydrocodeine and its active metabolite after single and multiple oral dosing. British Journal of Clinical Pharmacology. 48: 317–322.

88 Woods A et al. (1974) Medicines evaluation and monitoring group: central nervous system effects of pentazocine. British Medical Journal. 1: 305–307.

89 Borgbjerg FM et al. (1996) Experimental pain stimulates respiration and attenuates morphine-induced respiratory depression: a controlled study in human volunteers. Pain. 64: 123–128.

90 Regnard CFB and Badger C (1987) Opioids, sleep and the time of death. Palliative Medicine. 1: 107–110.

91 Collin E et al. (1993) Is disease progression the major factor in morphine 'tolerance' in cancer pain treatment? Pain. 55: 319–326.

92 Passik S and Portenoy R (1998) Substance abuse issues in palliative care. In: A Berger (ed) Principles and Practice of Supportive Oncology. Lippincott-Raven, Philadelphia, pp. 513–529.

93 Joranson D et al. (2000) Trends in medical use and abuse of opioid analgesics. Journal of the American Medical Association. 283: 1710–1714.

94 Twycross RG and Wald SJ (1976) Longterm use of diamorphine in advanced cancer. In: JJ Bonica and D Albe-Fessard (eds) Advances in Pain Research and Therapy. Vol 1. Raven Press, New York, pp. 653–661.

95 Twycross RG (1997) Oral Morphine in Advanced Cancer (3e). Beaconsfield Publishers, Beaconsfield.

96 Collins S et al. (1998) Peak plasma concentrations after oral morphine: a systematic review. Journal of Pain and Symptom Management. 16: 388–402.

97 Schug SA et al. (1992) A long-term survey of morphine in cancer pain patients. Journal of Pain and Symptom Management. 7: 259–266.

98 Twycross RG and Harcourt JMV (1991) The use of laxatives at a palliative care centre. Palliative Medicine. 5: 27–33.

99 Hanks GW et al. (1996) Morphine in cancer pain: modes of administration. British Medical Journal. 312: 823–826.

100 Smith GM et al. (1962) Subjective effects of heroin and morphine in normal subjects. The Journal of Pharmacology and Experimental Therapeutics. 136: 47–52.

101 Loan WB et al. (1969) Studies of drugs given before anaesthesia. XVII. The natural and semi-synthetic opiates. British Journal of Anaesthesia. 41: 57–63.

102 Wright CI and Barbour FA (1935) The respiratory effects of morphine, codeine and related substances. Journal of Pharmacology and Experimental Therapeutics. 54: 25–33.

103 Twycross RG (1977) Choice of strong analgesic in terminal cancer: diamorphine or morphine? Pain. 3: 93–104.

104 Ashby M et al. (1999) Opioid substitution to reduce adverse effects in cancer pain management. Medical Journal of Australia. 170: 68–71.

105 Pergolizzi J et al. (2008) Opioids and the management of chronic severe pain in the elderly: consensus statement of an International Expert Panel with focus on the six clinically most often used World Health Organization step III opioids (buprenorphine, fentanyl, hydromorphone, methadone, morphine, oxycodone). Pain Practice. 8: 287–313.

106 Krajnik M and Zylicz Z (1997) Topical opioids – fact or fiction? Progress in Palliative Care. 5: 101–106.

107 Krajnik M et al. (1998) Opioids affect inflammation and the immune system. Pain Reviews. 5: 147–154.

108 Smith HS (2008) Peripherally-acting opioids. Pain Physician. 11: S121–132.

109 Likar R et al. (1999) Dose-dependency of intra-articular morphine analgesia. British Journal of Anaesthesia. 83: 241–244.

110 Back NI and Finlay I (1995) Analgesic effect of topical opioids on painful skin ulcers. Journal of Pain and Symptom Management. 10: 493.

111 Krajnik M et al. (1999) Potential uses of topical opioids in palliative care – report of 6 cases. Pain. 80: 121–125.

112 Twillman R et al. (1999) Treatment of painful skin ulcers with topical opioids. Journal of Pain and Symptom Management. 17: 288–292.

113 Simonnet G (2008) Preemptive antihyperalgesia to improve preemptive analgesia. Anesthesiology. 108: 352–354.

114 Ren K and Dubner R (2008) Neuron-glia crosstalk gets serious: role in pain hypersensitivity. Current Opinion in Anaesthesiology. 21: 570–579.

115 Crain S and Shen K (2000) Antagonists of excitatory opioid receptor functions enhance morphine's analgesic potency and attenuate opioid tolerance/dependence liability. Pain. 84: 121–131.

116 Bartlett S et al. (1994) Pharmacology of morphine and morphine-3-glucuronide at opioid, excitatory amino acid, GABA and glycine binding sites. Pharmacology and Toxicology. 75: 73–81.

117 Zylicz Z and Twycross R (2008) Opioid-induced hyperalgesia may be more frequent than previously thought. Journal of Clinical Oncology. 26: 1564; author reply 1565.

118 Filitz J et al. (2008) Supra-additive effects of tramadol and acetaminophen in a human pain model. Pain. 133: 262–270.

119 Walker SM and Cousins MJ (1997) Reduction in hyperalgesia and intrathecal morphine requirements by low-dose ketamine infusion. *Journal of Pain and Symptom Management.* **14**: 129–133.

120 Bruera E et al. (1996) Opioid rotation in patients with cancer pain. *Cancer.* **78**: 852–857.

121 Lawlor P et al. (1998) Dose ratio between morphine and methadone in patients with cancer pain. *Cancer.* **82**: 1167–1173.

122 Begon S et al. (2002) Magnesium increases morphine analgesic effect in different experimental models of pain. *Anesthesiology.* **96**: 627–632.

123 Dubray C et al. (1997) Magnesium deficiency induces an hyperalgesia reversed by the NMDA receptor antagonist MK801. *Neuroreport.* **8**: 1383–1386.

124 Rauck RL et al. (2006) A randomized, double-blind, placebo-controlled study of intrathecal ziconotide in adults with severe chronic pain. *Journal of Pain and Symptom Management.* **31**: 393–406.

125 Gan TJ et al. (1997) Opioid-sparing effects of a low-dose infusion of naloxone in patient – administered morphine sulfate. *Anesthesiology.* **87**: 1075–1081.

126 Chindalore VL et al. (2005) Adding ultralow-dose naltrexone to oxycodone enhances and prolongs analgesia: a randomized, controlled trial of Oxytrex. *The Journal of Pain.* **6**: 392–399.

127 Eisenberg E et al. (2005) Efficacy and safety of opioid agonists in the treatment of neuropathic pain of nonmalignant origin: systematic review and meta-analysis of randomized controlled trials. *The Journal of the American Medical Association.* **293**: 3043–3052.

128 Eisenberg E et al. (2006) Efficacy of mu-opioid agonists in the treatment of evoked neuropathic pain: Systematic review of randomized controlled trials. *European Journal of Pain.* **10**: 667–676.

129 Vecht C et al. (1989) Initial bolus of conventional versus high-dose dexamethasone in metastatic spinal cord compression. *Neurology.* **39**: 1255–1257.

130 Loblaw D and Laperriere N (1998) Emergency treatment of malignant extradural spinal cord compression: an evidence-based guideline. *Journal of Clinical Oncology.* **16**: 1613–1624.

131 Anonymous (2000) Drug treatment of neuropathic pain. *Drug and Therapeutics Bulletin.* **38**: 89–93.

132 Collins S et al. (2000) Antidepressants and anticonvulsants for diabetic neuropathy and postherpetic neuralgia: a quantitative systematic review. *Journal of Pain and Symptom Management.* **20**: 449–458.

133 Backonja M (2001) Anticonvulsants and antiarrhythmics in the treatment of neuropathic pain syndromes. In: PT Hansson et al. (eds) *Neuropathic Pain: Pathophysiology and Treatment.* IASP, Seattle, pp. 185–201.

134 Sindrup S and Jensen T (2001) Antidepressants in the treatment of neuropathic pain. In: PT Hansson et al. (eds) *Neuropathic Pain: Pathophysiology and Treatment.* IASP, Seattle, pp. 169–183.

135 Dellemijn P et al. (1994) Medical therapy of malignant nerve pain. A randomised double-blind explanatory trial with naproxen versus slow-release morphine. *European Journal of Cancer.* **30A**: 1244–1250.

136 Ripamonti C et al. (1996) Continuous subcutaneous infusion of ketorolac in cancer neuropathic pain unresponsive to opioid and adjuvant drugs. A case report. *Tumori.* **82**: 413–415.

137 Dellemijn P (1999) Are opioids effective in relieving neuropathic pain? *Pain.* **80**: 453–462.

138 Stahl SM (2004) Anticonvulsants and the relief of chronic pain: pregabalin and gabapentin as alpha(2)delta ligands at voltage-gated calcium channels. *The Journal of Clinical Psychiatry.* **65**: 596–597.

139 Chabal C et al. (1992) The use of oral mexiletine for the treatment of pain after peripheral nerve injury. *Anaesthesiology.* **76**: 513–517.

140 Chong S et al. (1997) Pilot study evaluating local anesthetics administered systemically for treatment of pain in patients with advanced cancer. *Journal of Pain and Symptom Management.* **13**: 112–117.

141 McQuay H et al. (1996) A systematic review of antidepressants in neuropathic pain. *Pain.* **68**: 217–227.

142 McQuay H et al. (1995) Anticonvulsant drugs for the management of pain: a systematic review. *British Medical Journal.* **311**: 1047–1052.

143 Simpson DA (2001) Gabapentin and venlafaxine for the treatment of painful diabetic neuropathy. *Journal of Clinical Neuromuscular Diseases.* **3**: 53–62.

144 Gilron I et al. (2005) Morphine, gabapentin, or their combination for neuropathic pain. *The New England Journal of Medicine.* **352**: 1324–1334.

145 Enarson M et al. (1999) Clinical experience with oral ketamine. *Journal of Pain and Symptom Management.* **17**: 384–386.

146 Fine P (1999) Low-dose ketamine in the management of opioid nonresponsive terminal cancer. *Journal of Pain and Symptom Management.* **17**: 296–300.

147 Finlay I (1999) Ketamine and its role in cancer pain. *Pain Reviews.* **6**: 303–313.

148 Jackson K et al. (2001) 'Burst' ketamine for refractory cancer pain: an open-label audit of 39 patients. *Journal of Pain and Symptom Management.* **22**: 834–842.

149 Sola A and Bonica J (1990) Myofascial pain syndromes. In: J Bonica (ed) *The Management of Pain* (2e). Lea and Febiger, Philadelphia, pp. 352–367.

150 Mannix K et al. (2000) Using bisphosphonates to control the pain of bone metastases: evidence-based guidelines for palliative care. *Palliative Medicine.* **14**: 455–461.

151 Coluzzi P (1998) Sublingual morphine: efficacy reviewed. *Journal of Pain and Symptom Management.* **16**: 184–192.

APPENDIX 1: IASP PAIN DEFINITIONS

The International Association for the Study of Pain (IASP) has a series of definitions relating to pain, its pathogenesis, and its perception.[1] These can be accessed at www.iasp-pain.org.

In 2008, draft revised definitions were published,[2] and it is anticipated that these will be ratified in due course by the Council of IASP. The definitions below mostly come from the 2008 paper. Explanatory notes have been abbreviated, and the notes *in italics in parenthesis* are additions by the authors.

Allodynia
Pain in response to a non-nociceptive stimulus.

Note: The term allodynia was originally introduced to distinguish between hyperalgesia and hyperaesthesia. Allo means 'other' in Greek and is a common prefix for medical conditions that diverge from the expected. Odynia is derived from the Greek word 'odyne', which is used in 'pleurodynia' and 'coccydynia'. [*i.e. a synonym for '-algia' and '-algesia'*] It is important to recognize that allodynia involves a change in the quality of a sensation, whether tactile, thermal, or of any other sort. The original modality is normally non-painful, but the response is painful.

By contrast, hyperalgesia represents an augmented response in a specific mode, i.e. pain. With other cutaneous modalities, hyperaesthesia is the term which corresponds to hyperalgesia and, as with hyperalgesia, the quality is not altered. (Also see hyperalgesia and hyperpathia.)

Anaesthesia dolorosa
Pain in an area or region which is anaesthetic.

Analgesia
Absence of pain in response to stimulation which would normally be painful.

Causalgia
A syndrome of sustained burning pain, allodynia, and hyperpathia after a traumatic nerve lesion, often combined with vasomotor and sudomotor dysfunction impairment and later trophic changes.

Dysaesthesia
An unpleasant abnormal sensation, whether spontaneous or evoked.

Note: Compare with pain and with paraesthesia. Special cases of dysaesthesia include hyperalgesia and allodynia. Dysaesthesia should always be unpleasant whereas a paraesthesia should not be, although it is recognized that the borderline may present some difficulties when it comes to deciding as to whether a sensation is pleasant or unpleasant.

Hyperaesthesia
Increased sensitivity to stimulation, excluding the special senses.

Note: Hyperaesthesia may refer to various modes of cutaneous sensibility including touch and thermal sensation without pain, as well as to pain. The word is used to indicate both diminished threshold to any stimulus and an increased response to normally recognized stimuli.

Allodynia is the preferred term for pain after stimulation which is not normally painful. Hyperaesthesia includes both allodynia and hyperalgesia, but the more specific terms should be used whenever they are applicable.

Hyperalgesia
Increased pain sensitivity.

Note: Current evidence suggests that hyperalgesia is a consequence of perturbation of the nociceptive system with peripheral or central sensitization, or both.

Hyperpathia
A painful syndrome characterized by an abnormally painful reaction to a stimulus, particularly a repetitive stimulus, as well as an increased threshold.

Note: It may occur with allodynia, hyperaesthesia, hyperalgesia, or dysaesthesia. The pain is often explosive in character.

Hypoaesthesia
Decreased sensitivity to stimulation, excluding the special senses.

Note: Stimulation and locus to be specified. [Synonym: hypaesthesia.]

Hypoalgesia
Diminished pain in response to a generally painful stimulus.

Neuralgia
Pain in the distribution of a nerve or nerves.

Note: Particularly in Europe, common usage often implies a paroxysmal quality, but neuralgia should not be reserved for paroxysmal pains.

Neuropathy
A disturbance of function or pathological change in a nerve: in one nerve, mononeuropathy; in several nerves, mononeuropathy multiplex; if diffuse and bilateral, polyneuropathy.

Neuropathic pain
Pain arising as a direct consequence of a lesion or disease affecting the somatosensory system.

[Neuropathic pain is subdivided into peripheral neuropathic pain and central neuropathic pain depending on the site of the lesion or dysfunction impairment.]

Nociception
The neural processes of encoding and processing noxious stimuli.

Nociceptor
A sensory receptor that is capable of transducing and encoding noxious stimuli.

Nociceptive pain

Pain arising from activation of nociceptors.

Nociceptive stimulus

An actually or potentially tissue-damaging event transduced and encoded by nociceptors.

Pain

An unpleasant sensory and emotional experience associated with actual or potential tissue damage, or described in terms of such damage.

Note: Although pain most often has a proximate physical cause, some people report pain in the absence of tissue damage or any likely pathophysiological cause, generally for psychological reasons. There is generally no way to distinguish their experience from that due to tissue damage. If they regard their experience as pain and if they report it in the same ways as pain caused by tissue damage, it should be accepted as pain. This definition avoids tying pain to the stimulus.

Pain threshold

The minimal intensity of a stimulus that is perceived as painful.

Pain tolerance level

The maximum intensity of a stimulus that evokes pain and that a subject is willing to tolerate in a given situation.

Paraesthesia

An abnormal sensation, whether spontaneous or evoked.

Note: It is recommended that paraesthesia is used to describe an abnormal sensation which is not unpleasant, and dysaesthesia for an unpleasant one.

Sensitization

Increased responsiveness of neurones to their normal input or recruitment of a response to normally subthreshold inputs.

1 Merskey H and Bogduk N (eds) (1994) *IASP Task Force on Taxonomy. Classification of Chronic Pain.* IASP Press, Seattle.
2 Loeser JD and Treede RD (2008) The Kyoto protocol of IASP Basic Pain Terminology. *Pain.* **137**: 473–477.

APPENDIX 2: SUPPLEMENTARY PAIN DEFINITIONS

Acute pain[1]
A complex constellation of unpleasant sensory, perceptual and emotional experiences with associated autonomic, psychological and behavioural responses.

Chronic pain[1]
Pain which persists a month beyond the usual course of an acute disease or a reasonable time for an injury to heal, or is associated with a chronic pathological process which causes continuous pain or pain which recurs at intervals for months or years.

Cramp
A painful spasm of one or more skeletal muscles.

Myofascial pain
A muscle disorder characterized by the presence of one or more hypersensitive points (trigger points) within muscle and/or the surrounding connective tissue together with pain (often radiating into neighbouring areas or the adjacent limb), muscle spasm, tenderness, stiffness, limitation of movement, weakness and, occasionally, autonomic dysfunction impairment.

Plasticity
The ability of nociceptive neurones to vary their responsiveness to stimuli as a result of prolonged stimulation and/or chemical mediators of inflammation and/or neural injury.

Sensation threshold
The least stimulus at which a person perceives a sensation.

Note: this is uniform for all ethnic groups under laboratory conditions. Elsewhere, attention and suggestion radically modify the sensation threshold.

Spasm
A sustained involuntary muscle contraction.

---

1 Bonica J (1990) Definitions and taxonomy of pain. In: J Bonica (ed) *The Management of Pain* (2e). Lea and Febiger, Philadelphia, pp. 18–27.

3: ALIMENTARY SYMPTOMS

HALITOSIS

Halitosis is unpleasant or foul-smelling breath beyond socially acceptable levels.

Causes
Physiological
- ingestion of substances whose volatile products are excreted by the lungs or saliva, e.g. garlic, onions, alcohol
- normal putrefactive processes in the oral cavity.

Pathological[1,2]
- dry mouth
- poor oral and dental hygiene, e.g. food debris, coated tongue, gingivitis, peridontitis
- stomatitis
- necrosis and sepsis in the mouth, pharynx, nose, nasal sinuses or lungs
- severe infection
- gastro-oesophageal reflux
- gastric stagnation associated with gastroparesis or outflow obstruction
- hepatic or renal failure
- diabetic keto-acidosis
- smoking.

In the absence of local oral pathology, malodour is caused mainly by bacteria in saliva, the gingival crevice, the tongue surface, etc. metabolizing sulphur-containing amino acids into volatile sulphur compounds, e.g. hydrogen sulphide. The sulphur-containing amino acids are derived from salivary peptides and proteins, and their concentration increases as salivary flow decreases.[3] Patients with halitosis also have a different spectrum of bacteria in their mouths which exacerbates the production of volatile sulphur compounds.[4]

Evaluation

Clinical evaluation involves smelling air expelled from the nose and from the mouth, and comparing the two. Odour detectable from the mouth (but not the nose) suggests an oral cause, whereas odour from the nose (but not the mouth) suggests a problem in the nose or sinuses. Odour of similar intensity from both the mouth and nose suggests a systemic cause.

Management
Correct the correctable
Dental and oral hygiene
- clean teeth and tongue with toothbrush and toothpaste b.d.
- consider use of dental floss
- encourage fluid intake
- consider saliva substitutes and stimulants if the mouth is very dry (see p.64)
- offer refreshing mouthwashes
- gargles and/or mouthwashes on waking, after meals and at bedtime, particularly if there is a heavily furred tongue or necrotic cancer, e.g.:
  ▷ hydrogen peroxide 1.5%
  ▷ sodium bicarbonate mouthwash, compound BP
  ▷ chlorhexidine 0.2%
  ▷ povidone-iodine 1%
- modify diet, e.g. exclude garlic and onions
- stop smoking.

Infection
- treat oral candidosis (see p.70)
- send sputum for culture and prescribe the appropriate antibacterial
- if anaerobic infection, e.g. associated with necrotic cancer, prescribe metronidazole 400mg PO b.d.–t.d.s. for 10 days
- if pulmonary candidosis (rare), prescribe ketoconazole 200mg b.d. or fluconazole 100mg PO for 7 days.

Gastro-oesophageal reflux or stagnant gastric contents
Prescribe a prokinetic, e.g. metoclopramide 10mg SC stat and 40–100mg/24h by CSCI. If beneficial, convert to metoclopramide 10–20mg PO q.d.s.

DRY MOUTH (XEROSTOMIA)

Saliva contains electrolytes, immunoglobulins, proteins, enzymes, mucins, and nitrogenous products. The principal functions of saliva are:
- lubrication and cleansing of the mouth
- antimicrobial activity
- mastication, digestion and swallowing of food
- maintenance of teeth mineralization.

Three pairs of salivary glands (parotid, submandibular, and sublingual) produce over 90% of saliva, on average 600–1,000mL/day. This is often reduced in advanced disease and is the main cause of dry mouth, which occurs in 80% of patients with advanced cancer.[5]

Poor oral lubrication makes chewing and swallowing difficult and painful, and taste is impaired. These factors will all contribute to anorexia. Dentures may become problematic and speech affected, compounded by frustration and embarrassment. If dry mouth continues for a prolonged period, dental erosion and dental decay (caries) are increasingly likely.

Causes
There are multiple causes of dry mouth (Box 3.A) including drugs (Box 3.B). Smoking, alcohol (including in mouthwashes) and caffeine all dry the mouth.

Box 3.A Causes of dry mouth in advanced cancer

Cancer
Erosion of buccal mucosa
Replacement of salivary glands by cancer
Hypercalcaemia (→ dehydration)

Treatment
Local radiotherapy ⎱ affecting
Local radical surgery ⎰ salivary glands
Stomatitis associated
   with neutropenia
Drugs, particularly
   antimuscarinics
   opioids
   diuretics
   (see Box 3.B)

Oxygen without humidification

Debility
Anxiety
Depression
Mouth breathing
Dehydration
Infection
Zinc deficiency

Concurrent
Diabetes mellitus
   uncontrolled → dehydration
   autonomic neuropathy
Hypothyroidism
Auto-immune disease
Amyloid
Sarcoid

Caffeine
Alcohol
Smoking

Management
Prevent the preventable
- ideally, patients should have a dental check and any necessary treatment before commencing radiotherapy to the head and neck
- maintain good oral hygiene and mouth care before, during and after radiotherapy.

Correct the correctable
- review the drug regimen and stop or reduce the dose of antimuscarinic if possible
- substitute a drug with less or no antimuscarinic effects, e.g. an SSRI instead of amitriptyline, and haloperidol instead of prochlorperazine or chlorpromazine
- treat oral candidosis (see p.70).

Box 3.B   Drugs and dry mouth

Alpha-adrenergic antagonists (alpha-blockers) (for urinary hesitancy)	**Antihistamines** **Antihistiminic anti-emetics**	**Psychostimulants** Dexamfetamine Ecstasy Fenfluramine
Alpha-adrenergic agonists Clonidine Lofexidine	**Antimuscarinics** **Antimuscarinic bronchodilators**	**Other (psychotropics)** Buspirone Cannabinoids Diazepam Lithium Zopiclone
Analgesics Dihydrocodeine Ketorolac Morphine Nefopam Tramadol	**Antiparkinsonian drugs** **Antipsychotics** **Diuretics**	**Other (general)** Interferon alpha Interleukin-2 Sucralfate
Antidepressants Duloxetine MAOIs Maprotiline Mirtazapine Reboxetine SSRIs TCAs Trazodone Venlafaxine	**PPIs**	

Non-drug treatment
Short-lived relief may be obtained by frequent sips of water, preferably ice-cold, or mineral water. Mix carbonated with plain in equal parts to maintain freshness but decrease excessive gas content, or according to personal preference.

Mouth care
Debride the tongue if furred with, e.g.:
• a soft toothbrush and hydrogen peroxide 1.5% *or*
• a soft toothbrush and sodium bicarbonate mouthwash, compound BP
• 1/4 of 1g effervescent ascorbic acid placed on the tongue (avoid if mouth sore).

Artificial saliva
Artificial saliva is a poor substitute for natural saliva, and saliva stimulants should be used in preference. However, their use can be considered in patients who do not respond to, or are unable to tolerate saliva stimulants. For maximum effect, artificial saliva needs to be taken every 30–60min, and before and during meals. Proprietary artificial saliva products include:
• mucin-based lozenges and sprays (AS Saliva Orthana®); neutral pH
• hydroxyethylcellulose-based gels or sprays containing lactoperoxidase (Biotene Oralbalance®, BioXtra®); neutral pH.

Artificial salivas with a neutral pH are preferable for long-term use. Artificial salivas with an acidic pH should be avoided in dentate patients (demineralization of teeth) or in those with mucositis (increased pain).

Alternatives to proprietary preparations include:
- a small amount (e.g. 0.5mL) of butter, margarine or vegetable oil swished around the mouth with the tongue t.d.s and at bedtime may be helpful[6]
- locally-produced preparation comprising methylcellulose 10g and lemon essence 0.2mL in 1L of water
- pineapple chunks, contain ananase, a proteolytic enzyme, which cleans the mouth if sucked like a sweet; fresh pineapple contains more ananase than tinned pineapple, but either can be used.

In moribund patients the mouth should be moistened every 30min with water from a water spray, dropper or sponge stick or ice chips placed in the mouth. In addition:
- smear the lips with a suitable emollient, e.g. white soft paraffin (petroleum jelly, Vaseline®) q4h to prevent cracking
- use a room humidifier or air-conditioning when the weather is dry and hot.

Stimulate salivary flow
Acids in the mouth and chewing solids act as salivary stimulants, e.g.:
- acid drops, lemon drops, boiled sweets, strong candy
- chewing gum.

Chewing gum is as effective as, and preferred to, mucin-based artificial saliva. The gum should be sugar-free and, in patients with dentures, low-tack, e.g. Orbit® sugar-free gum.

Drug treatment with a saliva stimulant
For more information, see *PCF3*.

Can be given systemically, e.g. pilocarpine or bethanechol, or topically, e.g. SST® or Salivix®. However, the latter are acidic and long-term use should be avoided in dentate patients (demineralization of teeth) or in those with mucositis (increased pain).

Pilocarpine is a parasympathomimetic agent (predominantly muscarinic) with mild β-adrenergic activity which stimulates secretion from exocrine glands. About 90% of patients with drug-induced dry mouth respond to pilocarpine with benefit seen immediately.[7] In contrast, only about 50% of patients with dry mouth several weeks or months *after* radiotherapy respond to pilocarpine and benefit may not be apparent for up to 3 months.[7,8]

Bowel obstruction, asthma and COPD are contra-indications to the use of pilocarpine. The most common undesirable effect is sweating; others include nausea, flushing, urinary frequency, intestinal colic and weakness. Cheaper alternatives include the use of pilocarpine eyedrops PO and bethanechol.[9–12]

DROOLING

Drooling is a term used to describe the leakage of saliva from the mouth.[13] Although drooling most commonly occurs with a normal production of saliva, sialorrhoea (excessive saliva) is sometimes a causal factor. It can cause embarrassment, social isolation and impaired mood.[14]

Causes

Most cases of severe drooling are associated with neurological disorders which are interfering with swallowing (Box 3.C). These patients will also be at risk of aspiration pneumonia. The overall incidence in Parkinson's disease and in MND/ALS is about 40%. However, it is almost universal in those with severe swallowing difficulties.[14,15]

Apart from cancers of the head and neck, it is uncommon in advanced cancer.

Box 3.C Causes of drooling

Oral factors
Ill-fitting dentures
Oral cancer ± surgery → deformity
Dysphagia, e.g. cancer of the larynx
  or oesophagus
Episodic salivation associated with
  gastro-oesophageal reflux[16]
Idiopathic paroxysmal sialorrhoea[17]

Psychiatric[18]
Psychosis
Depression

Neurological disorders
Cancer of the pharynx/involving the
  base of the skull
Cerebral palsy
Cerebrovascular accident
MND/ALS
Parkinson's disease

Drugs
See Box 3.D

Box 3.D Drug-related hypersalivation[19]

Analgesics
Buprenorphine
Mefenamic acid
Ketamine

Antibacterials
Gentamicin
Kanamycin
Tobramycin

Anxiolytics/hypnotics
Alprazolam
Clonazepam
Zaleplon

Cardiac
Amiodarone
Guanethidine
Nicardipine

Other (psychotropics)
Clozapine
Haloperidol
Lamotrigine
Risperidone
Venlafaxine

Other (general)
Anticholinesterases
Iodides
Levodopa
Rivastigmine
Tacrine

Management

Correct the correctable

There may be little which can be done to correct the causes of drooling in advanced disease. Review the drug regimen and, if possible, stop or reduce the dose of drugs which can cause hypersalivation (Box 3.D). Modification of dentures may help.

Non-drug treatment

• head positioning, e.g. prevent jaw/chin from dropping, avoid a flexed neck
• exercises to improve the oral musculature
• chewing gum or sucking on hard candy will act as motor/tactile cues to increase the frequency of swallowing; however, will also stimulate saliva production
• suctioning
• irradiation of the salivary glands, e.g. with 4–10Gy (rarely indicated).[20]

Drug treatment

For more information, see PCF3.

Prescribe an antimuscarinic (Table 3.1), or switch from a drug the patient is already taking to an alternative with antimuscarinic properties, e.g. from sertraline to amitriptyline.

Table 3.1   Antimuscarinics for drooling

Drug	Typical starting dose
Glycopyrronium	200microgram t.d.s.
Hyoscine hydrobromide	1mg/72h TD
Propantheline	15mg PO b.d.–t.d.s.

The muscarinic receptors in salivary glands are very responsive to antimuscarinics and inhibition of salivation occurs at lower doses than required for other antimuscarinic effects.[21] This reduces, but does not eliminate, the likelihood of undesirable effects, e.g. blurred vision, urinary hesitancy/retention, drowsiness.

Local application of antimuscarinics has been tried in an attempt to minimize undesirable effects, but with disappointing results.[22–24]

However, there is an increasing role for neurobotulinum toxin (serotypes A and B) in drooling and sialorrhoea.[25] Produced by the bacterium Clostridium botulinum, it works pre-synaptically to inhibit acetylcholine release from cholinergic nerve endings resulting in chemical denervation. It is administered as one or more injections into the parotid ± submandibular glands, sometimes using ultrasound scan guidance. Saliva is reduced for 6–24 weeks and it appears well tolerated. Undesirable effects mainly relate to an excessively dry mouth, resulting in chewing difficulties and dysphagia.[26]

STOMATITIS

Stomatitis is a general term applied to diffuse inflammatory, erosive and ulcerative conditions affecting the mucous membranes lining the mouth (synonym: sore mouth). The term 'mucositis' tends to be restricted to stomatitis caused by chemotherapy or local radiotherapy. In contrast, aphthous ulcers are generally discrete small, round or ovoid ulcers with a definite margin, an erythematous halo and a yellow or grey floor.

Causes

Stomatitis is caused by dry mouth, superadded infection, mucositis, various deficiency states, trauma (Box 3.E) and drugs (Box 3.F).[27] Aphthous ulcers are caused through a combination of auto-immunity and opportunistic infection There may also be a genetic component, and stress, haematinic deficiency, neutropenia and immunosuppression may all be precipitants. It is important to determine the cause so that, if appropriate, specific as well as symptomatic treatment is given.

Box 3.E   Causes of stomatitis

Dry mouth (see p.62)

Drugs
Corticosteroids ⎫
Antibacterials   ⎬   candidosis
See Box 3.F   ⎭

Infection (associated with altered immunity)
Aphthous ulcers
Fungal
 candidosis
Bacterial
 Gram-negative
Viral
 cytomegalovirus
 Herpes simplex
 Varicella zoster

Mucositis
Local radiotherapy
Chemotherapy

Malnutrition
Hypovitaminosis
Anaemia
Protein deficiency

Trauma
Poor dentition
Ill-fitting dentures

Radiotherapy leads to the loss of basal keratinocytes, and a reduced ability to generate squamous epithelial cells. Mucositis results when the rate of loss exceeds the rate of generation. There is also a shift in oral flora to increased levels of Gram-negative enterobacteria and *Pseudomonas*. These exacerbate any tissue inflammation and injury.[28]

Evaluation

Generally there will be an obvious cause of diffuse stomatitis. Because the natural history differs, it is useful to differentiate between:
- minor aphthous ulcers (80%) are <5mm in diameter and heal in 1–2 weeks
- major aphthous ulcers are large ulcers which heal slowly over weeks or months with scarring
- herpetiform ulcers are multiple pinpoint ulcers which heal in <4 weeks.[29]

The differential diagnosis of mucositis includes viral or fungal disease and graft-versus-host disease.

Box 3.F   Drug-related oral ulceration[19]

Alimentary	**Chemotherapy**	**Other**
Pancreatin	Bleomycin	Alendronate
	Doxorubicin	Allopurinol
Analgesics	5-Fluoro-uracil	Emepromium
NSAIDs	Melphelan	Gold
	Mercaptopurine	Interferons
Antibacterials	Methotrexate	Interleukin-2
Aztreonam		Molgramostim
Clarithromycin	**Corticosteroids**	Penicillamine
Proguanil	Flunisolide	Potassium chloride
Vancomycin		
Zalcitabine	**Psychotropics**	
	Carbamazepine	
Cardiac	Olanzapine	
Captopril	Phenytoin	
Isoprenaline	Sertraline	
Losartan		
Nicorandil		
Phenindione		

Management
Correct the correctable
- review the drug regimen and, if possible, stop or reduce the dose of drugs which can cause stomatitis and/or a dry mouth
- mouth care before, during and after radiotherapy or chemotherapy treatment reduces the severity of mucositis
- check teeth and dentures; replace/reline ill-fitting dentures
- dry mouth (see p.62)
- candidosis (see p.70)
- aphthous ulcers (for more information, see *PCF3*).

Non-drug treatment
The following help to reduce pain when ulcers are present:
- avoid spicy foods and acidic fruit juices or carbonated drinks
- drink through a straw to bypass the mouth
- avoid sharp foods such as crisps.

Symptomatic drug treatment
For more information, see *PCF3*.

In addition to prophylactic measures and disease-specific treatment, there is a progression of symptomatic options:[30]
- *Step 1* topical NSAID
- *Step 2* topical local anaesthetic ± topical NSAID
- *Step 3* topical morphine ± systemic morphine
- *Step 4* concurrent use of 'burst' ketamine
- *Step 5* concurrent use of thalidomide.

ORAL CANDIDOSIS

Oral yeast carriage is present in about 1/3 of the general population. The prevalence in patients with advanced cancer is higher, sometimes nearly 90% and oropharyngeal candidosis is a common fungal infection in this group of patients.[31,32]

Candida albicans probably accounts for about 75% of the infections, and *Candida glabrata* for most of the rest.[32] *C. albicans* is inherently sensitive to antifungal drugs, but can acquire resistance to the azoles, whereas *C. glabrata* is inherently resistant to azoles.

Clinical features
Oral candidosis generally manifests as:
- white plaques on the buccal mucosa (thin and discrete) and/or tongue (thick and confluent) *or*
- a smooth red painful tongue and/or buccal mucosa *or*
- angular stomatitis.

Causes
Oral candidosis is associated with:
- poor performance status
- poor oral hygiene
- dry mouth
- dentures[33,34]
- AIDS, with CD4 T-helper cell count <200cells/mm^3.[35]

In relation to antibacterials (both topical and systemic) and corticosteroids (both inhaled and systemic), published data are equivocal.[33,34]

Management
Correct the correctable
Underlying causal factors should be corrected if possible, particularly poor oral hygiene and dry mouth (see p.62). Dentures must be thoroughly cleaned at least once daily using an appropriate antiseptic, e.g. chlorhexidine, sodium hypochlorite. They should also be soaked overnight in antiseptic, e.g. dilute sodium hypochlorite (Milton®); failure to do this leads to treatment failure.

Chlorhexidine inactivates nystatin.[36] If used with nystatin, the dentures must be thoroughly rinsed before re-insertion. In other circumstances, chlorhexidine mouthwashes can be used as an adjunctive antimicrobial treatment.[37]

Drug treatment
For more information, see *PCF3*.

Oropharyngeal candidosis generally responds to topical antifungal treatment. A systematic review concluded that there is no difference in efficacy between topical and systemic treatments.[38] When efficacy, lack of resistance, and cost are all taken into account, nystatin is clearly the antifungal drug of choice for oral candidosis in non-immunocompromised patients.

On the other hand, because they are more convenient (once daily administration), many patients are treated systemically with an azole antifungal, e.g. ketoconazole or fluconazole. Further, in AIDS, azoles are generally regarded as the treatment of choice.[35,39] However, organisms resistant to one or more azole do occur.

Most patients respond to a 10-day course of an antifungal but some need long-term treatment. Symptomatic relief often occurs within 2–3 days. In AIDS, particularly if infection extends to the oesophagus, higher doses for a prolonged period are necessary (Table 3.2).

Table 3.2 Summary of antifungal treatment recommendations

Class	Drug	Recommended regimen	Comments
Polyene group	Nystatin	Oral suspension 100,000units/mL; 1–5mL q.d.s. held in the mouth for 1min, and then swallowed. Tablets 500,000units; 1–2 q.d.s. for intestinal infection	Necessary to remove dentures before each dose, and clean before re-insertion
Azole group (Imidazoles)	Ketoconazole	*Official restriction: because of risk of hepatic impairment, use only if resistance to fluconazole.* Tablets 200mg; 1 tablet once daily for 2 weeks; if response inadequate, increase to 2 tablets once daily and continue until 1 week after cultures become negative	Suspension can be prepared locally[40]
	Miconazole	Oral gel 120mg/5mL; 5mL q.d.s. administered on a teaspoon; the patient spreads it around the mouth with the tongue. Can also be spread on denture fixings before insertion	Eventually swallowed so effect is mainly systemic
Azole group (Tiazoles)	Fluconazole	Capsules or oral suspension; 50mg once daily for 1 week, but 2 weeks if dentures worn; 100mg once daily for 2–4 weeks if immunocompromised (sometimes 100–200mg once daily indefinitely is needed); 150mg stat if debilitated and short prognosis	Best absorbed on an empty stomach
	Itraconazole	Capsules 100mg; oral solution 10mg/mL; 100mg once daily for 2 weeks but 200mg once daily if immunocompromised	

ABNORMAL TASTE

There are five basic tastes:
- sweet (sucrose)
- umami (amino acid, savoury)
- salt
- sour (acid)
- bitter (urea).

A 'fatty' taste, associated with free fatty acids, may represent a sixth taste category. Generally, sweet and amino acid tastes are associated with nutritionally rich food, and bitter tastes with noxious and toxic stimuli.

Flavour is the overall sensation arising from the ingestion and mastication of food, e.g. taste, touch and smell. When perceived positively it is associated with pleasure and gratification but, if disliked, it may be associated with disgust, nausea and aversion. About 1/4 of the population are 'supertasters' with a significantly greater sense of taste than usual. Many factors affect taste (Table 3.3).

Taste buds, each containing 50–100 taste receptor cells, are present on the lips, tongue (in the papillae), cheeks, soft palate, uvula, pharynx, upper oesophagus and larynx. The taste receptor cells have a life span of 10 days and are continually replaced. The facial, glossopharyngeal and vagus nerves transmit taste signals. Abnormalities of taste include:
- a reduction (hypogeusia) or loss (ageusia) of taste, due to an increase in taste threshold
- an unpleasant (parageusia) or altered taste (dysgeusia) which can be specific, e.g. in relation to bitterness but not to other tastes.

About 50% of patients with advanced cancer experience altered taste ± smell. It can impact on energy intake, survival, mood, social life and overall quality of life, e.g. leading to greater weight loss, frustration or sadness and interfering with cooking and meal times.[41,42]

Pathogenesis

The mechanisms underlying taste abnormalities in advanced cancer include:
- systemic inflammation
- nutritional deficiencies, e.g. zinc
- drugs (Box 3.G).

Some inflammatory cytokines, e.g. interferons, act directly on taste bud cells, interfering with their function and inducing apoptosis. This may cause abnormal cell turnover and skew the proportion of the different types of taste bud cell, resulting in a taste disorder.[43]

Zinc has an important role in cells with a high-rate of turnover, including taste bud and olfactory cells. Deficiency leads to taste and smell disturbance and also dry mouth, all of which can improve with replacement therapy.[44,45]

Serum zinc levels may be an unreliable indicator of deficiency. This probably explains why patients with idiopathic dysgeusia also improve with zinc.[46]

Drugs impair taste by affecting:
- the flow of saliva
- the chemical composition of saliva
- taste receptor function
- signal transduction.

Table 3.3 Factors affecting taste

Factor	Comment
Age	>70 years
Poor eyesight	Visual cues help whet the appetite and heighten the appreciation of taste
Sense of smell	Decreases with age
Mouth	Dry mouth Poor dentition and dental hygiene Tepid food
Drugs and chemicals	Smoking Alcoholism (also see Box 3.G, p.74)
Endocrine	Pregnancy Menopause Diabetes mellitus Hypothyroidism
Biochemical	Hyponatraemia
Systemic disease	Inflammation, e.g. infection, cancer Liver disease Kidney disease

CNS disease	Dementia
	Tumours, particularly if involving
	  cerebellopontine angle
	  jugular foramen
	  temporal lobe
	Epilepsy
	Multiple sclerosis

Psychological disorders	Depression

Chemotherapy interferes with the normal turnover of taste bud cells, resulting in loss of taste sensitivity. This generally improves 3–4 months after cessation of chemotherapy, although a permanent change in taste can occur. This is thought to be caused by the 'recoding' of taste as a result of the loss and replacement of large numbers of taste bud cells.[47]

Radiotherapy to the head and neck may affect taste via direct damage to the oral mucosa, taste buds and salivary glands causing dry mouth.[48] Smell may be impaired by radiation effects on the olfactory epithelium, olfactory bulb and possibly the orbitofrontal cortex.[49]

Hypogeusia is generally made worse by poor hygiene, dry mouth and oral candidosis.

Box 3.G Drugs affecting taste[19]

Alimentary
Colestyramine
Antimuscarinics
Omeprazole

Analgesics
Aspirin
Choline magnesium trisalicylate
Indometacin
Sulfasalazine

Antimicrobials
Amphotericin
Aztreonam
Cefamandole
Clarithromycin
Ethambutol
Ethionamide
Griseofulvin
Imipenem
Levofloxacin
Lincomycin
Lomefloxacin
Metronidazole
Ofloxacin
Pentamidine
Procaine penicillin
Rifabutin
Terbinafine
Tetracyclines

Cardiac
ACE inhibitors
Amiloride
Amrinone
Atorvastatin
Diltiazem
Dipyridamole
Hydrochlorothiazide
Lisinopril
Losartan
Lovastatin
Nifedipine
Nitroglycerin
Phenindione
Propafenone
Propranolol
Spironolactone
Tocainide
Valsartan

Chemotherapy
Azathioprine
Bleomycin
Carboplatin
Cisplatin
Doxorubicin
Etoposide
5-Fluoro-uracil
Interferon gamma
Methotrexate

Corticosteroids
Flunisolide
Hydrocortisone

Hypoglycaemics
Acarbose
Biguanides
Insulin
Rivastigmine

Metabolic
Calcitonin
Etidronate
Carbimazole
Propylthio-uracil
Thiamazole

Psychotropics
Amitriptyline
Amphetamines
Azelastine
Carbamazepine
Cetirizine
Clomipramine
Fluoxetine
Flurazepam
Fluvoxamine
Levodopa
Lithium
Pergolide
Phenytoin
Selegiline
Topiramate
Venlafaxine
Zopiclone

Other
Alcohol
Allopurinol
Baclofen
Benzocaine
Isotretinoin
Levamisole
Lidocaine
Penicillamine

Clinical features

These vary between individuals. However, many patients with cancer experience an enhanced sensitivity to sour and bitter tastes.[42] There may be vague complaints that:

'Food does not taste right'

'Everything tastes like cotton wool'.

Or specific complaints that:

'I can't take sweet things anymore'

'I've given up eating meat, it tastes so bitter'

'I find I have to add spoonfuls of sugar to everything'

'I have a persistent bad taste in my mouth'.

'I have a metallic taste in my mouth'

'I am more sensitive to certain odours'.

Food intake is often reduced, and this will be exacerbated if associated with nausea, early satiety and/or anorexia.

Management
Correct the correctable

- review the drug regimen and, if possible, stop or reduce the dose of drugs which can affect taste or cause a dry mouth
- improve mouth care and dental hygiene
- treat oral candidosis.

Non-drug treatment

The advice of a dietitian should be obtained, and an appropriate recipe book supplied. For those with reduced taste, the use of food enhancers may be useful in improving nutrition, physical function, taste and smell perception.[50] Patients undergoing chemotherapy should be warned about change in taste and smell. General advice includes:

- encourage tart foods, e.g. pickles, lemon juice, vinegar
- recommend food which leaves its own taste like fresh fruit, hard candy
- add or reduce sugar as appropriate
- reduce the urea content of diet by eating white meats, eggs, dairy products
- mask the bitter taste of food containing urea, e.g.:
  ▷ add wine and beer to soups and sauces
  ▷ marinate chicken, fish, meat
  ▷ use more and stronger seasonings
  ▷ eat food cold or at room temperature
  ▷ drink more liquids.

MUSCLE WASTING (SARCOPENIA) AND MALNUTRITION

With increasing age, normal homeostasis alters, leading to changes in body composition and food (energy) intake; this increases the likelihood of loss of body weight, skeletal muscle wasting (sarcopenia) and protein-energy malnutrition (Table 3.4).[51] These age-related changes will exacerbate disease-related cachexia.

An impaired ability of the gastric fundus to relax and accommodate food, together with delayed gastric emptying, leads to more rapid distension of the gastric antrum, causing fullness and early satiety (removal of the need or desire for food) along with prolonged satiation (a state of relative insensitivity to the need or desire for food).

Table 3.4 Examples of age-related changes leading to reduced body weight

Change	Cause(s)
↑ fat and ↓ skeletal muscle (>50 years)	↓ physical activity ↓ growth hormone ↓ testosterone/androgens ↓ resting metabolic rate
↓ food intake (>60 years)	↓ appetite ↓ sense of taste and smell ↑ satiety

Cytokine levels increase with age and may contribute to anorexia (see p.77). Other factors contributing to age-related malnutrition include difficulties with obtaining, preparing, chewing and swallowing food. Social isolation also plays a role; intake of energy from meals is about 1/3 less when eating alone compared with in company.

Screening for malnutrition
Whatever the cause of malnutrition, early detection and intervention is preferable and requires a pro-active approach. NICE guidance suggests that all patients should be screened for malnutrition when:
- admitted to hospital, and weekly thereafter
- admitted to care homes, and repeated if there is clinical concern
- first seen in outpatients, and repeated if there is clinical concern
- registering with a general practice.

In patients reporting weight loss, as a minimum, screening should include:
- the body mass index (BMI):

$$BMI = \frac{weight(kg)}{height^2(m)}$$

- percentage unintentional weight loss
- time over which nutrient intake has been unintentionally reduced and/or the likelihood of future impaired intake.[52]

A screening tool such as the Malnutrition Universal Screening Tool (MUST) can be used.[53] Nutritional support should be considered for patients with:
- BMI < 18.5kg/m^2
- unintentional weight loss > 10% in the last 3–6 months
- BMI < 20kg/m^2 and unintentional weight loss > 5%
- inadequate oral intake for > 5 days
- malabsorption, increased nutrient losses or increased requirements from catabolism.[52]

Ideally, those patients identified by the screening process should then have their nutritional status evaluated by an appropriately trained health professional (e.g. a dietitian) in order to produce a nutrition care plan, including monitoring.[54,55] Such an approach is considered appropriate for patients with a prognosis of at least 2–3 months, but is less relevant for patients at the end of life when management goals differ.

ANOREXIA

Eating may be motivated by hunger (manifesting as abdominal discomfort/pain, weakness, or irritability) and/or the seeking of pleasure (to satisfy an appetite). Both may become impaired with increasing age or disease.

Anorexia (loss of appetite) is common in advanced cancer. Despite this, many patients force themselves to eat to 'keep going' or to 'stay alive'. Nonetheless, anorexia generally leads to a reduction in food intake which contributes to the development of malnutrition and cachexia (see p.79), impairing quality of life and increasing morbidity and mortality.[56,57]

Pathogenesis

The regulation of food (energy) intake is complex, with the hypothalamus playing a key role. Fasting results in hormonal and other signals, e.g. ghrelin, malonyl-CoA, acting upon the hypothalamus to increase food intake by:

- stimulating orexigenic neurones (containing agouti-related protein (AgRP) and neuropeptide Y (NPY))
- inhibiting anorexigenic neurones (containing pro-opiomelanocortin, a precursor for α-melanocyte stimulating hormone (α-MSH)).

Melanocortin receptors, particularly melanocortin-4 (MC4-R), appear important in tonically inhibiting food intake and energy storage. Thus the orexigenic AgRP and NPY act as functional antagonists at MC4-R and the anorexigenic α-MSH is an agonist.

In cancer, and many other chronic diseases, there is an increased expression of cytokines, e.g., IL-1 and TNF-α, in the hypothalamus which ultimately:

- inhibit the hypothalamic response to fasting signals
- inhibit orexigenic neurones
- stimulate anorexigenic neurones.

This results in anorexia, increased energy expenditure and weight loss.[56,58]

Vagal afferent information arising from the GI tract, e.g. as a result of gastroduodenal distension, is processed by the brain stem and leads to satiety. Increased distension, caused by delayed gastric emptying, e.g. due to ageing, disease or drugs, will lead to anorexia and early satiety. Early satiety can also occur without concurrent anorexia ('I look forward to my meals but, then, after a few mouthfuls I feel full up and can't eat any more'); this is associated with various conditions, including:

- a small stomach (post-gastrectomy)
- hepatomegaly
- gross ascites.

Cytokines also contribute to an altered taste (see p.72) and smell. Patients can experience a persistent bad taste, taste distortion and an increased sensitivity to odours. These also impact adversely on nutritional intake, weight loss and quality of life.[42] One or more other factors may also contribute to anorexia (Table 3.5).

Management

Patients with anorexia and a prognosis of at least 2–3 months should be screened for malnutrition (see p.76).

Correct the correctable

When appropriate, identify and treat any causal factors (see Table 3.5). Early satiety in particular is common yet poorly identified and managed.[59]

Table 3.5 Causes of poor appetite in advanced cancer

Cause	Management possibilities
Unappetizing food	Choice of food by patient
Too much food provided	Small meals
Altered smell/taste	Adjust diet to counter smell/taste change
Dyspepsia	Antacid, antiflatulent, prokinetic
Nausea and vomiting	Anti-emetic
Early satiety	Prokinetic; 'small and often', snacks rather than meals
Gastric stasis	Prokinetic
Constipation	Laxatives
Sore mouth	Mouth care
Poor dentition, ill-fitting dentures	Dental review
Pain	Analgesics
Malodour	Treatment of malodour
Biochemical	
hypercalcaemia	Correction of hypercalcaemia (see p.215)
hyponatraemia	Demeclocycline 300mg b.d.–q.d.s. if caused by SIADH (see p.225)
uraemia	Anti-emetic
Secondary to treatment	
drugs	Modify drug regimen
radiotherapy chemotherapy	Anti-emetics
Disease process	Appetite stimulant
Anxiety	Active listening, explanation and support for patient and carer, including any specific issues relating to eating; anxiolytic
Depression	Empathic support, antidepressant
Social isolation, loneliness	Eat with others, attend a day centre

Non-drug treatment
General advice
See p.82.

Specific advice for those with a prognosis <2 months
Whose problem is it? The patient's or the family's?

Helping the patient and family accept and adjust to the reduced appetite is often the focus of management:

• listen to their fears; this can lead to discussion about the progressive impact of the illness

- explain that:
  - ▷ in the circumstances it is normal to be satisfied with less food
  - ▷ carer's can assist a fickle appetite by providing food when the patient is hungry (a microwave oven helps with this)
- a small helping looks better on a smaller plate
- offer specific dietary advice, particularly with early satiety
- discourage the 'he must eat or he will die' syndrome by emphasizing that a balanced diet is unnecessary at this stage in the illness:
  - ▷ 'Just give him a little of what he fancies'
  - ▷ 'I shall be happy even if he just takes fluids'
- recognize the 'food as love' and 'feeding him is my job' syndromes, encourage carer's to redirect their energies into other ways of caring and/or validate the importance of just 'being there'
- remember that eating is a social habit; people generally eat better at a table and when dressed.

Drug treatment
For more information, see PCF3.

For patients with early satiety, consider a trial of a prokinetic.

Appetite stimulants can increase calorie intake and as such may be indicated in selected patients for anorexia. If used, they should be closely monitored and stopped if no benefit is perceived after 1–2 weeks:
- corticosteroid, e.g. prednisolone 15–40mg each morning or dexamethasone 2–6mg each morning; useful in about 50% of patients but the effect generally lasts for only a few weeks[60–64]
- progestogen, e.g. megestrol acetate initially 80–160mg PO each morning; if response poor, consider doubling the dose after 2 weeks; maximum dose generally 800mg PO per 24h.[65,66]

Medroxyprogesterone acetate 400mg PO each morning–b.d. is an alternative in the UK and other countries where higher strength tablets are available (e.g. 100mg, 200mg and 400mg). Progestogens may be a more appropriate choice for long-term use than corticosteroids, but significant undesirable effects can occur. Starting doses should be low and titrated to the lowest effective dose.

Note: both progestogens and corticosteroids are best not regarded as 'anticachexia' drugs; any weight gain is likely to be due to an increase in fat and fluid retention, and the catabolism of skeletal muscle increased, particularly in inactive people.

CACHEXIA

Cachexia is common in cancer and other chronic diseases, impairing quality of life and increasing morbidity and mortality.[67] Unlike starvation where muscle mass is relatively preserved, in cachexia there is marked reduction in both skeletal muscle and body fat. Loss of skeletal muscle is associated with impaired physical function and quality of life, whereas loss of fat (the body's main energy store) is associated with reduced survival.

Cancer cachexia

Cancer cachexia is defined by a negative protein and energy balance driven by a variable combination of reduced food intake and abnormal metabolism. A key feature is ongoing loss of skeletal muscle mass which cannot be fully reversed by conventional nutritional support, leading to progressive functional impairment. It has been proposed that, in the absence of simple starvation, cancer cachexia is present when there is ongoing involuntary weight loss, which has resulted in either a weight loss $>5\%$ over the last 6 months, or a BMI of $<18.5kg/m^2$. Patients with lesser degrees of weight loss are considered to have pre-cachexia. Cachexia occurs in $>50\%$ of patients with advanced cancer, particularly of the lung and upper GI tract.[68]

Pathogenesis

Cancer cachexia is a complex paraneoplastic phenomenon caused by multiple factors (Box 3.H). The two main mechanisms are a reduced food intake (anorexia) and abnormal host metabolism resulting from substances produced by the cancer, e.g. proteolysis-inducing factor (PIF), or by the host in response to the cancer, e.g. cytokines.[69] One outcome of this is a chronic inflammatory state, the level of which relates to the degree and rate of weight loss.[70] Cytokines such as IL-1 and TNF-α act on the hypothalamus and skeletal muscle, and result in:

- anorexia
- inefficient energy expenditure
- loss of body fat
- wasting of skeletal muscle.

The management of cachexia requires the correction of both anorexia and the abnormal host metabolism; increasing nutritional intake alone is not enough.[69,71–73]

Box 3.H   Causal factors in cancer cachexia

Paraneoplastic

Cytokines and other substances produced by host cells and cancer, e.g. TNF-α, IL-1, IL-6, PIF, lead to:
- a pro-inflammatory state
- abnormal metabolism of:
  - ▷ protein → increased acute phase proteins, decreased skeletal muscle (catabolism ↑, anabolism ↓)
  - ▷ fat → increased lipolysis, fatty acid oxidation
  - ▷ carbohydrate → increased glucose production and recycling, insulin resistance and glucose intolerance
- increased metabolic rate → increased energy expenditure

Concurrent

Anorexia → deficient food intake
Vomiting
Diarrhoea
Malabsorption
Bowel obstruction
Debilitating effect of treatment:
- surgery
- radiotherapy
- chemotherapy

Ulceration ⎫ excessive loss of
Haemorrhage ⎬ body protein

Wasting of skeletal muscle results from cytokines and a cancer-derived PIF causing:

- increased catabolism, due to up-regulation of the ubiquitin-proteasome system and dysregulation of the dystrophin glycoprotein complex
- impaired anabolism, due to amino acid diversion to make acute-phase proteins and inhibition of muscle protein production and muscle cell proliferation and differentiation.[74]

The resultant weakness relates purely to the loss of muscle volume; muscle contractile function is not impaired.[75] This suggests that therapeutic exercise has a possible role.

Wasting of adipose tissue results from the actions of cancer and host-derived cytokines and lipid mobilizing factor/zinc α_2-glycoprotein leading to increased fat catabolism because of:

- impaired fat storage; there are increases in lipolysis, hypertriglyceridaemia, liver production of very-low density lipoprotein, fatty acid synthesis and futile cycling of fatty acids between liver and fat tissue
- enhanced metabolism of free fatty acids (FFA); particularly in brown adipose tissue, where their oxidation is 'uncoupled' from ATP production, releasing heat and wasting energy.[74]

Clinical features

The principal features of cancer cachexia are:

- marked weight loss
- anorexia
- weakness
- fatigue.

There may also be evidence of systemic inflammation, i.e. raised serum C-reactive protein level. Associated physical features include:

- altered taste sensation
- early satiety
- loose dentures causing pain and difficulty with eating
- pallor (anaemia)
- oedema (hypo-albuminaemia)
- pressure sores.

Psychosocial ramifications extend to:

- ill-fitting clothes which increase the sense of loss and displacement
- altered appearance which engenders fear and isolation
- difficulties in social and family relationships.

Management

Attending to nutritional needs is an integral part of good supportive care for patients receiving either curative or palliative anticancer treatments. It reduces symptoms from the cancer or its treatment, postoperative complications, infection rates, length of hospital stay and improves quality of life.[76] An emerging consensus is that the optimal management of cachexia requires a multiprofessional, multimodal approach which addresses both the reduced nutritional intake and the abnormal metabolism, and is offered *before* significant wasting has occurred.

However, in patients with a short prognosis (<2 months), helping the patient and family to accept and adjust to the reduced appetite and loss of weight is an appropriate focus of management.

For the management of concurrent anorexia, see p.77.

Prevent the preventable
Early detection and intervention is preferable and requires a pro-active approach. A sedentary lifestyle will contribute to the loss of muscle mass through disuse atrophy. Thus, patients should be encouraged to be as physically active as possible.

Correct the correctable
When appropriate, identify and treat any causal factors limiting food intake (see Table 3.5, p.78). If oral intake is to be improved, particular attention must be paid to:
- the ability to obtain and prepare food
- oral problems, e.g. dry mouth, mucositis, oral candidosis (see p.62, p.67, p.70 respectively).
- uncontrolled nausea and vomiting (see p.101)
- dysphagia (see p.85).

Non-drug treatment
For more information, see *PCF3*, Chapter 26, Oral nutritional supplements.

Because of abnormal metabolism, aggressive nutritional supplementation (enteral or parenteral) *alone* is of minimal value in *established* cancer cachexia.[77,78] When combined with chemotherapy or indometacin and insulin, nutritional supplementation (parenteral when necessary) has improved energy balance and survival.[79,80]

The aims of dietary advice vary according to the patient's prognosis:
- when <2 months, when cachexia is likely to be established, the focus should be on the psychosocial aspects of eating and drinking (see below)
- when ≥2 months, the focus should be on the prevention or slowing of the rate of weight loss in patients by ensuring sufficient intake of energy, protein, electrolytes vitamins, minerals and trace elements.

Dietary advice might include:
- meal patterns, e.g. eat small amounts frequently
- explanation to patients who have adopted a 'more healthy' diet (increased fruit and vegetables, reduced fat) that this can lead to a reduced overall energy intake
- encourage the increase in intake of energy-dense foods favoured by the patient
- replace water-based drinks, e.g. tea, coffee, with milk-based drinks, e.g. hot chocolate, malted drinks, milky coffee
- dietary fortification, e.g. use full-fat milk and cream, extra butter, margarine, oil and sugar (fats are the most concentrated source of energy)
- consider relaxing pre-imposed dietary restrictions, e.g. diabetic diet
- making use of microwave meals and convenience foods; quick and easy to prepare, often small portions, and high in fat and salt. The latter may help patients with a reduced sense of taste.

Generally, weight gain is more likely with nutritional supplements ± dietary advice than with dietary advice alone in patients with illness-related malnutrition.[81] Nonetheless, any increase in weight is likely to represent a gain in fat rather than muscle tissue.[82,83]

As cachexia progresses, the focus of treatment should shift from body weight to the amelioration of the psychosocial consequences for both the patient and the carer along with the physical complications (also see anorexia, p.77):

- weight loss is generally seen as indicative of disease progression and shortened survival which may bring to the fore a wide range of concerns
- trying to eat 'to stay alive' when difficult to do so or unsuccessful (i.e. weight loss continues) can become a burdensome and distressing activity for both the patient and (often more so) the carer, causing feelings such as anxiety, incomprehension, loss of control, anger, frustration, helplessness, rejection and guilt
- health professionals can help the patient and carer to come to terms with the situation by exploring their understanding of the situation, allowing venting of emotions, providing explanation, and helping to set realistic goals
- reline dentures to improve chewing and facial appearance; as a temporary measure, this can be done at the bedside and lasts about 3 months
- if affordable, buy new clothes to enhance self-esteem
- supply equipment to help maintain personal independence, e.g. raised toilet seat, commode, walking frame, wheelchair
- educate the patient and family about the risk of decubitus ulcers and the importance of skin care.[84–86]

Drug treatment

For more information, see *PCF3*.

Currently, there are no established drug treatments for cancer cachexia. Several drugs, targeting either the inflammatory response and/or the abnormal metabolism, have shown some efficacy in clinical trials,[87] including:

- *thalidomide*: 200mg at bedtime inhibits TNF-α and other cytokines, and reduces weight loss[88,89]
- *indometacin*: reduces inflammation and resting energy expenditure, and preserves body fat and performance status[90,91]
- *omega-3 polyunsaturated fatty acids*: eicosapentaenoic acid (EPA) has an anti-inflammatory effect and is available as a high-dose constituent of some oral nutritional supplements (e.g. ProSure®, Forticare®, Resource Support®) but it can be difficult for patients to ingest an effective amount (≥1.5g EPA/day), which may partly explain the lack of consistent benefit[92–94]
- *insulin*: increases survival, carbohydrate intake, body fat and metabolic efficiency during exercise, but not lean body mass or spontaneous physical activity[95]
- *ghrelin analogues*: ghrelin has multiple effects which include stimulating food intake and decreasing fat metabolism; an orally active analogue (RC-1291) increases total and lean body mass and muscle strength.[96]

A beneficial multimodal approach used at one centre is a combination of nutritional support (parenteral if necessary) with indometacin, epoetin, and insulin.[79,95] Positive results have also been seen in an ongoing study testing the combination of anti-oxidants together with a progestogen, an EPA-enriched oral nutritional supplement, l-carnitine, and thalidomide.[97] Such regimens require considerable determination by the patient.

The pharmaceutical industry has a growing interest in cachexia and muscle wasting, and several new drugs are in development.

DEHYDRATION

Terminally ill patients often lose interest in food as they physically deteriorate. Moribund patients often lose interest in hydration as well but are not distressed provided the mouth is cleaned and moistened regularly.[98,99]

On the other hand, patients who develop acute dehydration, for example as a result of vomiting, diarrhoea or polyuria, experience distressing thirst and generally need parenteral rehydration.[100] However, some patients prefer not to have an infusion even in these circumstances and generally their disinclination should be respected. Remember: the aim is comfort, not a perfect fluid balance chart with normal electrolytes (Box 3.I).

Box 3.I Parenteral hydration in palliative care

Indications
Generally all the following criteria should be met:
- the patient is experiencing symptoms (e.g. thirst, malaise, delirium) for which dehydration is the most likely cause
- increased oral intake not feasible
- anticipation that parenteral hydration will relieve the symptoms (e.g. in patients with severe dysphagia, vomiting or diarrhoea)
- the patient's general physical condition is relatively good (e.g. some patients with head and neck cancer)
- the patient is willing to have parenteral hydration
- the patient and relatives understand that the purpose is to relieve symptoms and not to cure.

It is advisable initially to give a provisional time limit for parenteral hydration, e.g. 2–3 days, after which it will be discontinued if not helpful.

Contra-indications
The patient requests not to have an invasive procedure.
The burdens of parenteral hydration outweigh the likely benefits.
The patient is moribund for reasons other than dehydration.

If it is not in the patient's best interests, parenteral hydration should not be introduced simply to satisfy relatives who insist that something must be done.

For some patients, intermittent SC infusion (hypodermoclysis) is preferable to continuous IV infusion. Either 5% glucose-saline or 0.9% saline can be infused. Amounts vary between 500mL and 2L/24h, given over 3–12h through a 25G needle.[101]

In a systematic review of five studies, the provision of hydration made no difference to patient outcomes in three, improved levels of sedation and myoclonus in one but increased symptoms related to fluid retention in the other.[102] Also see Box 3.K, p.89.

DYSPHAGIA

Dysphagia (difficulty in swallowing) is the presenting symptom in most pharyngeal and oesophageal cancers. At some stage, dysphagia occurs in almost all patients with head and neck cancer as a result of the cancer or its treatment.[103,104] This is not necessarily mechanical; nerve damage and fibrosis can cause severe dysphagia.[105]

Dysphagia is also a feature of other cancers which involve the mediastinum, neck, brain, or base of the skull, e.g. lung cancer and lymphoma. Non-obstructive dysphagia may also result from MND/ALS and other neurological diseases, e.g. dementia, stroke. Non-obstructive dysphagia associated with extreme weakness and/or cachexia is also common.

Dysphagia can lead to dehydration, malnutrition, and aspiration. Aspiration of oral or gastric contents does not always lead to coughing, but it increases the risk of:

- airway obstruction
- pneumonia
- abscess formation
- pulmonary fibrosis
- adult respiratory distress syndrome (non-cardiogenic pulmonary oedema).[106,107]

A reduced level of consciousness increases the risk of aspiration. Aspiration of larger quantities of fluids or food while eating may result in episodes of choking from acute obstruction of the pharynx, larynx or trachea (see p.360).

Physiology

Swallowing is a complex phenomenon, involving the brain stem, 5 cranial nerves, and 34 skeletal muscles.[108] It comprises four distinct phases, two voluntary and two reflexive:

- *oral preparatory phase*: food is mixed with saliva and chewed to reduce particle size
- *oral swallowing phase*: the lips are closed to prevent leakage and the anterior tongue retracts and elevates in a wave which pushes the bolus into the oropharynx
- *pharyngeal phase*: this is triggered by the bolus reaching the posterior tongue. The larynx closes, breathing stops, and a peristaltic wave moves the bolus into the oesophagus in less than 1 second. These complex actions are necessary to protect the airway because the pharynx is a shared passage for air and food
- *oesophageal phase*: reflex peristalsis carries the bolus into the stomach.

Causes

There are many causes of dysphagia in advanced cancer (Box 3.J). Two basic processes are involved:

- mechanical obstruction
- neuromuscular defects.

Dysphagia with severe odynophagia (painful swallowing) is occasionally caused by oesophageal spasm provoked by oesophagitis, e.g. radiation-induced or acid reflux.[109] In MND/ALS, increasingly severe dysphagia (and dysarthria) is due to pseudobulbar palsy (dysfunction of the lower cranial nerves).[110]

Evaluation

A detailed swallowing evaluation by a speech and language therapist will identify specific problems in relation to each stage of swallowing. A direct evaluation using videofluoroscopy or a fibre endoscope may sometimes be necessary.[111,112] Accurate evaluation facilitates the formulation of an individualized management plan.

Box 3.J   Causes of dysphagia in advanced cancer

Cancer
Mass lesion in mouth, pharynx, oesophagus or cardia of the stomach
Infiltration of pharyngo-oesophageal wall
→ damage to nerve plexus
External compression (mediastinal mass)
Perineural tumour spread (vagus and sympathetic)
Tumour spread across base of skull
→ cranial nerve palsies
Metastases in base of skull
→ cranial nerve palsies
Leptomeningeal infiltration
→ cranial nerve palsies
Cerebral metastatic disease
→ bulbar palsy
Paraneoplastic

Debility
Dry mouth
Pharyngo-oesophageal candidosis
Pharyngeal bacterial infection
Anxiety → oesophageal spasm
Drowsiness and disinterest
Extreme weakness (patient moribund)
Hypercalcaemia (rare)

Treatment
Surgery
   lingual
   buccal
Chemotherapy- or radiotherapy-induced mucositis
Post-radiation fibrosis
   difficulty in opening mouth and moving tongue
   prolonged oesophageal transit
   oesophageal stricture
Displacement of endo-oesophageal tube
Drugs (dystonic reaction)
   antipsychotics
   metoclopramide

Concurrent
Reflux oesophagitis
Benign stricture
Iron deficiency

The history together with clinical observation will generally indicate if the problem lies within the mouth or pharynx, or more distally in the oesophagus, and help to distinguish between dysphagia and odynophagia (painful swallowing). Remember:

- obstructing lesions cause dysphagia for solids initially with later progression to liquids
- neuromuscular disorders cause dysphagia for both solids and liquids at about the same time
- patients can almost always accurately identify the level of an obstruction.[108]

For problems arising within the mouth and pharynx, difficulties will arise *before*, *during* or *immediately after* a swallow. Clinical features may include:

- food loss from the mouth
- food sitting in the mouth
- food coming down the nose.

Coughing/choking before, during and/or immediately after the swallow suggests a pharyngeal problem.

For problems within the oesophagus, symptoms occur *after* a normal swallow; an endoscopy is generally indicated.

Explanation

Aspiration of food at mealtimes or of saliva at night may lead to distressing episodes of coughing or choking such that patients become extremely fearful of a recurrence. This fear should be validated and a strategy developed to give the patient confidence that he will not choke to death. Emphasize that:

- although aspiration leading to coughing is relatively common, the patient and family should be assured that it is *extremely rare* for aspiration to cause fatal choking
- there are measures which will reduce the frequency and intensity of aspiration or choking attacks.[110,113]

Management

Aspiration of water alone is well tolerated if it does not cause bouts of coughing, and patients should not be denied sips of water or ice chips to relieve a dry mouth or thirst.

Correct the correctable

When cancer is causing obstruction, possible ways of maintaining the lumen include:

- oesophageal stent (see p.90)
- radiotherapy (teletherapy or brachytherapy) $\pm$ chemotherapy
- LASER debridement, argon plasma coagulation
- trial of dexamethasone 12–16mg/24h.[105]

Non-drug treatment

Seek agreement between the patient, family and staff about feeding goals and treatment plans; this stems from an explanation of what is possible and what is not.

Ideally, a speech and language therapist should be involved before aspiration or choking becomes a major problem. They can advise the patient and carers about techniques to help prevent and manage episodes of aspiration/choking:

- about 'safe swallowing' (individualized to the specific swallowing problem)
- about keeping calm
- how to remove any obstructing material from the mouth
- emergency treatment of choking (see p.360).

Specific input from a dietitian may also be helpful, such as:

- how to maximize calorie intake in small volume meals, e.g.:
  - ▷ adding cream to soup, etc.
  - ▷ eating cold sour cream by the spoonful
  - ▷ oral nutritional supplements
- recommending suitable soft food cookbooks
- use of a liquidizer/blender
- general advice about mealtimes.

Support for the patient and carers will also be required to help them cope with the psychosocial consequences of dysphagia: disruption at meal times of the normal pattern of eating, drinking, and social interaction.

Feeding tubes

The provision of artificial nutrition or hydration is regarded as a medical treatment and is not part of basic care.[114,115] Artificial nutrition:

- may prolong life in patients with cancer who have difficulty swallowing due to a local cause, e.g. laryngeal cancer

- is contra-indicated in patients with cancer cachexia or those close to death because there is no evidence that it prolongs survival or improves quality of life.

Artificial hydration:
- is unlikely to influence survival for patients with advanced cancer and those close to death
- is unlikely to improve quality of life in those patients who have gradually reduced their fluid intake as part of the dying process; but it is debatable whether it has a limited role (generally on a trial basis) in:
  ▷ relieving distressing thirst in those close to death who have failed to obtain relief from good mouth care
  ▷ managing opioid-induced delirium
- exacerbates hypo-albuminaemia, oedema and ascites but does not prevent an increase in blood urea and creatinine as death approaches; i.e. the administered fluid ends up in the tissues, not the blood vessels[116]
- may improve quality of life in patients who suddenly become unable to take fluids, e.g. because of acute bowel obstruction.

The question of whether to use a feeding tube, arises more commonly in patients with neurological disorders, e.g. post-stroke and MND/ALS. Ideally, in such conditions, there should be discussion about artificial nutrition and hydration well in advance of the patient becoming unable to swallow. Options include:
- nasogastric tube, e.g. Clinifeed enteric tube; transnasal placement on the ward is possible if the oesophageal lumen > 1cm; not ideal for long-term use, i.e. >4 weeks
- feeding gastrostomy.[117]

Complications of tube feeding include:
- pain (post-insertion)
- haemorrhage
- pneumoperitoneum
- peritonitis
- peristomal infection
- mechanical obstruction
- tube migration
- peritubal leakage
- gastrocolonic fistula
- GI upset (vomiting, diarrhoea, constipation).

In MND/ALS, tube feeding is considered in patients who have experienced weight loss of > 10% of their baseline. Enteral tube feeding maintains nutrition, hydration and weight, and provides a route for drug administration. It has not been shown to improve quality of life or survival.[118] A percutaneous gastrostomy is the standard procedure, but a radiologically inserted gastrostomy may be more appropriate for patients with poor respiratory function (i.e. FVC <50% predicted); it does not require passage of a fibre-optic endoscope or sedation and can be done with the patient sitting rather than lying.[118] Occasionally a prophylactic tracheostomy is also necessary and appropriate in MND/ALS.[110]

Sensitive discussion is required around the decision to commence enteral tube feeding. Much depends on both the speed of deterioration and the opinion of the patient and family, together with those of the professional carers. Certain patients may benefit more than others, i.e. those with MND and dysphagia and dysarthria but little limb disability.[119] Some patients are relieved when a doctor sensitively confirms that they will not be forced to have a nasogastric tube or gastrostomy. If in doubt it is better to delay several days, or even weeks, before deciding to go ahead. It is easier not to start a treatment than to stop it. Ethical and practical guidelines on artificial nutrition (and hydration) are available, some specific to end of life care (Box 3.K).[114,115,120–124]

Box 3.K Summary of guidance on artificial nutrition and hydration (ANH) in end of life care[114]

See the guidance for full details and example case histories.

Artificial nutrition and hydration (ANH) is a medical treatment and the principles guiding decisions around its provision, withholding or withdrawal are as with any other medical treatment. It is not considered basic care, and it can be withheld or withdrawn if the clinician believes that its use is not in the patient's best interests. The only exception is when a patient is in a persistent vegetative state; in this case a court review is required.

Patients with capacity should be provided with sufficient information regarding the likely benefits and burdens of ANH to enable them to make an informed choice about consenting to or refusing ANH.

For patients without capacity (see Box 13.C, p.410):
• find out if there is an Advance Decision to Refuse Treatment (ADRT), Lasting Power of Attorney (LPA) or Court Appointed Deputy
• identify the person legally responsible for the decision to give or withdraw ANH; in the absence of an ADRT or LPA, this is likely to be the doctor responsible for the patient's care.

The responsible person should consider:
• the possible benefits and risks of ANH
• what is in the patient's best interests.

In order to achieve a consensus view, evaluation of best interests should:
• include the patient's participation where feasible
• ascertain what the patient's views might have been
• take into account the views of those close to the patient.

In the absence of any carers who can offer an opinion, then an Independent Mental Capacity Advocate (IMCA) may need to be consulted.

Ultimately:
• the responsible person should seek a consensus view, if necessary holding a case conference and/or obtaining a second opinion
• in complex cases, or if consensus can not be reached, advice should be sought on approaching the Court of Protection.

Drug treatment
For more information, see *PCF3*.

Dysphagia and odynophagia caused by oesophagitis and oesophageal spasm has been treated successfully with glyceryl trinitrate 400microgram SL 15min a.c.[109] If total obstruction leads to drooling, prescribe an antisecretory drug (see p.65).

Oral morphine has been used as an antitussive to reduce the likelihood of coughing from aspiration, e.g. of saliva, in patients with MND/ALS or similar neurological dysfunction.[125,126] Generally begin with small doses, e.g. morphine solution 5–6mg t.d.s. a.c. and at bedtime and titrate the dose as necessary. Some patients are able to take m/r tablets; most will ultimately need to convert to CSCI.[125] In one series, the median maximum dose of oral morphine was 60mg/24h; and for CSCI 180mg/24h.[125]

Patients can also be supplied with hyoscine hydrobromide 0.3mg SL to use if they are troubled by excessive saliva, and/or start to cough when drinking or eating and have difficulty in clearing matter from the trachea.[113] Hyoscine hydrobromide acts quickly, probably as a sedative. 'Sublingual' does not need to be literally under the tongue; placing it in a cheek or by the gums is equally satisfactory. Only about 1/3 of patients ever need to use SL hyoscine. The use of morphine ± hyoscine/glycopyrronium generally reduces the severity of coughing during drinking and eating, and at night, and thus reduces the associated distress.

In patients at risk of aspiration and choking, it is recommended that ampoules of the following drugs are kept in the patient's home for emergency use, and used if the patient becomes distressed as a result of a prolonged episode of coughing:
• diamorphine 5mg or morphine 10mg
• midazolam 10mg
• hyoscine hydrobromide 400–600microgram or glycopyrronium 200microgram.

As part of the Breathing Space Programme of the MND Association, a special box is available for MND/ALS patients to enable such medication to be kept at home in an obvious place. An information sheet about the programme and an application form for the box can be obtained by general practitioners from the MND Association (http://www.mndassociation.org/index.html).

OESOPHAGEAL STENTING

Self-expanding nitinol or stainless steel metal stents coated with a plastic membrane are used to relieve dysphagia and to close tracheo-oesophageal fistulas in patients with cancer of the oesophagus or proximal stomach. They can be constricted to a small diameter so that minimal pre-insertion dilation is required. They have effectively superseded flexible endo-oesophageal tubes, e.g. Celestin.

The procedure is generally carried out using IV sedation ± analgesia and takes about 30min. Using a fibre-optic endoscope, guide-wire and fluoroscopy, the stent is deployed across the stricture/fistula and, as a result of exposure to body temperature, slowly expands to its full diameter over hours–days.[127] Water-soluble contrast is used to check that the fistula is successfully sealed.

Stents differ in their properties and some are more suitable for certain situations than others, e.g. those with strong expansile forces are better suited for extrinsic oesophageal compression. On the other hand, a stent which can incorporate an antireflux valve may be more appropriate when the gastro-oesophageal junction is crossed.[128] Some are removable.

Most patients obtain rapid benefit but need to be careful about what and how they eat (Box 3.L and Box 3.M). Mortality from the procedure is low, but morbidity is relatively high:[127,129,130]
• chest pain requiring additional analgesia; generally settles after a 2–3 days

- bleeding
- oesophageal perforation
- fistula formation
- gastro-oesophageal reflux, aspiration
- airway compression.

Box 3.L Dietary recommendations for patients with an oesophageal stent

Protein-rich food

Eat	*Avoid*
Tender meat in gravy, otherwise minced or pureed	Tough or dry meats
Flaked fish in sauce	Any fish with bones or without sauce
Grated cheese/cheese in sauce	Lumps of hard cheese
Soft cheese: cottage/cream	Fried or hard boiled eggs
Soft boiled, poached and scrambled eggs, omelette	
Milk: full cream, evaporated, condensed	

Fruit and vegetables

Include	*Exclude*
Fruit juices	Dried fruit, e.g. raisins, sultanas, etc.
Peeled soft or stewed fruits (no pips)	Nuts
Puréed tinned fruit	Raw vegetables or salads, e.g. lettuce, tomato
Yoghurts (without chunks of fruit)/mousses	Stringy vegetables, e.g. celery, green beans, sweetcorn, peas, rhubarb, broccoli, cauliflower stalks
Soft well-cooked mashed vegetables	Fibrous or pithy fruits, e.g. grapefruit, orange, pineapple, grapes
	Fruit skins/pips, e.g. damson jam, peach, pear or apple skin

Starches

Eat	*Avoid*
Potato, mashed with butter, gravy, sauces or cream	Hard chips, roast, plain boiled or baked potatoes
Boiled white rice or spaghetti (rinsed well)	Potato crisps/snacks
Tinned spaghetti, macaroni, milk puddings	Wholegrain rice
Day-old wholemeal bread, crackers or crispbreads with plenty of butter/margarine	Fresh doughy bread, e.g. new white bread, doughy cakes, fruit cake
Soft crumbly biscuits, e.g. digestive, shortbread, chocolate-coated biscuits	French sticks, toast
	Hard flaky biscuits, e.g. water biscuits
Semisolid smooth breakfast cereals, e.g. porridge, Ready Brek®, All Bran®, Weetabix®	Puff pastry, Danish pastry
	Muesli, nutty cereals
	Shredded wheat, puffed wheat

Box 3.M   General advice to patients with an oesophageal stent

A metal stent has been put into your food pipe to help you eat and drink more easily.

Because this has an internal opening about the size of your index finger, you need to be careful with what you swallow; hard or lumpy food may block the stent.

Speak to your doctor about your medicines; tablets should be taken with plenty of water or some can be crushed; alternative soluble, liquid or capsular formulations are sometimes available.

Sit upright to eat.

Eat 'little and often', e.g. 6 snacks rather than 2–3 big meals.

Eat slowly; take small mouthfuls of food and chew well, avoid swallowing chunks of food.

Food should never be eaten dry; lubricate with butter, margarine, milk, gravy, sauce, etc.

Always sip a warm or fizzy drink with your meal.

Avoid ice/ice-cold drinks for at least 1 month after placement of a metal stent as the cold may cause the stent to alter shape and move out of place.

Drink more nourishing fluid and less tea, coffee, squash, water.

Drink alcohol in moderation; preferably adding a fizzy/carbonated mixer to your favourite tipple and sip it with your meals, e.g. gin and tonic, beer shandy, Bucks Fizz®.

If your stent becomes blocked, it may cause difficulty swallowing or regurgitation of food. Stop eating and try sipping a warm or fizzy drink, with standing up and walking around.

If this doesn't work, contact your doctor for further advice and help.

Although a blocked stent is distressing, it is not a serious medical problem.

Recurrent dysphagia occurs in 1/4–1/3 of patients due to:
- continued growth of the cancer around or within the stent
- overgrowth of granulation tissue
- food bolus impaction
- stent migration.

Partial or complete stent migration can occur. The stent can remain in the GI tract or be passed PR without problem. Rarely, the stent causes intestinal obstruction requiring surgical intervention; for this reason some clinicians remove migrated stents.[131,132]

For recurrent obstruction due to cancer, LASER debridement, argon plasma coagulation or repeat stent placement can be considered. For patients with a reasonable prognosis, brachytherapy is an option.[127]

Because of the relatively high rate of recurrent dysphagia, the use of metal stents as the *only* treatment for dysphagia is best suited to patients with a short prognosis, or other situations when anticancer therapies are inappropriate. In patients with a better prognosis, a stent can be placed for immediate relief, followed by radiotherapy/chemotherapy, which may give better long-term control with fewer complications, particularly when the stent is removed 4–6 weeks after the radiotherapy.[133]

Postoperative management after stent insertion
- a chest radiograph to exclude oesophageal perforation
- elevation on 2–3 pillows to prevent gastric reflux, particularly when the gastro-oesophageal junction is crossed by the stent
- prescription of a PPI
- fluids can be drunk after about 1h, when the topical local anaesthesia of the oropharynx has worn off
- most patients go home after an overnight stay, but some centres insert stents as a day case procedure
- a soft diet can be introduced the day after the procedure
- if the patient copes with a soft diet, more solid food can be introduced the next day; it must be chewed well and follow dietary recommendations (see Box 3.L, p.91)
- if there is discomfort continue with a soft diet, and try introducing solids again after 5–7 days.

Following general advice will also reduce the risk of the stent becoming blocked by food (see Box 3.M). However, despite improved swallowing, many patients continue to lose weight because of cachexia (see p.79).[134]

GASTRO-OESOPHAGEAL REFLUX

Heartburn and regurgitation are the archetypal symptoms of reflux of caustic gastric contents (acid, proteolytic enzymes, bile salts) into the oesophagus. Heartburn is generally described as a burning retrosternal discomfort, which may radiate to the neck, throat or back. However, a wide range of symptoms can occur, in part related to the vertical extent of the refluxate (Box 3.N).

Box 3.N Common symptoms associated with reflux

Gastro-oesophageal reflux
Heartburn
Regurgitation
Painful swallowing (odynophagia)
Non-cardiac chest pain
Transient dysphagia (for solid foods only)
Hiccup, belching
Water brash (episodic hypersalivation)
Cough ⎫
Wheezing ⎬ via a vagally mediated reflex

Laryngopharyngeal reflux
Cough ⎫
Wheezing ⎬ via macro- or micro-aspiration
Hoarseness ⎭
Throat clearing
'Lump in the throat' (globus)
Post-nasal drip
Episodes of difficult breathing or choking
Laryngitis/pharyngitis

About 1/5 of people intermittently experience typical reflux symptoms. They may be worse during or after meals and on talking, lying or bending forward. Endoscopically, gastro-oesophageal reflux disease is differentiated into erosive and non-erosive. The frequency and severity of symptoms does not predict the degree of mucosal damage; those with severe symptoms may have a normal endoscopy. Conversely those with minimal symptoms can present only when complications have developed, e.g. stricture formation, dysplasia with an increased risk of adenocarcinoma (Barrett's oesophagus). This may relate to the degree of oesophageal hypersensitivity, e.g. to acid, along with distinct responses of the oesophageal mucosa to acid exposure.[135]

Pathogenesis
The distal 5cm of the oesophagus is a high pressure zone (10–12mmHg) which acts as the lower oesophageal sphincter. A number of factors impair the function of the sphincter, leading to reflux (Box 3.O). Factors which increase the pressure gradient across the gastro-oesophageal junction (e.g. post-prandial gastric distension) also trigger transient relaxations of the sphincter. Delayed gastric emptying may predispose to reflux by increasing the volume of gastric contents available to be refluxed, or by contributing to gastric distension.[136]

Most reflux episodes are asymptomatic; episodes associated with typical symptoms have a more acidic refluxate and are more likely to occur after meals (particularly with a high fat content) or when lying flat.[137,138] Symptoms may also be associated with:
- impaired oesophageal motility (longer exposure time to caustic refluxate)
- acid breaching oesophageal mucosal defences (leading to cell damage, inflammation and sensory nerve stimulation)
- increased oesophageal sensitivity to acid (e.g. due to sensitization of visceral nerve pathways).

Box 3.O Factors which decrease the tone of the lower oesophageal sphincter

Dietary
Alcohol
Chocolate
Fat
Carminatives, e.g.
  mint, anise, dill
Carbonated beverages
Aerophagic habits, e.g.
  chewing gum
  sucking hard candy
Large meals
Acidic or spicy foods

Mechanical
Lying flat
Constricting abdominal garments
Obesity
Sliding hiatus hernia
Ascites

Drugs
Antimuscarinics
Benzodiazepines
Calcium-channel blockers
Nicotine
Nitrates and nitrites
Oestrogens
Pethidine (meperidine)
Theophylline

Many drugs decrease the tone of the lower oesophageal sphincter (Box 3.O). The onset of heartburn within 1–2 days of commencing a new drug should alert the doctor to this possibility. The use of morphine and other opioids may exacerbate reflux secondary to delayed gastric emptying.

Management
Correct the correctable
- stop or reduce the dose of causal drugs if possible
- change to a drug with less or no antimuscarinic effects, e.g. an SSRI instead of a TCA
- modify diet (Box 3.O)
- stop smoking
- abdominal paracentesis if marked ascites present
- weight reduction if obese (generally not applicable in advanced cancer).

Non-drug treatment
- avoid constricting garments and lying flat after meals
- elevate the head of the bed by 10cm
- lie in the left lateral position.[139]

Drug treatment
For more information, see *PCF3*.

The range of possibilities includes:
- occasional heartburn responds rapidly to OTC antacids or alginate-antacid combinations p.r.n.
- some H_2-receptor antagonists and PPIs are also available OTC for p.r.n. use; they take longer to work but have a longer duration of action[139,140]
- for frequent distressing symptoms, reduce gastric acid by prescribing a PPI regularly/long-term:[139,141,142]
  ▷ more effective than H_2-receptor antagonists
  ▷ heals erosive oesophagitis in >90% of patients
  ▷ prevents recurrence of oesophagitis in 80%
  ▷ eases symptoms in 1–2 weeks
  ▷ symptoms persist in 20–40%, possibly because of insufficient acid suppression (consider increasing the dose of the PPI or adding an H_2-receptor antagonist at night), bile or proteolytic enzyme reflux, oesophageal distension, oesophageal dysmotility and/or pain hypersensitivity
- the addition of a prokinetic, e.g. metoclopramide, can help by increasing the pressure of the lower oesophageal sphincter and enhancing gastric emptying.

Baclofen is a possible option in those failing to respond to the above. It reduces transient relaxations of the lower oesophageal sphincter, and thus reduces reflux episodes and symptoms:
- start with 5mg once daily (± PPI)
- increase over 10 days to 40–60mg/24h in divided doses, e.g. 10mg q.d.s., 20mg t.d.s.[139,143]

Further investigation, e.g. an endoscopy, is warranted in patients who fail to improve after 4–8 weeks of a PPI. In palliative care, the appropriateness of this will need to be considered on an individual basis.

DYSPEPSIA

Dyspepsia (literally 'bad digestion'; synonym: indigestion) refers to a constellation of symptoms related to the upper GI tract particularly after meals, e.g. discomfort/pain, fullness or bloating, early satiety, nausea or vomiting. It can relate to an organic disorder of the stomach or duodenum. Functional dyspepsia (without apparent organic cause) is common, affecting about 1/4 of the population.

Pathogenesis

There are many potential causes of dyspepsia in patients with advanced cancer (Box 3.P). The role of delayed gastric emptying (see p.98) and/or functional dyspepsia may be underestimated. In functional dyspepsia, symptoms may relate to:[144]

- visceral and central hypersensitivity, so that normal stimuli such as gastric distension leads to discomfort
- impaired gastric accommodation
- gastric and small intestinal dysmotility, most commonly causing delayed gastric emptying, but sometimes accelerated emptying
- duodenal hypersensitivity to fat or acid, possibly associated with delayed clearance
- psychological factors, e.g. stress, personality traits.

There appears to be a genetic predisposition to functional dyspepsia. An episode of infection or inflammation may contribute to its pathogenesis, and psychological factors to its progress and manifestations. There are similarities with irritable bowel syndrome which may co-exist or develop subsequently.

Box 3.P Causes of dyspepsia in advanced cancer

Cancer
Small stomach capacity
   large unresected stomach cancer
   massive ascites
Gatroparesis (paraneoplastic
   visceral neuropathy)

Treatment
Post-surgical
   post-gastrectomy
Radiotherapy
   lumbar spine
   epigastrium
Drugs
   physical irritant → gastritis,
     e.g. iron, tranexamic acid,
     PO bisphosphonates
   acid stimulant → gastritis,
     e.g. NSAIDs, corticosteroids
   delayed gastric emptying,
     e.g. antimuscarinics, opioids, cisplatin

Debility
Minimal food and fluid intake
Anxiety → aerophagia

Concurrent
Organic dyspepsia
   peptic ulcer
   Helicobacter pylori infection
   cholelithiasis
   renal failure
Functional dyspepsia

Evaluation

When appropriate, identify the underlying cause in order to provide specific treatment. Identify symptoms of reflux and treat appropriately. In functional dyspepsia, identify the predominant symptom and possible contributing factors, e.g. mood disturbance.

Management

Treat the underlying organic cause when appropriate.

In functional dyspepsia, symptoms relate poorly to the underlying cause, e.g. fullness, bloating and nausea can be associated with both delayed and accelerated gastric emptying. However, it is reasonable to try an initial approach based on the predominant symptom and its most likely cause, switching to an alternative approach if unsuccessful.

Correct the correctable

For example:
- stop or reduce the dose of causal drugs if possible
- drain ascites
- treat *H. pylori* infection (although the association with symptoms is unclear).

Non-drug treatment

Anecdotally, patients may benefit from:[145]
- eating 'small and often', i.e. 5–6 small meals/snacks during the day rather than 2–3 big meals
- avoiding late evening meals
- a low fat diet
- avoiding certain foodstuffs, e.g. onions, peppers, citrus fruits, coffee, carbonated drinks, spices.

Drug treatment

For more information, see *PCF3*.

Epigastric pain

Possible hypersensitivity:
- acid suppression with PPI:
  - ▷ most likely to benefit patients with concurrent heartburn
  - ▷ also used in NSAID-related gastritis
- TCAs.[144]

Fullness or bloating, early satiety, nausea and vomiting

Possible disordered gastric accommodation, motility and emptying:
- prescribe a prokinetic anti-emetic, e.g. metoclopramide, domperidone
- inconsistent benefit from other drugs, e.g. erythromycin
- if symptoms worsen with a prokinetic, accelerated gastric emptying may be the underlying cause; discontinue the prokinetic and consider a TCA with antimuscarinic effects or octreotide.[144]

Patients with a small stomach capacity may benefit from an antiflatulent after meals, to help clear space in an overfull stomach (see below).

Excessive belching (eructation)

- prescribe simeticone, an antifoaming agent (antiflatulent) available in several proprietary antacids, e.g. Asilone®
- depending on a patient's individual needs, give p.r.n., q.d.s., or both.

Concurrent anxiety/depression
- consider a TCA or SSRI.

GASTRIC STASIS

Gastric stasis (delayed gastric emptying) is common in advanced cancer. It accounts for about 25% of cases of nausea and vomiting.[146]

Clinical features

The clinical features of gastric stasis range from mild dyspepsia and anorexia to persistent severe nausea and large-volume vomiting (Box 3.Q). Gastric stasis is normally functional and is associated with one or more of the following conditions:
- functional dyspepsia (see p.96)
- constipation[147]
- drugs (opioids, antimuscarinics, aluminium hydroxide, levodopa)
- cancer of the head of the pancreas (disrupts duodenal transit)[148]
- paraneoplastic autonomic neuropathy
- retroperitoneal disease (→ nerve dysfunction)
- spinal cord compression
- diabetic autonomic neuropathy
- systemic disorders, amyloidosis, scleroderma
- neurological disease, e.g. Parkinson's
- post-surgical, e.g. gastric or oesophageal.

Box 3.Q   Clinical features of gastric stasis

Symptoms

Early satiety	Belching
Post-prandial fullness	Hiccup
Epigastric bloating	Nausea
Epigastric discomfort	Retching
Heartburn	Vomiting

Signs

Epigastric distension ⎫
Succussion splash ⎭ not invariable

A succussion splash requires > 400–500mL of fluid in the stomach and plenty of gas.

Bowel sounds, generally normal but may be decreased if the stasis is drug-induced.

If associated with autonomic neuropathy, there is often evidence of other autonomic abnormalities, e.g. orthostatic hypotension without a compensatory tachycardia.

Drug treatment

The use of metoclopramide generally leads to improvement and the resolution of the succussion splash.

Management
Correct the correctable
For example:
- treat constipation
- stop or reduce the dose of causal drugs if possible.

Non-drug treatment
Provide dietary advice, e.g.:
- eat 'small and often', i.e. 5–6 small meals/snacks during the day rather than 2–3 big meals
- avoid carbonated drinks which will increase stomach gas
- gastric electrical stimulation has been used for diabetic and idiopathic gastroparesis.[149]

Drug treatment
For more information, see PCF3.

Prescribe a prokinetic anti-emetic, e.g. metoclopramide, domperidone. Try to avoid the concurrent use of prokinetics and antimuscarinics; the latter block cholinergic receptors on intestinal muscle fibres, and thus will tend to antagonize the effect of prokinetic anti-emetics (Figure 3.1).[150] However, domperidone and metoclopramide will still exert an effect on the D_2-receptors in the chemoreceptor trigger zone (area postrema) in the brain stem.

Domperidone does not cross the blood–brain barrier, and should be used preferentially in patients with parkinsonism in whom central D_2-receptor antagonism is likely to be detrimental.

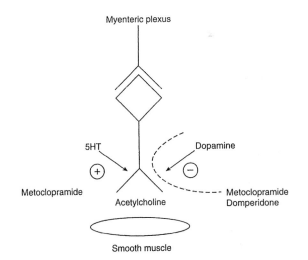

Figure 3.1 Schematic representation of drug effects on antroduodenal co-ordination via a post-ganglionic effect on the cholinergic nerves from the myenteric plexus.

$\oplus$ stimulatory effect of 5HT triggered by metoclopramide; $\ominus$ inhibitory effect of dopamine; ---- blockade of dopamine inhibition by metoclopramide and domperidone.

Erythromycin has a motilin-receptor agonist effect and can be tried if metoclopramide and domperidone fail to relieve. Erythromycin is typically given in a dose of 250mg PO b.d.–t.d.s. 30min a.c. (or 80–200mg IV in severe cases). Tolerance may develop with long-term use, but it has been used successfully for more than 1 year.

GASTRIC OUTFLOW OBSTRUCTION

Gastric stasis is occasionally associated with an organic obstruction:
• cancer of the gastric antrum
• external compression of the gastric antrum or duodenum by a cancer, e.g. of the pancreas.

The obstruction may not be complete. Even with no oral intake, the stomach needs to clear:
• swallowed saliva (normally 1,500mL/24h)
• basal gastric juices (1,500mL/24h).

Thus, if a patient is vomiting <2–3L/24h, something is probably getting passed the obstruction.

Management
Correct the correctable
• gastrojejunostomy, formed using open or laparoscopic surgery
• self-expanding metal stent.

A stent is less invasive and, at least in the short-term, may provide better relief than a gastrojejunostomy. However, further intervention is necessary in about 1/5 of patients in the 3 months after stent insertion, whereas this is almost never necessary after gastrojejunostomy. The stent can migrate or become occluded by cancer or food. Thus, a gastrojejunostomy may be a better option for patients with a prognosis of several months.[151]

Non-drug treatment
If the obstruction is partial, dietary advice may help, e.g.:
• take small amounts of a liquid or sloppy diet throughout much or all of the day, e.g. sips of a nutritional supplement drink
• avoid carbonated drinks which will fill the stomach with gas.

If a gastrojejunostomy or a stent is not appropriate or possible, a venting procedure is occasionally necessary, e.g.:
• nasogastric tube
• gastrostomy.

Drug treatment
For more information, see PCF3.

Generally this is directed at reducing the volume of gastric ± salivary secretions:[152,153]
• antimuscarinics, e.g.:
  ▷ hyoscine butylbromide 60–120mg/24h by CSCI
  ▷ glycopyrronium 600–1,200microgram/24h by CSCI
• somatostatin analogues, e.g. octreotide 250–500microgram/24h by CSCI; used alone or in addition to antimuscarinics at some centres, but are expensive

- H_2-receptor antagonists reduce both acid and gastric secretions, PPIs acid secretion alone; both can be given PO (in partial obstruction) or by injection, e.g. ranitidine, omeprazole, but greater caution is required with parenteral use of the latter.

NAUSEA AND VOMITING

Nausea is an unpleasant feeling of the need to vomit, often accompanied by autonomic symptoms, e.g. pallor, cold sweat, salivation, tachycardia and diarrhoea.

Retching is rhythmic, laboured, spasmodic movements of the diaphragm and abdominal muscles, generally occurring in the presence of nausea and often culminating in vomiting.

Vomiting is the forceful expulsion of gastric contents through the mouth.

Pathogenesis

The pathogenesis of nausea and vomiting is complex.[154–157] Emetogenic signals converge on the brain stem where there is a functional (rather than an anatomical) 'emetic pattern generator', often called the vomiting centre. The pattern generator comprises a collection of motor nuclei including the nucleus ambiguus, ventral and dorsal respiratory groups, and the dorsal motor nucleus of the vagus.

Closely related is another functional entity called the chemoreceptor trigger zone, in the area postrema in the floor of the 4th ventricle.[158] Because the area postrema lies outside the blood–brain barrier, it is 'bathed' in the systemic circulation. Dopamine receptors in the area postrema are stimulated by high concentrations of emetogenic substances such as calcium ions, urea, morphine and digoxin. The area postrema also receives input from the vestibular apparatus and the vagus.

Emetogenic signals from the GI tract are conducted rostrally in vagal and splanchnic afferents. The nucleus tractus solitarius is the main central connection of the vagus and lies partly in the deeper layers of the area postrema. It contains the greatest concentration of $5HT_3$-receptors in the brain stem.

Nausea is an expression of autonomic stimulation, whereas retching and vomiting are mediated via somatic nerves. Nausea is associated with atony of the stomach, lower oesophageal sphincter and pylorus, which facilitates the retrograde expulsion of the contents of the upper GI tract. Vomiting involves the co-ordinated activities of the GI tract, diaphragm and abdominal muscles. The expulsive effort of vomiting is produced by the primary and accessory muscles of respiration, notably the abdominal muscles, which pump out the contents of a flaccid upper GI tract. The emetic pattern generator co-ordinates the process, receiving and integrating input from several sources (Figure 3.2).[159]

Causes

Although there are many causes of nausea and vomiting in advanced cancer (Box 3.R), four account for most cases (Figure 3.3).[147] Although in physically fit people constipation rarely causes vomiting, in advanced cancer it is probably a common contributory factor.

Evaluation

Diagnosis is based on probability and pattern recognition.[160] First, clarify whether it is vomiting, and not just expectoration or regurgitation. Next, as with pain (see Box 2.A, p.17), ascertain the temporal and other characteristics of the nausea and vomiting.

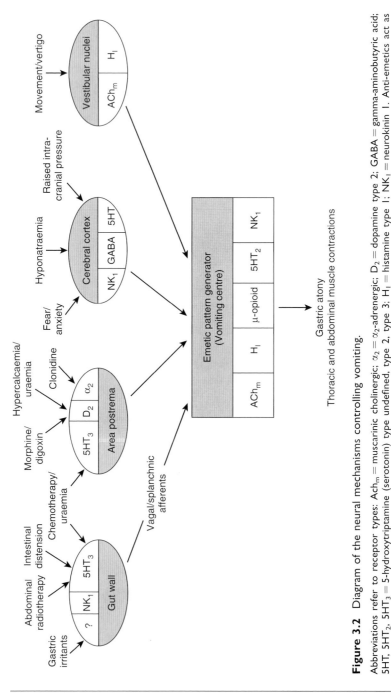

Figure 3.2 Diagram of the neural mechanisms controlling vomiting.

Abbreviations refer to receptor types: ACh_m = muscarinic cholinergic; α_2 = α_2-adrenergic; D_2 = dopamine type 2; GABA = gamma-aminobutyric acid; 5HT, $5HT_2$, $5HT_3$ = 5-hydroxytriptamine (serotonin) type undefined, type 2, type 3; H_1 = histamine type 1; NK_1 = neurokinin 1. Anti-emetics act as antagonists at these receptors, whereas the central anti-emetic effects of clonidine and opioids are agonistic.

Box 3.R Causes of nausea and vomiting in advanced cancer

Cancer
Gastroparesis (paraneoplastic visceral
    neuropathy)
Blood in stomach
Constipation
Faecal impaction
Bowel obstruction
Hepatomegaly
Gross ascites
Brain metastases
Raised intracranial pressure
Cough
Pain
Anxiety
Hypercalcaemia
Hyponatraemia
Renal failure

Debility
Constipation
Cough
Infection

Treatment
Chemotherapy
Radiotherapy
Drugs
    antibacterials
    aspirin
    carbamazepine
    corticosteroids
    digoxin
    iron
    irritant mucolytics
    lithium
    NSAIDs
    oestrogens
    opioids
    theophyllines

Concurrent
Functional dyspepsia
Peptic ulcer
Alcohol gastritis
Renal failure
Ketosis

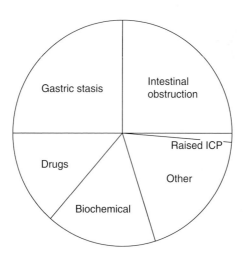

Figure 3.3 Common causes of nausea and vomiting in advanced cancer.[146]
ICP = intracranial pressure.

Again, as with pain, it is necessary to think simultaneously in several dimensions (see Figure 2.2, p.17):
- is the cancer the cause or something else?
- could a recently prescribed drug be the cause, e.g. an NSAID or an opioid?
- what is the likely underlying mechanism, e.g. delayed gastric emptying, hypercalcaemia, raised intracranial pressure?
- could there be a major psychological component?

Examine the abdomen. If constipation/faecal impaction is a possibility, do a rectal examination. If the cause is still not apparent:
- examine the CNS for signs of brain metastases or raised intracranial pressure
- consider checking the plasma concentrations of:
  - ▷ creatinine
  - ▷ calcium and albumin
  - ▷ any suspect drugs, e.g. carbamazepine, digoxin.

Generally, with attention to detail, it is possible to identify the most likely precipitating factor or main cause. It is this which dictates the management strategy.

Management
Correct the correctable
- cough → antitussive
- gastritis → reduction of gastric acid:
  - ▷ antacid
  - ▷ H_2-receptor antagonist
  - ▷ PPI
- consider stopping gastric irritant drugs:
  - ▷ antibacterial
  - ▷ corticosteroid
  - ▷ irritant mucolytic
  - ▷ NSAID
- constipation → laxatives (see p.111)
- raised intracranial pressure → corticosteroid
- hypercalcaemia → bisphosphonate (see p.215).

Non-drug treatment
- a calm environment away from the sight and smell of food, which can both be nauseating
- snacks, e.g. a few mouthfuls, and not big meals
- if the patient is the household cook, someone else may need to take on this role.

Drug treatment
For more information, see *PCF3*.
Guidelines: Nausea and vomiting in palliative care, p.106.

On the basis of putative sites of action it is possible to derive anti-emetics of choice for different situations (Table 3.6). The initial choice is often:
- metoclopramide (50%)
- haloperidol (25%).

Other commonly used drugs are:
- hyoscine butylbromide or glycopyrronium
- cyclizine
- levomepromazine.

Table 3.6 Classification of drugs used to control nausea and vomiting

Putative site of action	Class	Example
CNS		
Vomiting centre	Antimuscarinic	Hyoscine *hydrobromide*
	Antihistaminic antimuscarinic	Cyclizine[a]
	$5HT_2$-receptor antagonist	Levomepromazine, olanzapine
	NK_1-receptor antagonist	Aprepitant
Area postrema (chemoreceptor trigger zone)	D_2-receptor antagonist	Haloperidol, metoclopramide, domperidone, levomepromazine, prochlorperazine
	$5HT_3$-receptor antagonist	Granisetron, ondansetron
	NK_1-receptor antagonist	Aprepitant
Cerebral cortex	Benzodiazepine	Lorazepam
	Cannabinoid	Nabilone
	Corticosteroid	Dexamethasone
	NK_1-receptor antagonist	Aprepitant
GI tract		
Prokinetic	$5HT_4$-receptor agonist	Metoclopramide
	D_2-receptor antagonist	Metoclopramide, domperidone
	Motilin receptor agonist	Erythromycin
Antisecretory	Antimuscarinic	Hyoscine *butylbromide*, glycopyrronium
	Somatostatin analogue	Octreotide, lanreotide
Vagal $5HT_3$-receptor blockade	$5HT_3$-receptor antagonist	Granisetron, ondansetron
	NK_1-receptor antagonist	Aprepitant
Anti-inflammatory	Corticosteroid	Dexamethasone

a. phenothiazines also have H_1-receptor antagonistic and antimuscarinic properties.

$5HT_3$-receptor antagonists are of particular benefit in situations where there is a massive release of serotonin (5HT) from enterochromaffin cells or platelets, e.g. chemotherapy, abdominal radiation, obstruction (distension), renal failure.

Dexamethasone is often used as an 'add-on' anti-emetic when all else fails. It is also widely used for chemotherapeutic vomiting and may help in intestinal obstruction.[161,162] Dexamethasone possibly acts by reducing the permeability of the chemoreceptor trigger zone and of the blood-brain barrier to emetogenic substances, and by reducing the neuronal content of gamma-aminobutyric acid (GABA) in the brain stem. In obstruction, dexamethasone will also help by reducing inflammation at the site of the block, thereby increasing the lumen.

Guidelines: Management of nausea and vomiting

1 From the patient's history and physical examination, decide what is the most likely cause (or causes) of the nausea and vomiting. Take a blood sample if biochemical derangement is suspected.

2 Correct correctable causes/exacerbating factors, e.g. drugs, severe pain, cough, infection, hypercalcaemia. (*Remember: antibacterial treatment and correction of hypercalcaemia are not always appropriate in a dying patient.*) Anxiety exacerbates nausea and vomiting from any cause and may need specific treatment.

3 Prescribe the most appropriate anti-emetic stat, regularly and p.r.n. (see below). Give by SC injection or CSCI if continuous nausea or frequent vomiting.

Commonly used anti-emetics

Prokinetic anti-emetic (about 50% of prescriptions)
For gastritis, gastric stasis, functional bowel obstruction (peristaltic failure):
metoclopramide 10mg PO stat & q.d.s. or 10mg SC stat & 40–100mg/24h CSCI, & 10mg p.r.n. up to q.d.s.

Anti-emetic acting principally in chemoreceptor trigger zone (about 25% of prescriptions)
For most chemical causes of vomiting, e.g. morphine, hypercalcaemia, renal failure:
haloperidol 1.5–3mg PO stat & at bedtime, or 2.5–5mg SC stat & 2.5–10mg/24h CSCI, & 2.5–5mg p.r.n. up to q.d.s.
Metoclopramide also has a central action.

Antispasmodic and antisecretory anti-emetic
If bowel colic and/or need to reduce GI secretions:
hyoscine butylbromide 20mg SC stat, 60–120mg/24h CSCI (occasionally as high as 300mg/24h), & 20mg SC hourly p.r.n.

Anti-emetic acting principally in the vomiting centre
For raised intracranial pressure (with dexamethasone), motion sickness and in mechanical bowel obstruction:
cyclizine 50mg PO stat & b.d.–t.d.s. or 50mg SC stat & 150mg/24h CSCI, & 50mg p.r.n. up to b.d.

Broad-spectrum anti-emetic
For mechanical obstruction and when other anti-emetics are unsatisfactory:
levomepromazine 6–12.5mg PO/SC stat, at bedtime & p.r.n. up to q.d.s.

---

4 Initially, review anti-emetic dose each day; take note of p.r.n. use, and adjust the regular dose accordingly.

5 If little benefit despite upward titration of the dose, reconsider the likely cause(s), and review the route of administration and the choice of anti-emetic.

6 Some patients with nausea and vomiting need more than one anti-emetic.

continued

7 Prokinetics act through a cholinergic system which is competitively antagonized by antimuscarinics; concurrent use is best avoided.

8 A 5HT$_3$-receptor antagonist, e.g. granisetron 1–2mg stat & once daily, or ondansetron 8mg stat & b.d.–t.d.s PO/SC should be considered when there is a massive release of 5HT/serotonin from enterochromaffin cells or platelets, e.g. with chemotherapy, abdominal radiation, bowel distension, renal failure. Also consider with chemical causes of nausea and vomiting refractory to haloperidol and levomepromazine.

9 When all else fails, consider adding dexamethasone 8–16mg PO/SC stat & once daily for 7 days, and then review.

10 Continue the anti-emetic(s) unless the cause is self-limiting. Except in mechanical bowel obstruction (see below), consider changing to PO after 3 days of good control with CSCI.

More about bowel obstruction

11 Anti-emetics for inoperable bowel obstruction are best given by CSCI (for typical doses, see above), but levomepromazine can be given as a single SC dose at bedtime:

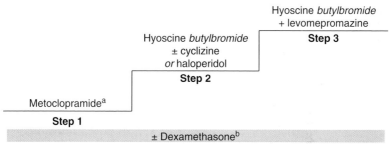

a. if colic, omit step 1
b. the place of dexamethasone in inoperable bowel obstruction is controversial.

12 If levomepromazine is too sedative, consider using olanzapine 1.25–2.5mg SC at bedtime instead; or revert to step 2 but give both cyclizine and haloperidol.

13 If hyoscine butylbromide is inadequate or to obtain more rapid relief, prescribe a somatostatin analogue (= an antisecretory agent without antispasmodic effects), e.g. octreotide 100microgram stat, 250–500microgram/24h CSCI, & 100microgram p.r.n. up to q.d.s.

BOWEL OBSTRUCTION

The focus here is on patients for whom available anticancer treatments have been exhausted. Obstruction of the alimentary tract can occur at any level. It is useful to think in terms of four syndromes, reflecting obstruction at high (proximal) or low (distal) levels:

- oesophageal, commonly the gastro-oesophageal junction (see oesophageal obstruction, p.90)
- gastric outlet and proximal small bowel
- distal small bowel
- large bowel.

Patients with disseminated intra-abdominal cancer, e.g. from colon or ovarian cancer, commonly have multiple sites of obstruction involving both small and large bowel. At each level, the obstruction can be functional (peristaltic failure) or mechanical (organic), or both. It can also be:

- partial or complete
- transient (acute) or persistent (chronic).

Some patients with partial bowel obstruction experience recurrent episodes which initially settle within a few days of resting the GI tract, i.e. nil by mouth and IV fluids. As the obstruction progresses, the frequency and duration of such episodes tend to increase, and eventually the obstruction may become complete and irreversible.

Causes
Bowel obstruction in advanced cancer may be caused by one or more of the following:
- the cancer itself
- past treatment, e.g. adhesions, post-radiation ischaemic fibrosis
- drugs, e.g. opioids, antimuscarinics
- debility, e.g. faecal impaction
- an unrelated benign condition, e.g. strangulated hernia.

Clinical features of intestinal obstruction
Abdominal pain associated with the underlying cancer is present in >90% of cases. Vomiting is invariable and intestinal colic is common in mechanical obstruction.[163] Distension is variable (more likely with distal obstruction) and bowel habit ranges from absolute constipation to diarrhoea secondary to bacterial liquefaction of retained faeces. Bowel sounds vary from absent in functional obstructions to hyperactive and audible (borborygmi) in some mechanical obstructions. Tinkling bowel sounds are uncommon.

In gastric outlet and proximal small bowel obstruction in particular, there may be vomiting with even small amounts of oral intake and retrosternal and epigastric discomfort from gastro-oesophageal reflux and gastric distension.

Evaluation
Evaluation is based on the patient's history and abdominal examination, together with information gleaned from surgical records, e.g. past laparotomy findings. Further investigations, e.g. abdominal radiograph, CT scan, endoscopy, can help to identify the level and nature of the obstruction and should be considered in all patients with an obstruction of unknown cause.

Management
High obstruction
Oesophageal obstruction
See p.90.

Pylorus/duodenum
Gastric cancer may obstruct the pylorus and pancreatic or duodenal cancer the duodenum (see gastric outflow obstruction, p.100). Functional obstruction of the stomach or duodenum can also occur, e.g. by cancer of the head of the pancreas causing impaired motility:
- try metoclopramide 60mg/24h by CSCI
- if beneficial, optimize the dose up to 100mg/24h
- if the vomiting is made worse, it indicates mechanical obstruction (see above); discontinue the metoclopramide
- occasionally, neostigmine is tried (see below)
- if none of the above is of benefit, discuss the use of a nasogastric tube or a venting gastrostomy with the patient.

With a high obstruction, it is generally not possible to stop vomiting completely with drugs; a practical goal is reducing the frequency to 2–3 times/24h.

Low obstruction
Distal small bowel/large bowel
Surgical intervention, e.g. palliative resection, bypass or colostomy, should be considered if the following criteria are all fulfilled:
- a single discrete mechanical obstruction seems likely, e.g. postoperative adhesions or an isolated cancer, e.g. carcinoid of the terminal ileum
- the patient's general performance status is good (i.e. independent and active) and disease is not widely disseminated
- the patient is willing to undergo surgery.

Surgical intervention is contra-indicated in each of the following circumstances:
- previous laparotomy findings preclude the prospect of a successful intervention
- diffuse intra-abdominal carcinomatosis as evidenced by diffuse palpable intra-abdominal tumours
- massive ascites which re-accumulates rapidly after paracentesis.[164]

Self-expanding metal stents ± subsequent surgery can be used for the relief of left-sided colorectal obstruction. Complications include perforation, incomplete stent expansion, pain, bleeding, stent migration and cancer overgrowth.[165,166]

In patients in whom an operative approach is contra-indicated, particularly when the obstruction is distal, the use of drugs can generally relieve symptoms without the need for a nasogastric tube and IV fluid. A series of drug changes over several days may be necessary before optimum relief is achieved. Management focuses primarily on the relief of pain and nausea and vomiting. An attempt can be made to reduce the obstruction, e.g. with corticosteroids, but evidence is limited.[167]

For the constant background cancer pain, morphine or diamorphine should be given regularly. If the patient is receiving parenteral metoclopramide or hyoscine butylbromide, the opioid can also be given by CSCI.

For those without colic and who are still passing flatus, a prokinetic is the initial drug of choice (see metoclopramide above). When metoclopramide is ineffective or poorly tolerated, neostigmine is occasionally used in some centres. A test dose of 1–2.5mg SC is given, and if tolerated, 5mg/24h CSCI up to a maximum of 20mg/24h. Such application is extrapolated from the use of neostigmine for acute colonic pseudo-obstruction.[168] For patients with severe colic, prokinetics are contra-indicated; instead, prescribe an antisecretory and antispasmodic drug, e.g. hyoscine butylbromide.

Bulk-forming, osmotic and stimulant laxatives should also be stopped. If constipation is a probable contributory factor, consider the use of a faecal softener, i.e. docusate sodium tablets 100–200mg b.d. $\pm$ a phosphate enema.

Corticosteroids benefit some patients with inoperable intestinal obstruction.[161] Because spontaneous resolution occurs in at least 1/3 of patients, it may be reasonable to treat the symptoms as suggested above and then, after 5–7 days, if the obstruction has not settled, a trial of corticosteroid for 3 days should be considered, e.g.:
• dexamethasone 10mg SC
• methylprednisolone 40mg IV over 1h.[162]

If there is improvement, either continue with the corticosteroid at a lower dose PO or stop and review the need for long-term treatment.

Corticosteroids probably act by reducing local oedema and improving the patency of the bowel lumen. They may also reduce pressure on intestinal nerves, thereby correcting neural dysfunction (and the associated functional obstruction). These actions are distinct from the specific anti-emetic effect of corticosteroids.[169]

In small bowel obstruction caused by adhesions, water-soluble contrast medium (e.g. Gastrografin® 100mL PO or via a nasogastric tube) is used to diagnose patients with a partial obstruction, suitable for a non-surgical approach as opposed to a complete obstruction which requires surgery. In the former, contrast will reach the caecum after 4–24h of administration (viewed by abdominal radiograph). In addition, some suggest that the contrast has a therapeutic effect, helping to clear a 'backlog' of intestinal contents across a narrowed lumen as a result of:
• the high osmolality promoting a shift of fluid into the lumen which leads to softening/dilution of the lumen contents, easing passage, together with an increase in the pressure gradient across the obstruction
• a reduction in bowel wall oedema
• an increase in intestinal motility.

In a small uncontrolled series of patients with cancer and bowel obstruction, benefit was reported with water-soluble contrast medium (e.g. amidotrizoato 50mL PO) given as part of a combined approach with IV metoclopramide, octreotide and dexamethasone.[170] However, a systematic review concluded that Gastrografin® improves surgical decision-making and reduces length of hospital stay but does not cause resolution of small bowel obstruction.[171] Undesirable effects of Gastrografin® include colic and severe pneumonia if aspirated. Thus, its administration is best reserved for patients with an empty stomach who are no longer vomiting (a nasogastric tube is one way to ensure this).

A persistent complete inoperable obstruction is a challenging prospect. Occasionally, two classes of drugs may be necessary, namely:
• somatostatin analogues, e.g. octreotide
• 5HT$_3$-receptor antagonists, e.g. granisetron, ondansetron, tropisetron.

Octreotide has an antisecretory effect throughout the alimentary tract. It is relatively expensive but is the preferred antisecretory drug at some centres. Octreotide is generally given by CSCI; typical doses are 250–500microgram/24h, sometimes more. In a double-blind RCT, hyoscine butylbromide (60–80mg/24h) and octreotide (600–800microgram/24h) provided equivalent relief of nausea and vomiting after 6 days.[172] However, benefit is achieved more quickly with octreotide (24h), compared with hyoscine butylbromide (72h).[153] A reduction in intestinal contents reduces distension and the likelihood of colic and vomiting. Some centres convert to the long-acting lanreotide which is given IM every 2 weeks; each injection costs over £500.

Generally, consider using octreotide when hyoscine butylbromide 200mg by CSCI fails to relieve the vomiting. However, it is not antispasmodic and if colic persists, it should be used concurrently with hyoscine butylbromide (or glycopyrronium).

Because raised intraluminal pressure results in the release of 5HT (serotonin) from the enterochromaffin cells in the bowel wall, some patients benefit from a 5HT$_3$-receptor antagonist. *A venting gastrostomy is rarely necessary for symptom relief in advanced cancer.*[173]

Inoperable patients managed by drug therapy should be encouraged to drink and eat small amounts of their favourite beverages and food. Some patients find that they can manage food best in the morning.

Antimuscarinics and diminished fluid intake often result in a dry mouth and thirst. These are generally relieved by conscientious mouth care. A few mL of fluid every 30min, possibly administered as a small ice cube, often brings relief. *IV hydration is rarely needed.*

CONSTIPATION

Constipation is common in advanced cancer, affecting 1/2 of palliative inpatients, and is rated severe by 1/6.[174,175] It is defined as the passage of hard faeces infrequently and with difficulty.[176] It is not possible to be more precise about frequency, although some would diagnose constipation if a patient defaecated twice or less per week, regardless of faecal consistency and difficulty in defaecation.[177] Increasing age, diminished food and fibre intake, lack of exercise and drugs are all contributory (Box 3.S).[178,179]

Box 3.S   Causes of constipation in advanced cancer

Cancer
Hypercalcaemia
Paraneoplastic visceral neuropathy
Bowel obstruction
Spinal cord compression

Drugs
Opioids
NSAIDs
Antimuscarinics
 antihistaminic anti-emetics
 phenothiazines
 TCAs
5HT$_3$-receptor antagonists
Vincristine
Diuretics
 dehydration
 hypokalaemia
Calcium or iron supplements

Debility
Inactivity
Poor nutrition
 decreased intake
 low residue diet
Poor fluid intake
Dehydration
 vomiting
 polyuria
 fever
Weakness
Inability to respond to an urge to
 defaecate because unable to get to
 a toilet unaided

However, some opioids are less constipating than equi-analgesic doses of morphine:

- buprenorphine
- fentanyl[180]
- methadone[181]
- tramadol.[182]

Constipation may be asymptomatic, but in some patients it can lead to:

- anorexia, nausea, vomiting, bowel obstruction
- abdominal distension, discomfort, pain
- rectal pain (constant or spasmodic)
- urinary dysfunction, e.g. hesitancy, retention, overflow incontinence
- rectal discharge, faecal leakage, overflow diarrhoea
- diminished sense of wellbeing, delirium.

Evaluation

Enquiring about the patient's normal (pre-morbid) bowel habit should be regarded as mandatory in palliative care, together with enquiry about present status. Even if a patient says that 'they're all right', it is wise to ask additional questions, such as:

'When did you last open your bowels?'

'And the time before that?'

'How many times have you opened your bowels in the last week?'

'Is it easy to pass your motions, or are they hard?'

'How big are the motions? Are they like rabbit pellets, or are they bigger?'

'Is the bulk normal, or are they a bit like your little finger?'

'Are you taking any medication for your bowels? When did you start taking it?'

'Have you taken any [laxative] suppositories?'

'Do you have to chip it out with your finger?'.

Abdominal examination may reveal hard faecal masses in the descending colon, possibly in the transverse colon, and occasionally in the ascending colon. An awareness that constipation can cause caecal distension and tenderness, or a more classical picture of bowel obstruction is important if the correct differential diagnosis is to be made.

Rectal examination can be done selectively, if indicated by the history and the abdominal examination. However, all patients with an anal discharge (see p.126), faecal leakage or diarrhoea (see p.120) should automatically have a digital rectal examination.

Sometimes it is not clear whether the primary disorder is obstruction with secondary constipation or primary constipation with secondary obstruction. It may be necessary to come to a 'working diagnosis' and treat accordingly; changing one's approach if the initial interventions lead to deterioration rather than relief.

Management

For most patients constipation responds to relatively simple measures such as laxatives. However, in a small proportion of patients constipation remains difficult to manage.

General measures
- when possible stop or reduce the dose of constipating drugs
- mobilize the patient if possible
- a prompt response to the patient's request for a commode or for help to get to the toilet
- use of a commode rather than a bedpan
- advise a position which increases abdominal pressure and aids defaecation:
  ▷ place feet on a foot stool to elevate the knees above the hips
  ▷ lean forward keeping the spine straight with elbows rested on the knees
- raise the toilet seat and install hand rails in the patient's home to increase toilet independence.

Diet
In patients well enough to tolerate an increased intake of food:
- add bran to diet
- increase fluid intake (at least 1.5L/24h, i.e. about 8 cupfuls)
- encourage fruit juices.

Drug treatment
For more information, see PCF3.
Guidelines: Opioid-induced constipation, p.117.

Because of anorexia and physical debility, laxatives are generally the mainstay of treatment of constipation in advanced cancer. Knowledge of the different classes of laxatives permits rational choices to be made and rational combinations to be used (Box 3.T).

Box 3.T Classification of commonly used bulking agents and laxatives

Bulk-forming drugs (fibre)
Ispaghula husk (e.g. Fybogel, Regulan)
Methylcellulose (Celevac)
Sterculia (e.g. Normacol)

Lubricants
Liquid paraffin/mineral oil[a]

Surface-wetting agents
Docusate sodium[a]
Poloxamer

Osmotic laxatives
Lactulose syrup
Macrogols/polyethylene glycols
 (Movicol®, Idrolax®)
Liquid paraffin and magnesium
 hydroxide emulsion BP
Magnesium hydroxide suspension
 (Milk of Magnesia)®
Magnesium sulphate (Epsom Salts®)

Contact (stimulant) laxatives
Bisacodyl
Dantron
Senna
Sodium picosulfate

---

a. docusate enhances the absorption of liquid paraffin; products containing both these substances are prohibited in some countries.

Surface wetting agents are effectively faecal softeners. Osmotic laxatives act primarily on the small bowel ('small bowel flushers'), whereas contact (stimulant) laxatives act either exclusively on the large intestine or on both small and large intestines (see below).

The best starting point varies from patient to patient. Sometimes it is appropriate to begin and continue with rectal measures or, with an inoperable partial bowel obstruction, use only a faecal softener.

About 90% of patients receiving morphine require a laxative.[178] Opioids induce constipation principally by enhancing intestinal ring contractions. This results in hypersegmentation, which impedes peristalsis. A contact (stimulant) laxative relaxes ring contractions, and is thus the logical management option (Figure 3.4).

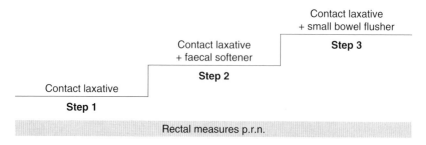

Figure 3.4 A treatment ladder with safety net (rectal measures) for opioid-induced constipation. Doses should be titrated upwards as necessary (see Guidelines, p.117). Many centres begin on Step 2.

Contact (stimulant) laxatives
Functionally, contact (stimulant) laxatives can be divided into two groups:
• those which act on both the small and large intestines, e.g. bisacodyl, dantron
• those which act only on the large intestine, e.g. senna, sodium picosulfate.

Given that opioids prolong transit times throughout the whole of the GI tract, there could be an advantage in prescribing dantron or bisacodyl rather than senna or sodium picosulfate. However, there is no RCT evidence to support such a view.

Patients receiving opioid analgesics often need a higher dose of a contact laxative than that recommended by the manufacturers. Many benefit from the addition of a faecal softener. In the UK, many palliative care units use co-danthrusate or co-danthramer, i.e. a combination of a contact laxative (dantron) and a faecal softener (docusate or poloxamer). Because of concern about possible carcinogenicity,[183,184] the licence for dantron-containing laxatives in the UK is now restricted to terminally ill patients.

Although the laxative requirement increases as the dose of morphine is increased in any given individual, there is no correlation between the dose of morphine and the effective dose of laxatives in patients as a whole.[185,186] Even so, knowledge of modal doses is helpful in targeting an appropriate starting dose:
• the modal dose of co-danthrusate for patients not taking morphine is 1–2 capsules at bedtime
• the modal dose of co-danthrusate for patients taking morphine is 2 capsules b.d.

Dantron-containing laxatives should be avoided in patients with persistent faecal leakage or incontinence because of the high risk of sustaining a peri-anal/perineal dantron skin burn (a characteristic sharply defined erythematous area).

Osmotic laxatives
These include various magnesium salts, non-absorbable carbohydrates, and the macrogols. All have a potential role in the management of constipation in palliative care

patients, and are sometimes used as sole agents. However, many patients prescribed lactulose for opioid-induced constipation remain constipated, probably because of a failure to titrate the dose upwards. Examination may reveal palpable 'faecal porridge' in the caecum but 'faecal rock cakes' in the descending colon, thus emphasizing the importance of reversing colonic hypersegmentation with a contact laxative.

On the other hand, the need for digital disimpaction of the rectum can be reduced by using macrogols.[187,188] These are supplied in sachets of powder which needs to be dispersed in water. For example, each sachet of macrogol 3350 (Movicol®) is taken in 125mL of water. The recommended dose is 8 sachets (1L) on day 1 and repeat on day 2 if necessary. However, most patients do not need a full second day's dose.

If using macrogols as the primary laxative, the dose ranges between 1–3 sachets/day. Although it is more expensive than lactulose, it is more effective and better tolerated.[189] Intestinal bacteria metabolize lactulose (but not macrogols) to produce gas which can lead to an unpleasant abdominal distension and flatus.

Bulk-forming drugs
Bulk-forming drugs have little to offer in the management of opioid-induced constipation, and may make matters worse by entrapping increased faecal bulk throughout a hypersegmented intestine, and possibly causing a symptomatic functional obstruction.

Opioid antagonists
SC methylnaltrexone, a peripherally-acting quaternary opioid antagonist, is marketed for use in patients with 'advanced illness' and opioid-induced constipation despite usual laxative therapy. About 50% of patients given methylnaltrexone have a bowel action <4h after a dose, without loss of analgesia or the development of opioid withdrawal symptoms.[190,191] Common undesirable effects include abdominal pain, diarrhoea, flatulence, and nausea.

Because constipation in advanced disease is generally multifactorial in origin,[178,179] methylnaltrexone is likely to augment rather than replace laxatives. Like most newly marketed drugs, methylnaltrexone is relatively expensive (£21 per 12mg vial). The manufacturer recommends:
- for patients weighing 38–61kg, start with 8mg on alternate days
- for patients weighing 62–114kg, start with 12mg on alternate days
- if outside this range, give 150microgram/kg on alternate days
- the interval between administrations can be varied, either extended or reduced, but not more than once daily.

The dose should be reduced in severe renal impairment (see p.118). Methylnaltrexone is contra-indicated in cases of known or suspected obstruction.

Prokinetics
Neostigmine has been successfully used to treat constipation failing to respond to usual measures:
- start with a 250microgram SC test dose
- if tolerated, administer b.d.–t.d.s.
- adjust dose upwards in 250microgram steps until a response is achieved
- median dose in eight patients was 500microgram, range 250–1,250microgram; two patients required only a single dose.[174]

For its use in functional bowel obstruction, see p.109.

Herbal preparations
There are many laxatives available OTC, including herbal remedies. For example, an Ayurvedic liquid herbal preparation *Misrakasneham*, contains 21 herbs, plus castor oil,

ghee and milk. It is as effective as senna 15–20mg, has a tolerable taste, requires only a small volume to be taken daily (2.5–10mL), and (in India) is cheaper.[192] Fresh baker's yeast has also been used to good effect.[192]

Rectal measures
One third of patients receiving morphine continue to need rectal measures either regularly or intermittently despite oral laxatives.[185,193] These comprise laxative suppositories, enemas and digital evacuation. Sometimes these measures are elective, e.g. in paraplegics and in the very old and debilitated (Box 3.U).

Suppositories take about 30min to dissolve after insertion. In patients who defaecate within 5min of the insertion of a bisacodyl suppository, the mechanism of action is ano-rectal stimulation and not pharmacological. A response after 20–30min reflects dissolution of the suppository, subsequent hydrolysis to the active metabolite, and a local action on the rectal musculature.

In the UK, most patients needing laxative suppositories receive both glycerol and bisacodyl (Box 3.U). Bisacodyl may result in some delayed rectal discharge or faecal incontinence. Carbalax® is used by some patients with chronic neurological dysfunction, e.g. paraplegia. It is in effect a gas enema and is safer than a large-volume phosphate enema.[194]

Osmotic micro-enemas contain mainly sodium citrate and sodium lauryl sulpho-acetate. The latter is a wetting agent (cf. docusate) whereas sodium citrate draws fluid into the bowel by osmosis, an action enhanced by sorbitol.

Box 3.U Rectal measures for the relief of constipation or faecal impaction

Suppositories
Glycerol 4g, has a hygroscopic and lubricant action. Also claimed to be a rectal stimulant but this is unsubstantiated.

Bisacodyl 10mg, after hydrolysis by enteric enzymes, stimulates propulsive activity.[195]

Carbalax®, a mixture of sodium bicarbonate and sodium phosphate which reacts in the rectum, releasing 200mL of carbon dioxide and stimulating evacuation by rectal distension.

Enemas
Surface-wetting micro-enemas, containing 90–120mg of docusate sodium/5mL.

Lubricant enema, arachis/peanut oil (130mL), generally instilled and left overnight before giving stimulant laxative suppository or other enema.

Osmotic micro-enemas, small volume (5mL) containing sodium citrate, sodium lauryl sulpho-acetate, glycerol and sorbitol.

Osmotic standard enemas, large volume (120–130mL) phosphate enemas.

Digital evacuation of faeces may occasionally be required:
- when other approaches have failed
- in faecal impaction
- in neurogenic bowel dysfunction, e.g. spinal cord injury (see p.272).

Guidelines: Opioid-induced constipation

Although some opioids are less constipating than morphine (e.g. buprenorphine, fentanyl, methadone, tramadol), most patients taking an opioid need a laxative. Thus, as a general rule, all patients prescribed an opioid should also be prescribed a laxative, with the aim of achieving a regular bowel action without straining every 1–3 days.

1 Ask about the patient's past (pre-morbid) and present bowel habit and use of laxatives; record the date of last bowel action.

2 Palpate for faecal masses in the line of the colon; examine the rectum digitally if the bowels have not been open for > 3 days or if the patient reports rectal discomfort or has diarrhoea suggestive of faecal impaction with overflow.

3 For inpatients, keep a daily record of bowel actions.

4 Encourage fluids generally, and fruit juice and fruit specifically.

5 When an opioid is prescribed, prescribe co-danthramer *strong* or co-danthrusate:

	Co-danthramer strong capsules	Co-danthramer strong suspension	Co-danthrusate capsules	Co-danthrusate suspension
Dantron	37.5mg/capsule	75mg/5ml	50mg/capsule	50mg/5ml
Start with:				
• prophylactic	1 at bedtime	2.5ml at bedtime	1 at bedtime	5ml at bedtime
• if constipated	2 at bedtime	5ml at bedtime	2 at bedtime	10ml at bedtime
If necessary, adjust every 2–3 days up to:	3 t.d.s.	10ml b.d. *or* 20ml at bedtime	3 b.d.	15ml b.d.
Total daily dose	337.5mg	300mg	300mg	300mg

6 It is sometimes appropriate to optimize a patient's existing laxative regimen, rather than automatically change to co-danthramer.

7 During dose titration and subsequently, if > 3 days since last bowel action, give suppositories, e.g. bisacodyl 10mg and glycerol 4g, or a micro-enema. If these are ineffective, administer a phosphate enema and possibly repeat the next day.

8 If co-danthramer/co-danthrusate causes intestinal colic, divide the total daily dose into smaller more frequent doses, e.g. change from co-danthramer strong 2 capsules b.d. to 1 capsule q.d.s. Alternatively, change to an osmotic laxative, e.g. macrogol 3350 (Movicol®) or macrogol 4000 (Idrolax®) 1–2 sachets each morning.

continued

9 If the maximum dose of co-danthramer/co-danthrusate is ineffective
- halve the dose and add an osmotic laxative, e.g macrogol 3350 (Movicol®) or macrogol 4000 (Idrolax®) 1 sachet each morning, and titrate as necessary or
- prescribe SC methylnaltrexone 8–12mg alternate days–once daily, according to the manufacturer's recommendations (see below).

10 An osmotic laxative, e.g. a macrogol, may be preferable in patients with a history of colic with colonic stimulants, e.g. bisacodyl, dantron, senna.

11 In patients with urinary or faecal incontinence, dantron-containing laxatives should be used with caution because of the risk of a contact skin burn in the perineum and surrounding areas.

Methylnaltrexone

- SC injection for use in patients with 'advanced illness' and opioid-induced constipation despite treatment with laxatives
- 50% of patients given methylnaltrexone have a bowel action within 4 hours, without loss of analgesia or the development of opioid withdrawal symptoms
- dose recommendations:
  - for patients weighing 38–61kg, start with 8mg on alternate days
  - for patients weighing 62–114kg, start with 12mg on alternate days
  - if outside this range, give 0.15mg/kg on alternate days
  - the interval between administrations can be varied, either extended or reduced, but not more than once daily
- in severe renal impairment (creatinine clearance <30mL/min), the dose should be reduced:
  - for patients weighing 62–114kg, reduce to 8mg
  - outside this range, reduce to *75microgram/kg*, rounding up the dose volume to the nearest 0.1mL
- methylnaltrexone is contra-indicated in cases of known or suspected GI obstruction
- common undesirable effects include abdominal pain, diarrhoea, flatulence, and nausea
- because constipation in advanced disease is generally multifactorial in origin, methylnaltrexone is likely to augment rather than replace laxatives
- methylnaltrexone is relatively expensive (£21 per 12mg vial).

Monitoring

If pain is regarded as the '5th vital sign', defaecation must surely count as the 6th. Its importance is reflected in the practice in many palliative care services of having 'bowel charts' to record information about patients' evacuations in greater detail than is possible on standard UK charts for vital signs, including details of rectal measures. As always, attention to detail brings it own rewards.

FAECAL IMPACTION

Faecal impaction means the lodging of faeces in the rectum (90%) or in the colon, occasionally as far back as the caecum.

Pathogenesis

Incomplete evacuation leads to accumulation of faeces in the rectum. The faeces become very firm because fluid is absorbed from them while they remain in contact with the bowel mucosa. Additional faecal material increases the size of the mass so that it becomes physically impossible for it to be evacuated. Bacterial liquefaction of more proximal faeces may result in overflow diarrhoea and faecal leakage.

Sometimes a soft impaction occurs. This is more likely if the impaction occurs despite the use of a bulk-forming drug or a faecal softener.

Causes

The causes of faecal impaction are similar to those of constipation (Box 3.V).

Box 3.V Causes of faecal impaction in advanced cancer	
Cancer Functional or partial mechanical bowel obstruction	**Debility** Weakness Immobility Cognitive impairment
Drugs Aluminium antacids Antimuscarinics Barium Opioids	**Concurrent** Anal stricture Anal fissure

Clinical features

The patient complains of constipation or of the frequent passage of small quantities of fluid faeces together with some or all of the following:
- anal discharge
- spasmodic rectal pain; may be agonizing
- abdominal colic
- abdominal distension
- delayed gastric emptying
- nausea and vomiting.

A debilitated or elderly patient may develop an agitated delirium. Rarely there may be bleeding or perforation as a result of pressure necrosis.[196]

Evaluation

A high level of suspicion is helpful in the diagnosis of faecal impaction and overflow. The patient may indicate that they have become progressively more constipated but then, 'They suddenly became loose. The trouble is I can't tell when my bowels are going to act, sometimes I have no warning'.

Abdominal examination frequently reveals hard faecal material in the descending and sigmoid colon; and the transverse and ascending colon may also be involved. A dilated caecum may also be noted. Although rectal examination generally confirms the presence of a large faecal mass, an empty rectum cannot rule out a high impaction. When doubt exists, possibly because the abdominal palpation is hard to interpret, an abdominal radiograph helps to confirm the presence and extent of any faecal retention.

Management
This partly depends on the degree of distress the impaction is causing the patient. For example, if someone is experiencing agonizing episodes of rectal pain and/or abdominal colic, has a distended anus with protruding hard faeces and faecal leakage, the best initial option could be IV midazolam sedation and digital disimpaction, i.e. disrupt the faecal mass by finger manipulation and remove piecemeal. However, in less extreme situations, laxatives (PO, PR, or both) are more appropriate.

Soft faeces
- bisacodyl 10–20mg PR once daily until there is no response
- contact with the rectal mucosa is essential for absorption
- give PO if mucosal contact impossible.

Hard faeces
Macrogols reduce the need for digital disimpaction (for more information, see PCF3).[187,188] Alternative approaches include:
- glycerol and bisacodyl suppositories, or osmotic enemas
- overnight retention enema of arachis oil (130mL) followed by a high phosphate enema the next day using a 45cm plastic catheter attached to the enema-giving set
- overnight retention enema of docusate sodium (300mg in 100mL, i.e. diluted oral syrup) or a proprietary docusate sodium micro-enema (contains 90–120mg) followed by a high phosphate enema the next day as above.

In all cases, steps must subsequently be taken to prevent a recurrence by establishing regular bowel evacuations.

DIARRHOEA

Diarrhoea is an increase in the frequency of defaecation and/or fluidity of the faeces. Sometimes it is defined as the passage of more than three unformed stools in 24h.[197] It is generally associated with an increase in faecal water and electrolyte excretion, and sometimes the passage of blood and pus. If severe, diarrhoea may manifest as faecal incontinence.

Causes
There are many potential causes (Box 3.W) but the most common are:
- laxative overdose
- faecal impaction with overflow
- partial bowel obstruction.[193]

Other relatively common causes include:
- gastro-enteritis, mainly viral
- radiation enteritis

- drugs (Box 3.X)
- steatorrhoea.

Steatorrhoea is excess fat in faeces (>20g/24h). Generally, the faeces are pale in colour, bulky and float making them difficult to flush away. Causes of steatorrhoea include:
- pancreatic cancer
- chronic pancreatitis
- obstructive jaundice
- post-gastrectomy
- blind loop syndrome
- bowel ischaemia.

Radiation enteritis results from mucosal damage, prostaglandin release and bile salt malabsorption, leading to:
- diarrhoea
- abdominal pain, including colic
- rectal urgency
- tenesmus
- nausea and vomiting
- weight loss
- bleeding (occasionally).

Generally, the onset is within 6 weeks of therapy and it settles after 2–6 months. Occasionally, the onset is months or years after exposure because of progressive radiation-induced endarteritis resulting in bowel ischaemia. This can result in ulceration, fibrosis and stricture or fistula formation. There may be associated malabsoption and bacterial overgrowth.[197]

Box 3.W   Causes of diarrhoea in advanced cancer ('*LOOSED*')

Length of bowel (shortened)
Bowel resection, colostomy
Ileostomy, ileocolic fistula

Overflow
Faecal impaction (see p.119)
Bowel obstruction (see p.108)

Osmotic
Non-absorbable sugars, e.g. lactulose, sorbitol-containing solutions
Enteral feeds
Magnesium salts

Enhanced motility
Diet (see Box 3.Z, p.124)
Constitutional
Anxiety
Irritable bowel syndrome
Hyperthyroidism
Steatorrhoea
Carcinoid syndrome
Islet cell tumours, e.g. VIPoma
Visceral neuropathy, e.g. diabetic, paraneoplastic
Coeliac plexus block[199]
Lumbar sympathectomy

Drugs (see Box 3.X)

Secretory
Infective, e.g. gastro-enteritis, *C. difficle* diarrhoea, cholera, bacterial overgrowth
Injury, e.g. radiotherapy, chemotherapy, ulcerative colitis
Cholegenic

Box 3.X   Drug-induced diarrhoea in advanced cancer

Common	**Occasional**	**Chemotherapy**
Antacids	Anticholinesterases	Capecitabine
magnesium salts	neostigmine	Cytarabine
Antibacterials, e.g.	Caffeine	Docetaxel
erythromycin	Hypoglycaemics	Doxorubicin
penicillins	sulphonylureas, e.g.	Etoposide
sulphonamides	chlorpropamide	5-FU
tetracyclines	biguanides, e.g.	Irinotecan
Iron	metformin	Methotrexate
Laxatives	NSAIDs	Mitomycin
Mefenamic acid	Oestrogens	Oxaliplatin
Misoprostol	diethylstilboestrol	
SSRIs	>3mg/day	**Targeted cancer drugs**
	Sorbitol[a]	Tyrosine kinase
	Theophylline	inhibitors, e.g.
		erlotinib
		gefitinib
		Overflow[b]
		Aluminium hydroxide
		Antimuscarinics
		Opioids

a. a non-absorbable disaccharide used as a sweetener in 'sugar-free' liquid medicines
b. all drugs which predispose to constipation may lead to overflow diarrhoea.

Diarrhoea, along with fever, abdominal pain, nausea and vomiting, is also a feature of neutropenic enterocolitis (synonyms: necrotizing enterocolitis or typhlitis), a life-threatening complication of chemotherapy, particularly with high-dose myelo-ablative regimens. There is bacterial or fungal infection of the bowel wall associated with necrosis. Urgent treatment is required to avoid death from sepsis or perforation.[197]

Diarrhoea is common in AIDS; pathogens are identifiable in about 1/2 the cases.[198]

Clostridium difficile diarrhoea
This is a complication of antibacterial therapy, particularly broad-spectrum antibacterials. It is caused by colonization of the bowel by C. difficile and the production of toxins A and B which cause the mucosal damage. Failure to mount an immune response is associated with colonization and toxin production. Risk factors include:
- increasing age
- severe underlying disease
- immunosuppression
- treatment in an intensive care unit
- long inpatient stay in hospital
- long duration of causal antibacterial treatment
- multiple antibacterials
- non-surgical GI procedures
- nasogastric tube
- anti-ulcer medication.[200]

Symptoms generally begin within 1 week of starting antibacterial therapy or shortly after stopping, but may occur up to 1 month later (Box 3.Y). A pseudomembranous colitis is present in severe cases, with sloughing of the inflamed colonic epithelium, manifesting as foul-smelling diarrhoea mingled with mucus and blood. *C. difficile* diarrhoea has a mortality of up to 25% in elderly frail patients.[201]

Box 3.Y *Clostridium difficile* diarrhoea

Causal antibacterials[202]
Most prevalent
Ampicillin
Amoxicillin   *Highest incidence*
Cephalosporins   Clindamycin
Ciprofloxacin   Lincomycin
Clarithromycin
Erythromycin

Clinical features
Watery diarrhoea + mucus ± blood
Abdominal pain and tenderness
Fever and malaise
± Dehydration and delirium

Cholegenic diarrhoea
Active absorption of bile acids occurs mainly in the distal ileum. Non-absorbed bile acids are metabolized in the colon by bacterial enzymes to form unconjugated α-dihydroxy bile acids which stimulate fluid and electrolyte secretion. This results in cholegenic diarrhoea which is often explosive and watery, and poorly responsive to standard antidiarrhoeals. Cholegenic diarrhoea is uncommon in cancer patients but may occur following resection:
- of > 100cm of ileum, leading to bile salt (and disaccharide) malabsorption, *or*
- the ileocaecal valve, allowing bacterial invasion of the small intestine with consequential severe diarrhoea; this responds to metronidazole.

Evaluation
A carefully elicited history and clinical examination is often sufficient to determine the most likely cause of diarrhoea. A careful review of medication is important, and will generally indicate whether too much laxative is the cause. A high level of suspicion in high-risk patients who develop diarrhoea (> 300mL of liquid faeces in 24h) is needed to diagnose *C. difficile* diarrhoea. If appropriate, consider:
- blood tests for urea and electrolytes (hypokalaemia and renal failure)
- abdominal radiograph (faecal impaction, obstruction)
- laboratory detection of faecal *C. difficile* toxin. Absence of toxin in a single stool sample does not exclude infection. If in doubt, test three samples of faeces at 12h intervals. Endoscopy and rectal biopsy are of value, although a trial of therapy is more practical
- faecal microscopy and culture; possibly indicated if the history and examination do not point to a likely cause and diarrhoea occurring within 3 days of inpatient admission.[203]

Management
Prevention of C. difficile diarrhoea
Adhere to local guidelines concerning environmental measures and antibacterial prescribing.

Correct the correctable
- review diet, and modify if indicated (Box 3.Z). Stop alcohol and high-osmolar dietary supplements. If diarrhoea is chemotherapy-induced, stop all lactose-containing products[204]
- review medication, including laxatives, and modify if indicated. If diarrhoea is due to laxative overdose, reduce laxative dose but do not prescribe anti-diarrhoeal drug
- consider antibacterial treatment if infective cause or if bacterial overgrowth seems likely
- if patient has C. difficile diarrhoea, stop causal antibacterial if possible, and treat with metronidazole, vancomycin or other recommended antibacterial according to local guidelines.[205]

Box 3.Z Laxative foods	
Beans	Raw fruit (fresh or dried)
Coleslaw	Sauerkraut
Greens	Spicy foods
Lentils	Wholegrain cereals
Nuts	Wholemeal foods
Onions	

Non-drug treatment
If diarrhoea is severe or persistent, it is important to prevent dehydration. Options include an oral rehydration solution, e.g. Dioralyte® 200–400mL or, if unavailable, flat Coke or lemonade after each loose motion. If the patient is nauseated, vomiting or dehydrated, parenteral rehydration may be necessary.

Occasionally, if chronic diarrhoea is unresponsive to dietary and appropriate drug treatment (see below) and is causing faecal incontinence, an anal plug may be helpful (Conveen®, UK). This is a small foam tampon, available in two sizes (small and large), with a long string for easy removal. When inserted, it is the size of a large suppository but expands over 30sec after contact with moisture and forms a self-retaining plug. It can be left in place for up to 12h and is removed by pulling on its cloth tail. However, it must be removed (and discarded) before defaecation, and subsequently replaced by a new one. The plug is particularly useful if attending a special occasion and, in fitter patients, can be used when swimming.

Drug treatment
For more information, see PCF3.

After excluding faecal impaction, obstruction and colitis (ulcerative, infective or antibacterial-related), and if there is no specific treatment (Box 3.AA), prescribe a non-specific antidiarrhoeal drug.

> **Box 3.AA** Drugs for treating diarrhoea
>
> | **Specific treatment** | **Non-specific treatment** |
> |---|---|
> | Steatorrhoea | Opioids |
> | pancreatin supplements | codeine |
> | Cholegenic diarrhoea | diphenoxylate |
> | colestyramine (an anion exchange | loperamide |
> | resin) | morphine |
> | *C. difficile* diarrhoea | Absorbants |
> | metronidazole | hydrophilic bulking agents |
> | vancomycin | pectin |
> | Ulcerative colitis | Adsorbants |
> | corticosteroids | activated charcoal |
> | mesalazine | chalk |
> | sulfasalazine | kaolin |
> | Infection | Mucosal PG inhibitors |
> | appropriate antibacterial | bismuth subsalicylate |
> | | NSAIDs[206] |
> | | Somatostatin analogues |
> | | octreotide |

Opioids are generally used as they are more potent and have a faster onset of action. The following regimens are approximately equivalent:

- loperamide 2mg b.d
- diphenoxylate 2.5mg (in Lomotil®) q.d.s.
- codeine phosphate 60mg t.d.s.–q.d.s.

Loperamide is about 3 times more potent than diphenoxylate and 50 times more potent than codeine. It is longer acting and generally needs to be given only b.d. Loperamide 4mg is the normal initial dose for acute diarrhoea, followed by 2mg after each loose bowel action. It is uncommon to need more than 16mg/24h.[207] Kaolin and morphine mixture BP is an alternative traditional remedy.

Mild–moderate radiation enteritis and mild–moderate chemotherapy-induced diarrhoea generally responds adequately to opioids, but in severe cases (particularly if complicated by nausea/vomiting, dehydration, fever, and/or sepsis) octreotide 250–1,500microgram/24h by CSCI should be given (although not all cases respond).[204,208]

Irinotecan-induced diarrhoea may respond to neomycin.[209] Thalidomide 400mg/day has been used for otherwise resistant chemotherapy-induced diarrhoea.[210]

In AIDS, PO morphine (or morphine/diamorphine by CSCI) may be necessary to achieve control. These have both peripheral and central constipating effects, whereas loperamide acts only peripherally. Octreotide by CSCI may also be necessary.

ANAL DISCHARGE

A discharge from the anus can be:
- more or less continuous or intermittent
- spontaneous or related to the passage of flatus
- faecal or mucoid in consistency
- clear or opaque ± blood-stained.

In addition to soiling clothes, a discharge can result in:
- malodour, leading to embarrassment and social isolation, and lowered mood and morale
- peri-anal maceration
- pruritus.

Causes
- patulous anus
- haemorrhoids
- following evacuation induced with laxative suppositories (transient)
- rectal tumour
- radiation coloproctitis.

Differential diagnosis
An anal discharge needs to be differentiated from faecal incontinence, either of solid faeces or of leakage associated with diarrhoea or secondary to impaction (see p.119). Faecal incontinence is more likely in the elderly, particularly nursing home residents with cognitive impairment or decreased mobility who are reliant on others to get to a toilet.[211] Faecal incontinence can also occur in association with pelvic floor dysfunction and anal sphincter incompetence secondary to nerve damage caused by childbirth, diabetes mellitus or degenerative spine disease, etc. If the patient has been taking a dantron-containing laxative, faecal leakage may be complicated by an area of sharply demarcated peri-anal skin erythema.

An 'anal discharge' can also occur with an ileorectal or rectovesical fistula. However, the volume of the 'discharge' is likely to alert the clinician to the correct diagnosis.

Management
Correct the correctable
Where applicable:
- reduce tumour size:
  ▷ radiotherapy
  ▷ fulguration (surgical diathermy)
  ▷ transanal resection
  ▷ LASER treatment
- reduce peritumour or post-radiation inflammation:
  ▷ prednisolone suppositories 5mg b.d.
  ▷ prednisolone retention enema 20mg every 2–3 days
- reduce mucous discharge from a rectal tumour:
  ▷ NSAID
  ▷ octreotide.[212]

Non-drug treatment
Protect the skin of the perineum and genitalia:
- use only soft absorbent toilet paper
- wash anal area with a soft cloth after each bowel movement and as necessary
- use water only; *do not use soap*
- pat dry with a soft cloth; *do not rub*
- if above measures do not keep the area dry, protect skin with a barrier ointment, e.g. Cavilon No Sting Barrier Film® (this is sprayed on and does not sting on broken skin), or Morhulin® (zinc oxide 38%) or Comfeel® barrier cream (for more information, see *PCF3*)
- monitor carefully for small blisters suggestive of fungal infection; treat with clotrimazole 1% solution or cream b.d.–t.d.s.
- use cotton underclothes and change at least once daily
- incontinence aids, e.g. pads, anal plug (see p.124).

Drug treatment
If anal hygiene fails to relieve peri-anal pruritus, prescribe a systemic antihistamine.

ASCITES

A small amount of fluid (50–100mL) is present in the peritoneal cavity for lubrication. It is produced by capillaries and is removed by lymphatics in the peritoneum. Excessive accumulation of fluid (ascites) results from the excess production and/or reduced resorption of fluid.

When mild, ascites is asymptomatic but, when severe, it is distressing (Box 3.BB).

Box 3.BB Clinical features of ascites	
Abdominal distension	Nausea and vomiting
Abdominal discomfort/pain	Breathlessness
Early satiety, anorexia	Inability to sit upright
Dyspepsia, acid reflux	Leg oedema

Cancer accounts for about 10% of all cases of ascites.[213] Ovarian cancer has the highest incidence; 30% at presentation and 60% in advanced disease.[214] Non-cancer causes include cirrhosis (commonest overall), heart failure, kidney disease and pancreatitis.

Ascites is associated with a poor prognosis; in cancer, the mean survival is about 5 months after detection:
- worse in patients with an unknown primary and with a GI cancer
- better with cancer of the ovary
- best with lymphoma.[215]

In cirrhosis, median survival is about 2 years.[216]

Pathogenesis
There are two main causal mechanisms for ascites associated with cancer:
- peritoneal carcinomatosis
- extensive liver metastases (Table 3.7).

Table 3.7 Main causes of malignant ascites and implications for treatment

Feature	Peritoneal carcinomatosis	Extensive liver metastases
Pathophysiology	Obstruction of lymphatics in the peritoneum or regional lymph nodes by cancer Cytokine production, e.g. VEGF, by peritoneal and cancer cells which promote: • increasing capillary permeability • local cancer growth by enhancing angiogenesis	Similar to cirrhosis, i.e. portal hypertension + hypo-albuminaemia Portal hypertension leads to: • an increase in nitric oxide levels → splanchnic/peripheral vasodilation → decrease in effective arterial blood volume → ↑ renin, aldosterone, sympathetic nervous system activity • renal retention of sodium → expansion of plasma volume → increased peritoneal fluid Hypo-albuminaemia → reduced plasma oncotic pressure → increased peritoneal fluid
Typical example	Ovarian cancer	Liver metastases from colon cancer
Serum:ascites albumin gradient (see Table 3.8, p.130)	<11g/L (Ascitic albumin concentration relatively high because ascites = *exudate*)	≥11g/L (Ascitic albumin concentration relatively low because ascites = *transudate*.)
Response to diuretic therapy	None, or mild response if secondary hyperaldosteronsim has developed	More likely
Recurrent paracentesis or indwelling drain	Mainstay of treatment	Only if diuretics ineffective/not tolerated
Intra-abdominal therapy, e.g. chemotherapy, corticosteroids	May be beneficial	Unlikely to benefit

Determining which mechanism is operative in the individual patient guides the approach to management (see below).

Evaluation

The most diagnostically sensitive clinical findings are ankle oedema, increased abdominal girth and dullness and bulging of the flanks.[216] However, clinical examination can be unreliable. Useful investigations include:

- *ultrasound*: can identify ⩾100mL fluid, loculations and distinguish between distension due to fluid, cancer, organomegaly or bowel distension
- *cytological, microbiological and biochemical examination*: carried out when there is diagnostic uncertainty.

The ascitic total protein content is a reflection of the serum protein concentration and portal pressure. The difference between the level of albumin in the serum and ascitic fluid (serum:ascites albumin gradient) along with other features can help identify the cause of the ascites (Table 3.8). The presence of more than one cause may lead to a mixed picture.[216]

Other tests include:

- *cytology*: positive in up to 2/3 of cancer-related ascites
- *lymphocyte count*: high in peritoneal carcinomatosis, tuberculosis, fungal infection, following diuresis and (rarely) haematological cancer
- *neutrophil count*: a high count (⩾250 cells/microL) suggests infection (see p.136)
- *RBC count*: haemorrhagic ascites (RBC count of > 50,000 cells/microL) is generally due to a traumatic tap but can occur in cancer, cirrhosis and heart failure; to correct the neutrophil count of bloody ascitic fluid, take 1 neutrophil away for every 250 RBC
- *glucose and LDH*: aid the diagnosis of secondary bacterial peritonitis (see p.136)
- *amylase*: ascitic level > 1,000 units/L or ascites:serum amylase ratio increasing up to 0.6 suggests pancreatic disease
- *triglycerides*: milky-coloured fluid with triglyceride level > 2.2mmol/L (200mg/dL) confirms chylous ascites; can occur in cancer, cirrhosis and certain infections, e.g. tuberculosis
- *bilirubin*: ascitic level > 100micromol/L (> 6mg/dL) or ascites:serum bilirubin ratio > 1 suggests a biliary leak.

Management
Correct the correctable

If appropriate and successful, chemotherapy will control ascites. This can be either systemic or intraperitoneal. A range of other intraperitoneal agents are under investigation, e.g. anti-VEGF or anti-VEGF-receptor antibodies.

Non-drug treatment
Paracentesis
Guidelines: 'Blind' paracentesis of ascites in cancer patients, p.133.

Paracentesis is appropriate for patients with:

- an unknown diagnosis
- a tense distended abdomen in need of rapid relief
- ascites which is unlikely to respond to diuretic therapy, i.e. predominantly peritoneal (an *exudate* with relatively high albumin concentration) or chylous ascites
- ascites that has failed to respond to diuretic therapy

Table 3.8 Differential diagnosis of ascites

Serum:ascites albumin gradient	< 11g/L		≥ 11g/L	
	≥25g/L	<25g/L		
Total ascitic fluid protein			Normal or reduced	Elevated
JVP	–	–	–	Elevated
Possible diagnoses	Peritoneal carcinomatosis TB Pancreatic ascites Bacterial peritonitis	Protein-losing enteropathy Nephropathy Malnutrition	Liver metastases Cirrhosis Alcoholic hepatitis Hepatic failure Budd-Chiari syndrome Portal vein thrombosis Hypothyroidism	Heart failure Constrictive pericarditis Pulmonary hypertension

- intolerance to diuretic therapy
- possible bacterial peritonitis.

The only absolute contra-indications to paracentesis are clinically evident fibrinolysis or DIC (see p.250).

The amount of ascites drained will depend on whether the procedure is primarily diagnostic or therapeutic. For therapeutic paracentesis, practice varies. In a survey of the management of ascites in ovarian cancer, most centres:[217]
- used a Bonanno® suprapubic catheter (80%) or IV cannula (15%)
- did not routinely give fluid replacement (85%)
- drained to dryness, using controlled (60%) or free drainage (40%).

Controlled drainage was reported variably as:
- draining a specific volume (0.5–8L, median 2L) before discontinuing
- draining a certain volume per hour (0.5–2L, median 1L) or per day (1–6L, median 2L).

About 1/2 routinely asked radiologists to insert the drain or mark an entry site using ultrasound guidance. This happened less in palliative care settings (about 30%), possibly reflecting the condition of the patients and/or lack of proximity to a radiology department. However, ultrasound-guided paracentesis may be associated with greater success and fewer complications and is increasingly used where it is readily available.

Ultrasound-guided paracentesis should be used if:
- severe bowel distension
- widespread intra-abdominal cancer deposits
- previous extensive abdominal/pelvic surgery
- difficult previous paracentesis
- pregnancy.[216]

Most patients (90%) obtain symptom relief from paracentesis; sometimes after the removal of a relatively small volume, e.g. 1–2L.[218] Complications of paracentesis include:[216,219]
- abdominal discomfort; may require additional analgesics
- bleeding, sufficient to require transfusion (<1%):
  ▷ risk of bleeding is low even in patients with coagulopathy and/or thrombocytopenia; although sometimes given, prophylactic fresh-frozen plasma or platelet transfusion is not generally necessary
  ▷ risk of bleeding increases with worsening renal impairment because of associated platelet dysfunction; and because of varices in patients with portal hypertension if midline puncture below the umbilicus
- bowel or bladder puncture:
  ▷ risk reduced by ensuring the bladder is empty, avoiding scars (possible underlying adherent bowel) and the use of ultrasound guidance
- persistent small volume leak at the site of puncture (<1%):
  ▷ the risk can be minimized by use of a small-gauge needle and making a Z-track (i.e. using skin traction to misalign the puncture sites through skin, fascia and muscle)
  ▷ if there is a leak, ask the patient to lie on their side with the puncture site uppermost and firmly apply a thick gauze dressing
  ▷ if the leak persists consider a purse-string suture or the use of medical glue (e.g. Dermabond®)
  ▷ a colostomy bag is occasionally needed for large volume leakage

- hypotension:
  - ▷ large volume paracentesis can lead to haemodynamic changes resulting in hypovolaemia, hypotension and, in severe cases, collapse and renal failure
  - ▷ risk is minimized by limiting paracentesis to ≤5L in patients with cirrhosis receiving diuretics, and any patient with serum creatinine >250micromol/L (indicative of renal failure), albumin <30g/L or sodium <125mmol/L
- pulmonary embolism; possibly due to the release of pressure from abdominal veins
- local infection or peritonitis; the risk is minimal with an aseptic technique.

With cirrhotic ascites, if drainage of >5L is required:
- stop diuretics used for ascites 48h before procedure, during paracentesis, and immediately afterwards
- administer volume expanders, e.g. IV dextran 70, 150mL for every litre of ascites drained
- monitor pulse and blood pressure every 30min during paracentesis, then hourly for 6h.

With cancer-related ascites, removal of >5L is less problematic. However, in the presence of any of the above abnormalities in creatinine, albumin or sodium, it makes sense to take a similar approach as in cirrhotic ascites.

Indwelling catheters
For patients requiring frequent paracentesis and who have a prognosis of at least 1 month, an indwelling tunnelled drain can be considered, e.g. Pleurx® catheter. To reduce the risk of infection, this catheter contains a one-way valve and a polyester cuff which promotes fibrosis in the SC tissue; the latter also helps to secure the catheter.

Patients are taught to drain off fluid using special Pleurx® drainage sets with vacuum bottles, initially up to 2L every day for 1–2 weeks (to reduce complications of leakage while awaiting healing around the cuff), and then as required, generally alternate days.[220]

An indwelling catheter can reduce the frequency of hospital visits/admissions, which may be of particular benefit to frail patients who have to travel long distances. The overall complication rate (i.e. infection, loculation, persistent leakage) is similar to intermittent drainage (about 8%).[220]

Peritoneovenous shunt
Shunts contain a one-way valve allowing fluid to be drained from the peritoneal cavity into the superior vena cava. They are indicated for patients who are relatively fit with rapidly recurring ascites despite drainage and diuretic therapy.[221]

Their main advantage is the avoidance of protein and fluid depletion associated with frequent paracentesis. Contra-indications to their use include haemorrhagic ascites, and heart failure. Potential complications include pulmonary oedema, embolism, DIC, infection, cancer emboli. Many occlude, lasting a mean of 10 weeks in cancer patients.[219]

Patients with breast or ovarian cancer with an expected survival of 1–3 months appear to fare best. Patients with GI cancer have a poor response rate and are not considered good candidates for shunts.[219]

The use of shunts is likely to decline as the use of indwelling drains increases.

Guidelines: 'Blind' paracentesis of ascites in cancer patients

Although the rapid drainage of large volumes of cirrhotic (transudative) ascites can be detrimental, i.e. cause hypotension/cardiovascular shock and/or exacerbate/precipitate hepatic encephalopathy, free drainage is generally safe in malignant (exudative) ascites.

Indications for paracentesis
- to aid diagnosis of the underlying cause
- to relieve symptoms caused by tense ascites:
  ▷ abdominal discomfort or pain
  ▷ breathlessness secondary to splinting of the diaphragm
  ▷ acid regurgitation, nausea and/or vomiting.

'Blind' vs. ultrasound-guided
'Blind' paracentesis is more frequent in a hospice setting, possibly reflecting the condition of the patients and/or lack of proximity to a radiology department. However, when feasible, ultrasound-guided paracentesis is preferable, and is essential with:
- previous extensive abdominal surgery
- pregnancy
- severe bowel distension
- peritoneal carcinomatosis with multiple palpable tumours
- difficult previous paracentesis.

Pre-paracentesis investigations
- *blood tests*: if frail, dehydrated, on diuretics, bruising easily, or receiving chemotherapy check biochemistry, FBC, clotting screen. Some centres do no routine blood tests if patient fit enough for day case paracentesis
- if diagnostic, also measure plasma albumin, LDH and glucose
- *vital signs*: pulse and BP.

Equipment
- clean trolley; sterile gloves, gauze and drapes
- iodine or alcohol solution for cleansing of the skin
- local anaesthetic, e.g. lidocaine 1% 5–10mL; 10mL syringe, 25G (orange) and 21G (green) needles
- for a *diagnostic* paracentesis, use a 50mL syringe with a 21G (green) needle
- for a *therapeutic* paracentesis, use an appropriate catheter, e.g. 8–10Fr Flexima® pigtail, Bonanno®, Safe-T-Centesis® together with tubing and drainage bag/bottle
- suture (if catheter not self-retaining); not necessary if procedure limited to a few hours
- adhesive dressing to cover site of insertion and anchor catheter
- tubes or bottles required for diagnostic tests (see below).

Diagnostic tests
- *ascitic fluid*: microscopy, culture, differential cell count, cytology, albumin, LDH, glucose, amylase or triglyceride as appropriate.

Positioning
After emptying their bladder, the patient should adopt a comfortable supine position. However, use a lateral decubitus position for diagnostic taps of small volume ascites.

continued

Choose the drain site
Confirm that the chosen site is dull to percussion. Insert the drain:
- in a lower quadrant, 2–3cm lateral to the anterior rectus muscle border *or*
- midline 2cm below umbilicus (unless the patient has portal hypertension).

Avoid:
- going too far lateral
- areas of superficial infection
- obvious cancer
- previous scarring
- engorged veins.

Procedure
1 Clean the skin with an iodine or alcohol solution using sterile gauze and drape the puncture site to create a sterile field.

2 Infiltrate the skin and subcutaneous tissues with local anaesthetic using a 10mL syringe with an 25G (orange) needle, then 21G (green). Attempt to aspirate as the needle is advanced through the abdominal wall. Withdraw the needle when ascitic fluid is aspirated.

3 Diagnostic *paracentesis*: with a 50mL syringe attached to a 21G (green) needle, enter the anaesthetized puncture site at a perpendicular angle. Slowly advance the needle through the soft tissue, aspirating while advancing:
- to lessen the risk of leakage after the procedure in patients with a thin abdominal wall, make a 'Z-tract', i.e. apply traction on the skin with one hand to prevent superimposition of the puncture holes through the skin, muscle, and fascia
- the needle will 'give' as it enters the peritoneal cavity. Stop advancing and aspirate 20–50mL for diagnostic tests. Remove the needle while aspirating and remove the skin traction once the needle has been completely withdrawn
- apply pressure to the puncture site for 2–3 minutes, to ensure no excessive bleeding or fluid leakage; then apply a dry gauze bandage to the site.

4 *Therapeutic paracentesis*: insert an appropriate catheter and (if not self-retaining) secure with dressing ± suture. Connect with tubing to a drainage bag/bottle:
- if a day case, allow free drainage of ascites for up to 6 hours, then remove the drain
- some centres limit drainage to 4–6L over 6–12 hours. Removing more does not generally increase relief, although it may extend the interval between paracenteses
- in patients with concurrent hepatic failure, creatinine > 250micromol/L, albumin < 30g/L or sodium < 125mmol/L, limit paracentesis to 4–6L because of the risk of hypovolaemia/hypotension. If drainage of > 6L is necessary in these patients:
  ▷ discontinue diuretics used for ascites 48 hours before procedure
  ▷ during the paracentesis or shortly afterwards administer volume expanders, e.g. IV dextran 70, 150mL for every 1L of ascites drained.

Monitoring
- if the patient experiences increasing discomfort, feels faint or unwell, stop the drainage and check pulse and BP
- with patients at risk of hypovolaemia/hypotension, monitor pulse and BP every 30 minutes during paracentesis, then hourly for 6 hours after its completion
- give patients treated as day case instructions on who to contact if problems arise.

Recurrent ascites
- repeat paracentesis as necessary
- if hyperaldosteronism is a contributory factor, e.g. with massive liver metastases, consider prescribing spironolactone
- if there is need for frequent drainage (more than every 2 weeks), consider:
  ▷ an indwelling drain, e.g. Pleurx® catheter, for the patient to drain intermittently
  ▷ intra-abdominal corticosteroids if ascites associated with peritoneal carcinomatosis, e.g. triamcinolone acetonide 8mg/kg (maximum 520mg).

Drug treatment

For more information, see *PCF3*.

Hyperaldosteronism often occurs with ascites associated with portal hypertension (a *transudate* with a relatively low albumin concentration), i.e.:

- cirrhosis
- hepatocellular cancer
- extensive liver metastases.[222,223]

Most evidence comes from cirrhosis, but spironolactone, an aldosterone antagonist, in a median daily dose of 200–300mg is successful in the majority of patients with these conditions (90% in cirrhosis).[219,222–226] Elimination of ascites may take 10–28 days (Box 3.CC).

Box 3.CC   Diuretic treatment for ascites

Monitor body weight and renal function.

Start with spironolactone 100–200mg each morning with food; give in divided doses if it causes nausea and vomiting.

If necessary, increase by 100mg every 3–7 days to achieve a weight loss of 0.5–1kg/24h (<0.5kg/24h when peripheral oedema absent).

A typical maintenance dose is 200–300mg once daily; maximum dose 400–600mg once daily.[222,223,226,227]

If not achieving the desired weight loss with spironolactone 300–400mg once daily, consider adding furosemide 40–80mg each morning.

In cirrhosis, furosemide is generally increased in 40mg steps every 3 days to a maximum of 160mg once daily.[225,226,228,229]

If Na^+ falls <120mmol/L, temporarily stop diuretics.

If K^+ falls to <3.5mmol/L, temporarily stop or decrease the dose of furosemide.

If K^+ rises to >5.5mmol/L, halve the dose of spironolactone; if >6mmol/L, temporarily stop spironolactone.

If creatinine rises >150micromol/L, temporarily stop diuretics.[225]

Even if paracentesis becomes necessary, diuretics should be continued as they reduce the rate of recurrence.[225]

A diuretic-induced reduction in plasma volume can increase the activity of various closely related neurohumoral systems, e.g. the renin-aldosterone-angiotensin system, sympathetic nervous system, ADH secretion, which results in impaired renal perfusion and increased sodium and water resorption. These changes reduce the effect of the diuretic and contribute to renal impairment.

In patients with cirrhosis receiving spironolactone ± furosemide, improved renal function and diuresis is seen with co-administration of octreotide 300microgram SC b.d. or clonidine 75microgram PO b.d.[230,231]

In peritoneal carcinomatosis or chylous ascites, a response to spironolactone is less likely.[224] Consider its use only when secondary hyperaldosteronism is also present (suggested by ankle oedema) or as a therapeutic trial; discontinue if ineffective.

In peritoneal carcinomatosis, after a preliminary paracentesis, depot corticosteroids have been instilled to reduce the rate of ascitic fluid formation. Evidence is limited, but in an open study, mean interval between paracenteses increased from 9 days to 18 days:
- in the UK, give triamcinolone acetonide 8mg/kg, up to a maximum of 520mg (13 vials) or
- triamcinolone hexacetonide (not UK) 10mg/kg, up to a maximum of 640mg[232,233] or
- methylprednisolone 10mg/kg, up to a maximum of 640mg (8 vials).

Octreotide is also reported to reduce the rate of formation of malignant ascites.[212,234] It may interfere with ascitic fluid formation through a reduction in splanchnic blood flow or as a result of a direct tumour antisecretory effect. Octreotide may also help improve the efficacy of diuretics as in cirrhosis.[230] Octreotide could be considered in patients with rapidly accumulating ascites due to peritoneal carcinomatosis or massive liver metastases failing to respond to diuretic therapy. Octreotide may also help resolve chylous ascites.[235,236]

Infected ascites

Infection can arise in ascitic fluid, either with no apparent intra-abdominal source, i.e. spontaneous bacterial peritonitis, or secondary to a perforated viscus or intra-abdominal abscess.

Spontaneous bacterial peritonitis may be caused by bacteria (e.g. *Escherichia coli*, *Klebsiella pneumoniae* and *Pneumococcus*) gaining access to the systemic circulation because of impaired immune defences. It occurs in 10–30% of hospital inpatients with liver cirrhosis and ascites, and has a poor prognosis (30% die in hospital, and another 20% die within 1 year).

Table 3.9 Management of patients with suspected bacterial peritonitis

Diagnosis	Ascitic fluid analysis	Management
Spontaneous bacterial peritonitis	≥250 neutrophils/microL and/or positive culture for a single organism	Antibacterials
Variant spontaneous bacterial peritonitis	≥250 neutrophils/microL + negative culture	Antibacterials
Monomicrobial non-neutrocytic bacterascites	<250 neutrophils/microL + positive culture for a single organism	If symptomatic or extraperitoneal infection, give antibacterials. If asymptomatic, repeat paracentesis within 24h and give antibacterials if bacterascites persists
Secondary bacterial peritonitis/polymicrobial bacterascites	Positive culture for multiple organisims	Antibacterials; consider other investigations (see Table 3.10)

A high index of clinical suspicion is required because peritonism, an elevated WBC, fever or abdominal pain are not always present. Patients may present with confusion or a non-specific deterioration.

A diagnostic paracentesis should be undertaken and ascitic fluid put immediately into culture bottles. As a Gram stain is often negative in early spontaneous bacterial peritonitis, the cell count and culture are used to guide management (Table 3.9).[216]

Distinguishing spontaneous from secondary bacterial peritonitis is important (Table 3.10). Both are treated with antibacterials, but secondary bacterial peritonitis will require imaging to search for the underlying cause, which may require surgical intervention.[216]

Table 3.10 Features which help to distinguish between spontaneous and secondary bacterial peritonitis[216]

	Bacterial peritonitis	
Feature	Spontaneous	Secondary
Fever	±	+
Peritonism	±	+
Free intraperitoneal gas	−	+
Ascitic fluid		
Glucose <2.78mmol/L	−	+
LDH >225units/L	−	+
Total protein >10g/L	±	+
Gram stain	−	+
Culture	monomicrobial	polymicrobial

1 Tangerman A (2002) Halitosis in medicine: a review. *International Dental Journal.* **52 Suppl 3**: 201–206.
2 Porter SR and Scully C (2006) Oral malodour (halitosis). *British Medical Journal.* 333: 632–635.
3 Sopapornamorn P *et al.* (2007) Relationship between total salivary protein content and volatile sulfur compounds levels in malodor patients. *Oral Surgery, Oral Medicine, Oral Pathology, Oral Radiology and Endodontics.* 103: 655–660.
4 Haraszthy VI *et al.* (2007) Identification of oral bacterial species associated with halitosis. *Journal of the American Dental Association.* 138: 1113–1120.
5 Davies A and Beighton D (2001) Xerostomia in patients with advanced cancer. *Journal of Pain and Symptom Management.* 22: 820–825.
6 Kusler D and Rambur B (1992) Treatment for radiation-induced xerostoma: An innovative study. *Cancer Nursing.* 15: 191–195.
7 Davies A *et al.* (1998) A comparison of artificial saliva and pilocarpine in the management of xerostomia in patients with advanced cancer. *Palliative Medicine.* 12: 105–111.
8 Rieke JW *et al.* (1995) Oral pilocarpine for radiation-induced xerostomia: integrated efficacy and safety results from two prospective randomized clinical trials. *International Journal of Radiation Oncology Biology Physics.* 31: 661–669.
9 Everett H (1975) The use of bethanechol chloride with tricyclic antidepressants. *American Journal of Psychiatry.* 132: 1202–1204.
10 Epstein J *et al.* (1994) A clinical trial of bethanechol in patients with xerostomia after radiation therapy. A pilot study. *Oral Surgery, Oral Medicine and Oral Pathology.* 77: 610–614.
11 Taylor SE (2003) Efficacy and economic evaluation of pilocarpine in treating radiation-induced xerostomia. *Expert Opin Pharmacother.* 4: 1489–1497.
12 Davies AN and Vriens J (2005) Oral transmucosal fentanyl citrate and xerostomia. *Journal of Pain and Symptom Management.* 30: 496–497.
13 Lucas V and Schofield L (2000) Treatment of drooling. *European Journal of Palliative Care.* 7: 5–7.

14 Chou KL et al. (2007) Sialorrhea in Parkinson's disease: A review. Movement Disorders. 22: 2306–2313.
15 Newick P and Laughton-Hewer R (1984) Motor neurone disease – can we do better? British Medical Journal. 289: 539–542.
16 Mandel L and Tamari K (1995) Sialorrhea and gastrooesophageal reflux. Journal of the American Dental Association. 126: 1537–1541.
17 Lieblich S (1989) Episodic supersalivation (idiopathic paroxysmal sialorrhoea). Description of a new clinical syndrome. Oral Surgery, Oral Medicine and Oral Pathology. 68: 159–161.
18 Cohen G et al. (1990) Salivary complaints; a manifestation of depressive illness. NY State Dental Journal. 56: 31–33.
19 Scully C and Bagan JV (2004) Adverse drug reactions in the orofacial region. Critical Reviews in Oral Biology and Medicine. 15: 221–239.
20 Neppelberg E et al. (2007) Radiotherapy reduces sialorrhea in amyotrophic lateral sclerosis. European Journal of Neurology. 14: 1373–1377.
21 Ali-Melkkila T et al. (1993) Pharmacokinetics and related pharmacodynamics of anticholinergic drugs. Acta Anaesthesiologica Scandinavica. 37: 633–642.
22 Hyson HC et al. (2002) Sublingual atropine for sialorrhea secondary to parkinsonism: a pilot study. Movement Disorders. 17: 1318–1320.
23 De Simone GG et al. (2006) Atropine drops for drooling: a randomized controlled trial. Palliative Medicine. 20: 665–671.
24 Thomsen TR et al. (2007) Ipratropium bromide spray as treatment for sialorrhea in Parkinson's disease. Movement Disorders. 22: 2268–2273.
25 Benson J and Daugherty KK (2007) Botulinum toxin A in the treatment of sialorrhea. Ann Pharmacother. 41: 79–85.
26 Fuster Torres MA et al. (2007) Salivary gland application of botulinum toxin for the treatment of sialorrhea. Medicina Oral, Patología Oral y Cirugía Bucal. 12: E511–517.
27 Davies A and Finlay I (eds) (2005) Oral Care in Advanced Disease. Oxford University Press, Oxford.
28 Sciubba JJ et al. (2006) Oral complications of radiotherapy. Lancet Oncology. 7: 175–183.
29 Scully C and Shotts R (2000) ABC of oral health: mouth ulcers and other causes of orofacial soreness and pain. British Medical Journal. 321: 162–165.
30 Turhal N et al. (2000) Efficacy of treatment to relieve mucositis-induced discomfort. Support Care Cancer. 8: 55–58.
31 Davies AN et al. (2002) Oral yeast carriage in patients with advanced cancer. Oral Microbiology and Immunology. 17: 79–84.
32 Finlay I and Davies A (2005) Fungal infections. In: A Davies and I Finlay (eds) Oral Care in Advanced Disease. Oxford University Press, Oxford, pp. 55–71.
33 Davies AN et al. (2006) Oral candidosis in patients with advanced cancer. Oral Oncology. 42: 698–702.
34 Davies AN et al. (2008) Oral candidosis in community-based patients with advanced cancer. Journal of Pain and Symptom Management. 35: 508–514.
35 Greenspan D (1994) Treatment of oropharyngeal candidiasis in HIV-positive patients. Journal of the American Academy of Dermatology. 31: S51–S55.
36 Barkvoll P and Attramadal A (1989) Effect of nystatin and chlorhexidine digluconate on Candida albicans. Oral Surgery, Oral Medicine and Oral Pathology. 67: 279–281.
37 Ellepola AN and Samaranayake LP (2001) Adjunctive use of chlorhexidine in oral candidoses: a review. Oral Diseases. 7: 11–17.
38 Worthington HV et al. (2007) Interventions for treating oral candidiasis for patients with cancer receiving treatment. Cochrane Database of Systematic Reviews. 1: CD001972.pub 001973.
39 DeWit S et al. (1989) Comparison of fluconazole and ketoconazole for oropharyngeal candidiasis in AIDS. Lancet. 1: 746–748.
40 Allen L (1993) Ketoconazole oral suspension. US Pharmacist. 18: 98–101.
41 Bernhardson BM et al. (2007) Chemosensory changes experienced by patients undergoing cancer chemotherapy: a qualitative interview study. Journal of Pain and Symptom Management. 34: 403–412.
42 Hutton JL et al. (2007) Chemosensory dysfunction is a primary factor in the evolution of declining nutritional status and quality of life in patients with advanced cancer. Journal of Pain and Symptom Management. 33: 156–165.
43 Wang H et al. (2007) Inflammation activates the interferon signaling pathways in taste bud cells. Journal of Neuroscience. 27: 10,703–10,713.
44 Tanaka M (2002) Secretory function of the salivary gland in patients with taste disorders or xerostomia: correlation with zinc deficiency. Acta Oto-laryngologica Supplementum. 134–141.
45 Henkin RI et al. (1999) Efficacy of exogenous oral zinc in treatment of patients with carbonic anhydrase VI deficiency. The American Journal of Medical Sciences. 318: 392–405.
46 Heckmann SM et al. (2005) Zinc gluconate in the treatment of dysgeusia–a randomized clinical trial. Journal of Dental Research. 84: 35–38.

47 Berteretche MV et al. (2004) Decreased taste sensitivity in cancer patients under chemotherapy. *Support Care Cancer.* **12**: 571–576.

48 Ruo Redda MG and Allis S (2006) Radiotherapy-induced taste impairment. *Cancer Treatment Reviews.* **32**: 541–547.

49 Holscher T et al. (2005) Effects of radiotherapy on olfactory function. *Radiotherapy and Oncology.* **77**: 157–163.

50 Schiffman SS et al. (2007) Combination of flavor enhancement and chemosensory education improves nutritional status in older cancer patients. *The Journal of Nutrition, Health & Aging.* **11**: 439–454.

51 Chapman IM (2007) The anorexia of aging. *Clinics in Geriatric Medicine.* **23**: 735–756, v.

52 National Collaborating Centre for Acute Care (2006) *Nutrition Support in Adults: Oral Nutrition Support, Enteral Tube Feeding and Parenteral Nutrition* (No. 32). National Institute for Clinical Excellence, London.

53 Malnutrition Advisory Group (2003) The Malnutrition Universal Screening Tool. BAPEN, UK. Available from: www.bapen.org.uk/must_tool.html

54 Davies M (2005) Nutritional screening and assessment in cancer-associated malnutrition. *European Journal of Oncology Nursing.* **9 (suppl 2)**: S64–73.

55 Thoresen L and de Soysa AK (2006) The nutritional aspects of palliative care. *European Journal of Palliative Care.* **13**: 194–197.

56 Laviano A et al. (2005) Therapy insight: Cancer anorexia-cachexia syndrome–when all you can eat is yourself. *Nature Clinical Practice Oncology.* **2**: 158–165.

57 Lis C et al. (2009) Can anorexia predict patient satisfaction with quality of life in advanced cancer? *Supportive care in cancer.* **17**: 129–135.

58 Wilcock A (2006) Anorexia: a taste of things to come? *Palliative Medicine.* **20**: 43–45.

59 Churm D et al. (2009) A questionnaire study of the approach to the anorexia-cachexia syndrome in patients with cancer by staff in a district general hospital. *Support Care Cancer.*

60 Moertel C et al. (1974) Corticosteroid therapy for preterminal gastrointestinal cancer. *Cancer.* **33**: 1607–1609.

61 Bruera E et al. (1985) Action of oral methylprednisolone in terminal cancer patients: a prospective randomized double-blind study. *Cancer Treatment Reports.* **69**: 751–754.

62 Bruera E et al. (1998) Effectiveness of megestrol acetate in patients with advanced cancer: a randomized, double-blind, crossover study. *Cancer Prevention Control.* **2**: 74–78.

63 Willox JC et al. (1984) Prednisolone as an appetite stimulant in patients with cancer. *British Medical Journal.* **288**: 27.

64 Twycross RG and Guppy D (1985) Prednisolone in terminal breast and bronchogenic cancer. *Practitioner.* **229**: 57–59.

65 Donnelly S and Walsh TD (1995) Low-dose megestrol acetate for appetite stimulation in advanced cancer. *Journal of Pain and Symptom Management.* **10**: 182–183.

66 Vadell C et al. (1998) Anticachectic efficacy of megestrol acetate at different doses and versus placebo in patients with neoplastic cachexia. *American Journal of Clinical Oncology.* **21**: 347–351.

67 Laviano A et al. (2003) Cancer anorexia: clinical implications, pathogenesis, and therapeutic strategies. *The Lancet Oncology.* **4**: 686–694.

68 Bruera E and Higginson I (1996) *Cachexia-Anorexia in Cancer Patients.* Oxford University Press, Oxford.

69 Gordon JN et al. (2005) Cancer cachexia. *QJM: Monthly Journal of the Association of Physicians.* **98**: 779–788.

70 Scott HR et al. (2002) The systemic inflammatory response, weight loss, performance status and survival in patients with inoperable non-small cell lung cancer. *British Journal of Cancer.* **87**: 264–267.

71 Davis MP et al. (2004) Appetite and cancer-associated anorexia: a review. *Journal of Clinical Oncology.* **22**: 1510–1517.

72 Ramos EJ et al. (2004) Cancer anorexia-cachexia syndrome: cytokines and neuropeptides. *Current Opinion in Clinical Nutrition and Metabolic Care.* **7**: 427–434.

73 Laviano A et al. (2005) Therapy insight: Cancer anorexia-cachexia syndrome–when all you can eat is yourself. *Nature Clinical Practice Oncology.* **2**: 158–165.

74 George J et al. (2007) Cancer cachexia syndrome in head and neck cancer patients: Part II. Pathophysiology. *Head & Neck.* **29**: 497–507.

75 Weber M-A et al. (2008) Morphology, metabolism, microcirculation, and strength of skeletal muscles in cancer-related cachexia. *Acta Oncologica.* **19**: 1–9.

76 Marin Caro MM et al. (2007) Nutritional intervention and quality of life in adult oncology patients. *Clinical Nutrition.* **26**: 289–301.

77 Arends J et al. (2006) ESPEN guidelines on enteral nutrition: non-surgical oncology. *Clinical Nutrition.* **25**: 245–259.

78 Barber M et al. (1998) Current controversies in cancer. Should cancer patients with incurable disease receive parenteral or enteral nutritional support? *European Journal of Cancer.* **34**: 279–285.

79 Lundholm K et al. (2004) Palliative nutritional intervention in addition to cyclooxygenase and erythropoietin treatment for patients with malignant disease: Effects on survival, metabolism, and function. *Cancer.* **100**: 1967–1977.

80 Shang E et al. (2006) The influence of early supplementation of parenteral nutrition on quality of life and body composition in patients with advanced cancer. JPEN: Journal of Parenteral and Enteral Nutrition. **30**: 222–230.

81 Baldwin C and Parsons TJ (2004) Dietary advice and nutritional supplements in the management of illness-related malnutrition: systematic review. Clinical Nutrition. **23**: 1267–1279.

82 Bruera E and MacDonald N (1988) Nutrition in cancer patients: an update and review of our experience. Journal of Pain and Symptom Management. **3**: 133–140.

83 Bosaeus I and Bosaeus I (2008) Nutritional support in multimodal therapy for cancer cachexia. Supportive Care in Cancer. **16**: 447–451.

84 Strasser F et al. (2007) Fighting a losing battle: eating-related distress of men with advanced cancer and their female partners. A mixed-methods study. Palliative Medicine. **21**: 129–137.

85 Hopkinson JB et al. (2008) Management of weight loss and anorexia. Annals of Oncology. **19 Suppl 7**: vii289–293.

86 Shragge JE et al. (2006) The management of anorexia by patients with advanced cancer: a critical review of the literature. Palliative Medicine. **20**: 623–629.

87 Argiles JM et al. (2008) Novel approaches to the treatment of cachexia. Drug Discovery Today. **13**: 73–78.

88 Khan ZH et al. (2003) Oesophageal cancer and cachexia: the effect of short-term treatment with thalidomide on weight loss and lean body mass. Alimentary Pharmacology & Therapeutics. **17**: 677–682.

89 Gordon JN et al. (2005) Thalidomide in the treatment of cancer cachexia: a randomised placebo controlled trial.[see comment]. Gut. **54**: 540–545.

90 Lundholm K et al. (2004) Evidence that long-term COX-treatment improves energy homeostasis and body composition in cancer patients with progressive cachexia. International Journal of Oncology. **24**: 505–512.

91 Lundholm K et al. (1994) Anti-inflammatory treatment may prolong survival in undernourished patients with metastatic solid tumours. Cancer Research. **54**: 5602–5606.

92 Wilcock A (2005) Cachexia and omega-3 polyunsaturated fatty acids: the beginning of the end or the end of the beginning? Palliative Medicine. **19**: 500–502.

93 Colomer R et al. (2007) N-3 fatty acids, cancer and cachexia: a systematic review of the literature. British Journal of Nutrition. **97**: 823–831.

94 Dewey A et al. (2007) Eicosapentaenoic acid (EPA, an omega-3 fatty acid from fish oils) for the treatment of cancer cachexia. Cochrane Database of Systematic Reviews. CD004597.

95 Lundholm K et al. (2007) Insulin treatment in cancer cachexia: effects on survival, metabolism, and physical functioning. Clinical Cancer Research. **13**: 2699–2706.

96 Garcia J et al. (2007) A phase II randomized, placebo-controlled, double-blind study of the safety and efficacy of RC-1291 (RC) for the treatment of cancer cachexia. ASCO Annual Meeting Proceedings Part 1. Journal of Clinical Oncology. **(supplement) 25**: 9133.

97 Mantovani G et al. (2008) Randomized phase III clinical trial of five different arms of treatment for patients with cancer cachexia: interim results. Nutrition. **24**: 305–313.

98 Burge F (1993) Dehydration symptoms of palliative care cancer patients. Journal of Pain and Symptom Management. **8**: 454–464.

99 Meares C (1994) Terminal dehydration: A review. American Journal of Hospice and Palliative Care. **11 (3)**: 10–14.

100 Dunphy K et al. (1995) Rehydration in palliative and terminal care: if not – why not? Palliative Medicine. **9**: 221–228.

101 Fainsinger R et al. (1994) The use of hypodermoclysis for rehydration in terminally ill cancer patients. Journal of Pain and Symptom Management. **9**: 298–302.

102 Good P et al. (2008) Medically assisted hydration for adult palliative care patients. Cochrane Database of Systematic Reviews. Art No,: CD006273.

103 Garcia-Peris P et al. (2007) Long-term prevalence of oropharyngeal dysphagia in head and neck cancer patients: Impact on quality of life. Clinical Nutrition. **26**: 710–717.

104 Logemann JA et al. (2006) Site of disease and treatment protocol as correlates of swallowing function in patients with head and neck cancer treated with chemoradiation. Head & Neck. **28**: 64–73.

105 Carter R et al. (1982) Pain and dysphagia in patients with squamous carcinomas of the head and neck: the role of perineural spread. Journal of the Royal Society of Medicine. **75**: 598–606.

106 Terry P and Fuller S (1989) Pulmonary consequences of aspiration. Dysphagia. **3**: 179–183.

107 Garon (1997) A randomized control study to determine the effects of unlimited oral intake of water in patients with identified aspiration. Journal of Neurological Rehabilitation. **11**: 139–148.

108 Logemann JA (1983) Evaluation and Treatment of Swallowing Disorders. College Hill Press, San Diego.

109 McDonnell F and Walsh D (1999) Treatment of odynophagia and dysphagia in advanced cancer with sublingual glyceryl trinitrate. Palliative Medicine. **13**: 251–252.

110 Oliver D et al. (eds) (2006) Palliative Care in Aamyotrophic Lateral Sclerosis from Diagnosis to Bereavement (2e). Oxford University Press, Oxford.

111 Bastian RW (1998) Contemporary diagnosis of the dysphagic patient. Otolaryngolic Clinics of North America. **31**: 489–506.

112 Farrell Z and O'Neill D (1999) Towards better screening and assessment of oropharyngeal swallow disorders in the general hospital. *Lancet.* **354**: 355–356.

113 O'Brien T et al. (1992) Motor neurone disease: a hospice perspective. *British Medical Journal.* **304**: 471–473.

114 National Council for Palliative Care and The Association of Palliative Medicine for Great Britain & Ireland (2007) Artificial Nutrition and Hydration – Guidance in End of Life Care for Adults. Available from: www.ncpc.org.uk/publications/index.html

115 Morita T et al. (2007) Development of a national clinical guideline for artificial hydration therapy for terminally ill patients with cancer. *Journal of Palliative Medicine.* **10**: 770–780.

116 Morita T et al. (2006) Artificial hydration therapy, laboratory findings, and fluid balance in terminally ill patients with abdominal malignancies. *Journal of Pain and Symptom Management.* **31**: 130–139.

117 Moran B and Frost R (1992) Percutaneous endoscopic gastrostomy in 41 patients: indications and clinical outcome. *Journal of the Royal Society of Medicine.* **85**: 320–321.

118 Radunovic A et al. (2007) Clinical care of patients with amyotrophic lateral sclerosis. *Lancet Neurology.* **6**: 913–925.

119 Britton J et al. (1997) The use of percutaneous endoscopic gastrostomy (PEG) feeding tubes in patients with neurological disease. *Journal of Neurology.* **244**: 431–434.

120 McCamish M and Crocker N (1993) Enteral and parenteral nutrition support of terminally ill patients: practical and ethical perspectives. *The Hospice Journal.* **9**: 107–129.

121 Bozzetti F (1996) Guidelines on artificial nutrition versus hydration in terminal cancer patients. *Nutrition.* **12**: 163–167.

122 NCHSPCS (1997) Artificial hydration (AH) for people who are terminally ill. *European Journal of Palliative Care.* **4**: 124–128.

123 General Medical Council (2002) Withholding and withdrawing life-prolonging treatments: good practice in decision making. Available from: www.gmc-uk.org

124 British medical Association (2007) *Withholding and Withdrawing Life-prolonging Medical Treatment. Guidance for decision making* (3e). Blackwell Publishing, Oxford, UK.

125 Oliver D (1998) Opioid medication in the palliative care of motor neurone disease. *Palliative Medicine.* **12**: 113–115.

126 Oliver D et al. (2000) *Palliative Care in Amyotrophic Lateral Sclerosis (Motor Neurone Disease).* Oxford University Press, Oxford.

127 Dua KS (2007) Stents for palliating malignant dysphagia and fistula: is the paradigm shifting? *Gastrointestinal Endoscopy.* **65**: 77–81.

128 Power C et al. (2007) Superiority of anti-reflux stent compared with conventional stents in the palliative management of patients with cancer of the lower esophagus and esophago-gastric junction: results of a randomized clinical trial. *Disease of the Esophagus.* **20**: 466–470.

129 Keller R et al. (2007) Self-expanding metal stents for malignant esophagogastric obstruction: experience with a new design covered nitinol stent. *Journal of Gastrointestinal and Liver Disease.* **16**: 239–243.

130 Verschuur EM et al. (2007) Esophageal stents for malignant strictures close to the upper esophageal sphincter. *Gastrointestinal Endoscopy.* **66**: 1082–1090.

131 Ko HK et al. (2007) Fate of migrated esophageal and gastroduodenal stents: experience in 70 patients. *Journal of Vascular and Interventional Radiology.* **18**: 725–732.

132 Govender P et al. (2007) Small bowel obstruction–an unusual complication of oesophageal stent migration. *The British Journal of Radiology.* **80**: 767–768.

133 Shin JH et al. (2005) Comparison of temporary and permanent stent placement with concurrent radiation therapy in patients with esophageal carcinoma. *Journal of Vascular and Interventional Radiology.* **16**: 67–74.

134 Lecleire S et al. (2006) Undernutrition is predictive of early mortality after palliative self-expanding metal stent insertion in patients with inoperable or recurrent esophageal cancer.[see comment]. *Gastrointestinal Endoscopy.* **64**: 479–484.

135 Fox M and Forgacs I (2006) Gastro-oesophageal reflux disease. *British Medical Journal.* **332**: 88–93.

136 Boeckxstaens GE (2007) Review article: the pathophysiology of gastro-oesophageal reflux disease. *Alimentary Pharmacology & Therapeutics.* **26**: 149–160.

137 Portale G et al. (2007) When are reflux episodes symptomatic? *Diseases of the Esophagus.* **20**: 47–52.

138 Shapiro M et al. (2007) Assessment of dietary nutrients that influence perception of intra-oesophageal acid reflux events in patients with gastro-oesophageal reflux disease. *Alimentary Pharmacology & Therapeutics.* **25**: 93–101.

139 Richter JE (2007) The many manifestations of gastroesophageal reflux disease: presentation, evaluation, and treatment. *Gastroenterology Clinics of North America.* **36**: 577–599, viii–ix.

140 Tran T et al. (2007) Meta-analysis: the efficacy of over-the-counter gastro-oesophageal reflux disease therapies. *Alimentary Pharmacology & Therapeutics.* **25**: 143–153.

141 Dore MP et al. (2007) Effect of antisecretory therapy on atypical symptoms in gastroesophageal reflux disease. *Digestive Diseases and Sciences.* **52**: 463–468.

142 Khan M et al. (2007) Medical treatments in the short term management of reflux oesophagitis. Cochrane Database of Systematic Reviews. CD003244.

143 Sifrim D et al. (2007) Review article: acidity and volume of the refluxate in the genesis of gastro-oesophageal reflux disease symptoms. Alimentary Pharmacology & Therapeutics. 25: 1003–1017.

144 Camilleri M (2007) Functional dyspepsia: mechanisms of symptom generation and appropriate management of patients. Gastroenterology Clinics of North America. 36: 649–664, xi–x.

145 Saad RJ and Chey WD (2006) Review article: current and emerging therapies for functional dyspepsia. Alimentary Pharmacology & Therapeutics. 24: 475–492.

146 Lichter I (1993) Results of antiemetic management in terminal illness. Journal of Palliative Care. 9 (2): 19–21.

147 Tjeersdma H et al. (1993) Voluntary suppression of defecation delays gastric emptying. Digestive Diseases and Sciences. 38: 832–836.

148 Barkin J et al. (1986) Pancreatic carcinoma is associated with delayed gastric emptying. Digestive Diseases and Sciences. 31: 265–267.

149 Abrahamsson H and Abrahamsson H (2007) Treatment options for patients with severe gastroparesis. Gut. 56: 877–883.

150 Schuurkes JAJ et al. (1986) Stimulation of gastroduodenal motor activity: dopaminergic and cholinergic modulation. Drug Development Research. 8: 233–241.

151 Jeurnink SM et al. (2007) Stent versus gastrojejunostomy for the palliation of gastric outlet obstruction: a systematic review. BMC Gastroenterology. 7: 18.

152 De-Conno F et al. (1991) Continuous subcutaneous infusion of hyoscine butylbromide reduces secretions in patients with gastrointestinal obstruction. Journal of Pain and Symptom Management. 6: 484–486.

153 Mercadante S et al. (2000) Comparison of octreotide and hyoscine butylbromide in controlling gastrointestinal symptoms due to malignant inoperable bowel obstruction. Support Care Cancer. 8: 188–191.

154 Borison HL and Wang SC (1953) Physiology and pharmacology of vomiting. Pharmacological Reviews. 5: 193–230.

155 Borison H and McCarthy L (1983) Neuropharmacologic mechanisms of emesis. In: J Laszlo (ed) Antiemetics and Cancer Chemotherapy. Williams and Wilkins, Baltimore, pp. 6–20.

156 Andrews P et al. (1998) Neuropharmacology of emesis and its relevance to anti-emetic therapy. Support Care Cancer. 6: 197–203.

157 Pleuvry B (2006) Physiology and pharmacology of nausea and vomiting. Anaesthesia & intensive care medicine. 7: 473–477.

158 Borison H et al. (1984) Role of the area postrema in vomiting and related function. Federal Proceedings. 43: 295–298.

159 Twycross RG et al. (1997) The use of low dose levomepromazine (methotrimeprazine) in the management of nausea and vomiting. Progress in Palliative Care. 5: 49–53.

160 Bentley A and Boyd K (2001) Use of clinical pictures in the management of nausea and vomiting: a prospective audit. Palliative Medicine. 15: 247–253.

161 Feuer D and Broadley K (1999) Systematic review and meta-analysis of corticosteroids for the resolution of malignant bowel obstruction in advanced gynaecological and gastrointestinal cancers. Annals of Oncology. 10: 1035–1041.

162 Laval G et al. (2000) The use of steroids in the management of inoperable intestinal obstruction in terminal cancer patients: do they remove the obstruction? Palliative Medicine. 14: 3–10.

163 Baines M (1987) Medical management of intestinal obstruction. Bailliere's Clinical Oncology. 1: 357–371.

164 Krebs H and Goplerud D (1987) Mechanical intestinal obstruction in patients with gynecologic disease: a review of 368 patients. American Journal of Obstetrics and Gynecology. 157: 577–583.

165 Watt AM et al. (2007) Self-expanding metallic stents for relieving malignant colorectal obstruction: a systematic review. Annals of Surgery. 246: 24–30.

166 Song HY et al. (2007) A dual-design expandable colorectal stent for malignant colorectal obstruction: results of a multicenter study. Endoscopy. 39: 448–454.

167 Mercadante S et al. (2007) Medical treatment for inoperable malignant bowel obstruction: a qualitative systematic review. Journal of Pain and Symptom Management. 33: 217–223.

168 Eisen GM et al. (2002) Acute colonic pseudo-obstruction. Gastrointestinal Endoscopy. 56: 789–792.

169 Harris A and Cantwell B (1986) Mechanisms and treatment of cytotoxic-induced nausea and vomiting. In: C Davis et al. (eds) Nausea and Vomiting: Mechanisms and Treatment. Springer-Verlag, Berlin, pp. 78–93.

170 Mercadante S et al. (2004) Aggressive pharmacological treatment for reversing malignant bowel obstruction. Journal of Pain and Symptom Management. 28: 412–416.

171 Abbas S et al. (2007) Oral water soluble contrast for the management of adhesive small bowel obstruction.[update of Cochrane Database Syst Rev. 2005; (1): CD004651; PMID: 15674958]. Cochrane Database of Systematic Reviews. CD004651.

172 Mystakidou K et al. (2002) Comparison of octreotide administration vs conservative treatment in the management of inoperable bowel obstruction in patients with far advanced cancer: a randomized, double-blind, controlled clinical trial. Anticancer Research. 22: 1187–1192.

www.palliativedrugs.com

173 Ashby M et al. (1991) Percutaneous gastrostomy as a venting procedure in palliative care. *Palliative Medicine.* **5**: 147–150.

174 Rubiales AS et al. (2006) Neostigmine for refractory constipation in advanced cancer patients. *Journal of Pain and Symptom Management.* **32**: 204–205.

175 Goodman M et al. (2005) Constipation management in palliative care: a survey of practices in the United Kingdom. *Journal of Pain and Symptom Management.* **29**: 238–244.

176 Larkin PJ et al. (2008) The management of constipation in palliative care: clinical practice recommendations. *Palliative Medicine.* **22**: 796–807.

177 Thompson WG et al. (1999) Functional bowel disorders and functional abdominal pain. *Gut.* **45 Suppl 2**: II43–47.

178 Sykes N (1998) The relationship between opioid use and laxative use in terminally ill cancer patients. *Palliative Medicine.* **12**: 375–382.

179 Davis MP (2008) Cancer constipation: Are opioids really the culprit? *Supportive Care in Cancer.* **16**: 427–429.

180 Radbruch L et al. (2000) Constipation and the use of laxatives: a comparison between transdermal fentanyl and oral morphine. *Palliative Medicine.* **14**: 111–119.

181 Daeninck P and Bruera E (1999) Reduction in constipation and laxative requirements following opioid rotation to methadone: a report of four cases. *Journal of Pain and Symptom Management.* **18**: 303–309.

182 Wilder-Smith C and Bettiga A (1997) The analgesic tramadol has minimal effect on gastrointestinal motor function. *British Journal of Clinical Pharmacology.* **43**: 71–75.

183 Muller S et al. (1996) Genotoxicity of the laxative drug components emodin, aloe-emodin and danthron in mammalian cells: Topoisomerase II mediated? *Mutation Research.* **371**: 165–173.

184 Mueller S and Stopper H (1999) Characterization of the genotoxicity of anthraquinones in mammalian cells. *Biochimica et Biophysica Acta.* **1428**: 406–414.

185 Twycross RG and Harcourt JMV (1991) The use of laxatives at a palliative care centre. *Palliative Medicine.* **5**: 27–33.

186 Fallon M and Hanks G (1999) Morphine, constipation and performance status in advanced cancer patients. *Palliative Medicine.* **13**: 159–160.

187 Culbert P et al. (1998) Highly effective new oral therapy for faecal impaction. *British Journal of General Practice.* **48**: 1599–1600.

188 Culbert P et al. (1998) Highly effective oral therapy (polyethylene glycol/electrolyte solution) for faecal impaction and severe constipation. *Clinical Drug Investigation.* **16**: 355–360.

189 Attar A et al. (1999) Comparison of a low dose polyethylene glycol electrolyte solution with lactulose for treatment of chronic constipation. *Gut.* **44**: 226–230.

190 Portenoy RK et al. (2008) Subcutaneous methylnaltrexone for the treatment of opioid-induced constipation in patients with advanced illness: a double-blind, randomized, parallel group, dose-ranging study. *Journal of Pain and Symptom Management.* **35**: 458–468.

191 Thomas J et al. (2008) Methylnaltrexone for opioid-induced constipation in advanced illness. *The New England Journal of Medicine.* **358**: 2332–2343.

192 Ramesh P et al. (1998) Managing morphine-induced constipation: a controlled comparison of an Ayurvedic formulation and senna. *Journal of Pain and Symptom Management.* **16**: 240–244.

193 Twycross RG and Lack SA (1986) *Control of Alimentary Symptoms in Far Advanced Cancer.* Churchill Livingstone, Edinburgh, pp. 173–174.

194 Goldman M (1993) Hazards of phosphate enemas. *Gastroenterology Today.* **3**: 16–17.

195 von Roth W and von Beschke K (1988) Pharmakokinetik und laxierende wirkung von bisacodyl nach gabe verschiedener zubereitungsformen. *Arzneimittel Forschung Drug Research.* **38**: 570–574.

196 Wald A (2008) Management and prevention of fecal impaction. *Current Gastroenterology Reports.* **10**: 499–501.

197 Cherny N (2008) Evaluation and management of treatment-related diarrhea in patients with advanced cancer: a review. *Journal of Pain and Symptom Management.* **36**: 413–423.

198 Rolston K et al. (1989) Diarrhea in patients infected with the human immunodeficiency virus. *American Journal of Medicine.* **86**: 137–138.

199 Dean AP and Reed WD (1991) Diarrhoea – an unrecognised hazard of coleliac plexus block. *Australian and New Zealand Journal of Medicine.* **21**: 47–48.

200 Bignardi GE (1998) Risk factors for Clostridium difficile infection. *The Journal of Hospital Infection.* **40**: 1–15.

201 Pepin J et al. (2004) Clostridium difficile-associated diarrhea in a region of Quebec from 1991 to 2003: a changing pattern of disease severity. *Canadian Medical Association Journal.* **171**: 466–472.

202 Thomas C et al. (2003) Antibiotics and hospital-acquired Clostridium difficile-associated diarrhoea: a systematic review. *The Journal of Antimicrobial Chemotherapy.* **51**: 1339–1350.

203 Chitkara YK et al. (1996) Development and implementation of cost-effective guidelines in the laboratory investigation of diarrhea in a community hospital. *Archives of Internal Medicine.* **156**: 1445–1448.

204 Benson AB et al. (2004) Recommended guidelines for the treatment of cancer treatment-induced diarrhea. *Journal of Clinical Oncology.* **22**: 2918–2926.

205 Durai R (2007) Epidemiology, pathogenesis, and management of Clostridium difficile infection. *Digestive Diseases and Sciences.* **52**: 2958–2962.

206 Mennie A et al. (1975) Treatment of radiation-induced gastrointestinal distress with acetylsalicylate. Lancet. **2**: 942–943.

207 Cascinu S et al. (2000) High-dose loperamide in the treatment of 5-fluorouracil-induced diarrhea in colorectal cancer patients. Support Care Cancer. **8**: 65–67.

208 Yavuz M et al. (2000) A randomized study of the efficacy of octreotide versus diphenoxylate on radiation-induced diarrhea. ASCO Online. **Visited 21**: Abstract 2370.

209 Sharma R et al. (2005) Management of chemotherapy-induced nausea, vomiting, oral mucositis, and diarrhoea. The Lancet Oncology. **6**: 93–102.

210 Govindarajan R et al. (2000) Effect of thalidomide on gastrointestinal toxic effects of irinotecan. Lancet. **356**: 566–567.

211 Crane SJ et al. Chronic gastrointestinal symptoms in the elderly. Clinics in Geriatric Medicine. **23**: 721–734.

212 Harvey M and Dunlop R (1996) Octreotide and the secretory effects of advanced cancer. Palliative Medicine. **10**: 346–347.

213 Runyon B (1994) Care of patients with ascites. New England Journal of Medicine. **330**: 337–342.

214 Hird V et al. (1989) Malignant ascites: review of the literature, and an update on monoclonal antibody-targeted therapy. European Journal of Obstetrics, Gynaecology and Reproductive Biology. **32**: 37–45.

215 Parsons S et al. (1996) Malignant ascites. British Journal of Surgery. **83**: 6–14.

216 McGibbon A et al. (2007) An evidence-based manual for abdominal paracentesis. Digestive Diseases and Sciences. **52**: 3307–3315.

217 Macdonald R et al. (2006) Ovarian cancer and ascites: A questionnaire on current management in the United kingdom. Journal of Palliative Medicine. **9**: 1264–1270.

218 McNamara P (2000) Paracentesis – an effective method of symptom control in the palliative care setting? Palliative Medicine. **14**: 62–64.

219 Becker G et al. (2006) Malignant ascites: systematic review and guideline for treatment. European Journal of Cancer. **42**: 589–597.

220 Rosenberg S et al. (2004) Comparison of percutaneous management techniques for recurrent malignant ascites. Journal of Vascular and Interventional Radiology. **15**: 1129–1131.

221 Osterlee J (1980) peritoneovenous shunting for ascites in cancer patients. British Journal of Surgery. **67**: 663–666.

222 Greenway B et al. (1982) Control of malignant ascites with spironolactone. British Journal of Surgery. **69**: 441–442.

223 Fernandez-Esparrach G et al. (1997) Diuretic requirements after therapeutic paracentesis in non-azotemic patients with cirrhosis. A randomized double-blind trial of spironolactone versus placebo. Journal of Hepatology. **26**: 614–620; erratum 1430.

224 Pockros P et al. (1992) Mobilization of malignant ascites with diuretics is dependent on ascitic fluid characteristics. Gastroenterology. **103**: 1302–1306.

225 Moore KP et al. (2003) The management of ascites in cirrhosis: report on the consensus conference of the International Ascites Club. Hepatology. **38**: 258–266.

226 Santos J et al. (2003) Spironolactone alone or in combination with furosemide in the treatment of moderate ascites in nonazotemic cirrhosis. A randomized comparative study of efficacy and safety. Journal of Hepatology. **39**: 187–192.

227 Fogel M et al. (1981) Diuresis in the ascitic patient: a randomized controlled trial of three regimens. Journal of Clinical Gastroenterology. **3**: 73–80.

228 Gines P et al. (1987) Comparison of paracentesis and diuretics in the treatment of cirrhotics with tense ascites. Gastroenterology. **93**: 234–241.

229 Sharma S and Walsh D (1995) Management of symptomatic malignant ascites with diuretics: two case reports and a review of the literature. Journal of Pain and Symptom Management. **10**: 237–242.

230 Kalambokis G et al. (2006) The effects of treatment with octreotide, diuretics, or both on portal hemodynamics in nonazotemic cirrhotic patients with ascites. Journal of Clinical Gastroenterology. **40**: 342–346.

231 Lenaerts A et al. (2006) Effects of clonidine on diuretic response in ascitic patients with cirrhosis and activation of sympathetic nervous system. Hepatology. **44**: 844–849.

232 Mackey J et al. (2000) A phase II trial of triamcinolone hexacetanide for symptomatic recurrent malignant ascites. Journal of Pain and Symptom Management. **19**: 193–199.

233 Jenkin RP et al. (2008) The use of intraperitoneal triamcinolone acetonide for the management of recurrent malignant ascites in a patient with non-Hodgkin's lymphoma. Journal of Pain and Symptom Management. **36**: e4–5.

234 Caims W and Malone R (1999) Octreotide as an agent for the relief of malignant ascites in palliative care patients. Palliative Medicine. **13**: 429–430.

235 Widjaja A et al. (1999) Octreotide for therapy of chylous ascites in yellow nail syndrome. Gastroenterology. **116**: 1017–1018.

236 Ferrandiere M et al. (2000) Chylous ascites following radical nephrectomy: efficacy of octreotide as treatment of ruptured thoracic duct. Intensive Care and Medicine. **26**: 484–485.

4: RESPIRATORY SYMPTOMS

BREATHLESSNESS

Breathlessness is the subjective experience of breathing discomfort. It comprises qualitatively distinct sensations which vary in intensity. The experience derives from interactions among multiple physiological, psychological, social and environmental factors and may induce secondary physiological and behavioural responses.[1] Breathlessness on exertion is a normal (physiological) experience, occurring at lower levels of exertion with physical deconditioning and increasing age. It becomes pathological when it limits activities of daily living or is associated with mood disturbance, e.g. anxiety.

Breathlessness is common in patients with advanced cancer, particularly those with involvement of the lungs. About 1/2 of the patients with incurable lung cancer report breathlessness interfering with physical activities and 1/4 with their mood, enjoyment of life and relationships.[2]

Patients with lung cancer commonly report that breathlessness:[3,4]
- is intermittent, occurring in episodes lasting 5–15min precipitated, for example, by exertion, bending over, talking, anxiety, and associated with feelings of exhaustion
- restricts general activities of daily living and social functioning leading to a loss of independence and of role, resulting in frustration, anger and depression
- induces feelings of anxiety, fear, panic, hopelessness and impending death (Figure 4.1).

Explanations for breathlessness in the absence of lung involvement include limb $\pm$ respiratory muscle weakness related to physical deconditioning or cachexia. Even in patients who are breathless on exertion, limb muscle fatigue is frequently reported as contributing to the limitation of activities of daily living.[6]

The prevalence of breathlessness in other advanced diseases ranges between 90–95% (COPD), 60–90% (heart disease) and 10–60% (AIDS and renal disease).[7]

The incidence of breathlessness increases as death nears; it is present in 70% of patients with cancer in the last few weeks before death and is severe in 25% of patients in their last week of life.[8] Breathlessness is an independent predictor of survival second only to performance status.[9]

Pathogenesis
Involuntary rhythmic respiration is generated by the central pattern generator in the brain stem and is primarily concerned with the regulation of arterial carbon dioxide (and thus

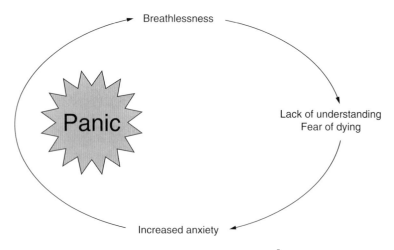

Figure 4.1 Breathlessness is a common trigger for panic.[5]

acid–base balance) and maintenance of adequate arterial oxygen. It is modulated by various neurotransmitters and neuromodulators relaying information from:
- higher centres, e.g. level of arousal, emotion, motor cortex activity, temperature
- chemoreceptors, e.g. hypoxia, hypercapnia, acidosis
- airways, e.g. distortion or collapse
- respiratory muscles, e.g. weakness, fatigue (Table 4.1).

The voluntary control of respiration allows the central pattern generator to be overridden temporarily to allow activities such as talking, swallowing and coughing. Generally, sensations associated with breathing do not reach consciousness because they are filtered or gated out. Cognitive awareness occurs when their intensity exceeds a threshold allowing them to pass through the gate and/or the threshold is lowered by the background physiological or cognitive/behavioural/mood state, e.g. level of attention, anxiety (Figure 4.2).

During exertion, there is an increase in the effort or work of breathing reflecting the increased motor command to the inspiratory muscles. In health, this will be matched by an appropriate increase in ventilation, signalled by changes in pressure, airflow or movement of the lungs and chest wall. Thus, breathing is generally perceived as comfortable and appropriate for the level of exertion.

In situations where the mechanical response of the respiratory system cannot meet the demands of the motor command, a mismatch exists (known as neuromechanical dissociation).[1,11] Such a mismatch may arise with:
- increased ventilatory drive, e.g. exercise, limb muscle dysfunction or weakness, mood disturbance (anxiety, panic disorder, depression)
- respiratory muscle abnormalities, e.g. neuromuscular diseases
- abnormal ventilatory impedance, e.g. an increased resistive and/or elastic load
- reduced ventilatory efficacy, e.g. diseases of the lung parenchyma and pulmonary vasculature.

Table 4.1 Neurotransmitters and neuromodulators involved in the control of breathing[10]

Substance	Effect on respiration
Neurotransmitters responsible for respiratory rhythm	
Glutamate	Stimulates central generation and transmission of respiratory rhythm
GABA	Transmission of phasic waves of inhibition
Glycine	Transmission of phasic waves of inhibition
Neuromodulators responsible for shaping respiratory pattern	
Acetylcholine	Stimulatory or inhibitory
Serotonin/5HT	Mainly inhibitory
Noradrenaline (norepinephrine)	Mainly stimulatory
Adrenaline (epinephrine)	Mainly stimulatory
Dopamine	Mainly stimulatory (respiratory frequency)
Opioids	Inhibitory (interfere with the effect of glutamate)
Substance P	Mainly stimulatory (tidal volume)
Somatostatin	Inhibitory
Cholecystokinin	Stimulatory or inhibitory
Thyrotropin-releasing hormone	Stimulatory

In these situations, the effort of breathing will be disproportionately high for the level of ventilation and, once a threshold intensity is reached, this will be perceived as abnormal and unpleasant. The latter determines the emotional response (e.g. fear, distress), which in turn leads to a behavioural response, e.g. cessation of activity, seeking help, pursed lip breathing, in order to alleviate the breathlessness and thus the fear and distress.

These responses will be influenced by the patient's previous experience, expectation, personality, level of attention, behavioural style and emotional state. For some, extreme fear will precipitate panic which, via the autonomic nervous system, leads to respiratory and circulatory responses. These may further increase respiratory discomfort.[11]

Causes
Breathlessness in advanced cancer is often multifactorial (Box 4.A). Most patients will have:[12,13]

- parenchymal or pleural disease
- a history of smoking
- abnormal spirometry (mixed > restrictive > obstructive pattern)
- weak inspiratory muscles.

About 1/2 are hypoxic and about 1/5 have evidence of concurrent cardiac ischaemia or arrhythmia.[12] Although inspiratory muscle weakness, a history of smoking and a raised $PaCO_2$ all appear to exacerbate breathlessness, anxiety is the only feature to consistently correlate with breathlessness.[12,14,15]

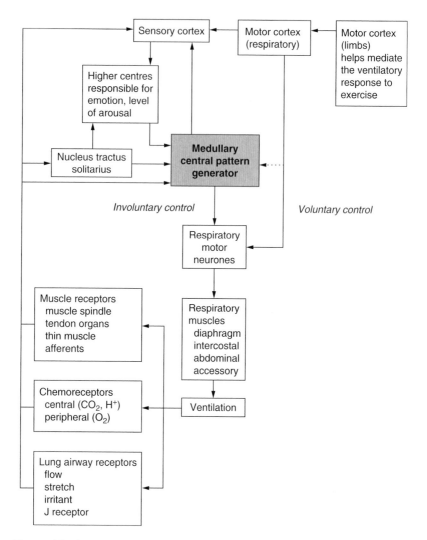

Figure 4.2 A simple model of the control of breathing and respiratory sensation.

Evaluation

The history, examination and appropriate investigation(s) will identify pulmonary, cardiac or neuromuscular abnormalities (Box 4.B). A comprehensive evaluation will also include an evaluation of the patient's knowledge, beliefs and behaviours associated with their breathlessness and cancer, and the impact it has upon them.[16]

Try to determine the cause of any recent deterioration because rapid changes often provide an opportunity for corrective treatment, such as pleural aspiration or antibacterials.

Box 4.A Causes of breathlessness

Cancer
Pleural effusion
Obstruction of a large airway
Replacement of lung by cancer
Lymphangitis carcinomatosa
Cancer micro-emboli in the pulmonary
　vascular bed
Cardiac metastases or direct invasion
Pericardial effusion
Phrenic nerve palsy
SVC obstruction
Massive ascites
Abdominal distension
Cachexia
　respiratory muscle weakness

Treatment
Pneumonectomy
Radiation-induced fibrosis
Chemotherapy-induced
　pneumonitis
　fibrosis
　cardiomyopathy
Progestogens
　stimulate ventilation
　increase sensitivity to CO_2

Debility
Anaemia
Atelectasis
Pulmonary embolism
Pneumonia
Empyema
Muscle weakness

Concurrent
COPD
Asthma
Heart failure
Acidosis
Fever
Pneumothorax
Anxiety
Panic attack
Panic disorder
Depression

Management
Breathlessness in advanced cancer can be divided into three types:
- breathlessness on exertion (prognosis = months−years)
- breathlessness at rest (prognosis = weeks−months)
- terminal breathlessness (prognosis = days−weeks).[7]

The relative importance of the three treatment categories (correct the correctable, non-drug treatment, drug treatment) changes as the patient's condition deteriorates (Figure 4.3).

Correct the correctable
Particularly while the patient is still ambulant, consideration should be given to the identification and correction of correctable causes (Table 4.2):
- is the breathlessness caused by the cancer?
- can the cancer be modified?
- can the impact of the cancer be modified?

Non-drug treatment
Non-drug treatment begins by exploring the patient's experience of breathlessness (Box 4.C). Open acknowledgement of the fear and feelings of terror and panic

---

Box 4.B   Evaluation of the breathless patient with cancer[17]

History
Speed of onset.
Associated symptoms, e.g. pain, cough, haemoptysis, sputum, stridor, wheeze.
Exacerbating and relieving factors.
Symptoms suggestive of hyperventilation:
• poor relationship of breathlessness to exertion
• presence of hyperventilation attacks
• breathlessness at rest
• rapid fluctuations in breathlessness within minutes
• fear of sudden death during an attack
• breathlessness varying with social situations.
Past medical history, e.g. history of cardiovascular disease.
Drug history, e.g. drugs precipitating fluid retention or bronchospasm.
Symptoms of anxiety or depression.
Social circumstances and support networks.
Level of independence:
• ability to care for themselves
• coping strategies.
What does the breathlessness mean to the patient?
How do they feel when they are breathless?

Examination
Central cyanosis (a bluish tinge to the tongue and oral mucous membranes) indicates arterial hypoxaemia. It is visible when *tissue* microcirculation has a de-oxygenated Hb of ~4–5g/dL; this occurs when *arterial* de-oxygenated Hb is ~1.5g/dL. When Hb is normal, this is seen when SaO_2 falls to about 90% at a PaO_2 of about 7.7kPa (58mmHg). In anaemia, PaO_2 must be lower to achieve the required de-oxygenated Hb. Thus, cyanosis is not a very sensitive sign; *it may be absent in severe anaemia despite hypoxaemia, and conversely be present in polycythaemia despite normal arterial oxygen.*
Observe the patient walking a set distance or carrying out a specific task.
Does hyperventilation reproduce symptoms?

Investigations
Common
Chest radiograph.
Haemoglobin concentration.
Less common
Ultrasound scan (useful for differentiating between pleural effusion and solid tumour).
Oxygen saturation (may be useful if evaluating value of oxygen).
Peak flow/simple spirometry (evaluating response to bronchodilators or corticosteroids).
ECG.
Echocardiography.
CT pulmonary angiography.

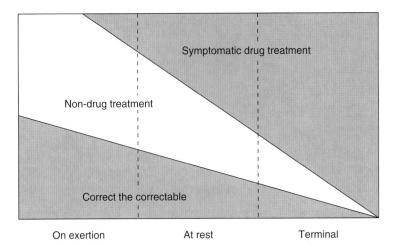

Figure 4.3 Treatment for severe breathlessness in advanced cancer.

associated with the acute exacerbations, e.g. when climbing stairs, is the key to enable the patient (and the family) to cope better. The patient must be assured that they will not die during an attack. Emphasize that 'Although you may feel you're suffocating, you've always recovered, and you always will'.

Breathing retraining, panic management and activity pacing all ease breathlessness in patients with lung cancer.[20,21] Any health professional with an interest can be trained to offer these techniques, although generally nurses, occupational therapists and physiotherapists have taken the lead.

Breathing retraining
Shallow, rapid breathing is an ineffective and inefficient pattern of breathing that contributes to anxiety and panic. Breathing retraining aims to:
• promote a relaxed and gentle breathing pattern
• minimize the work of breathing
• establish a sense of control over breathing that aids confidence in coping with breathless episodes.

Approaches include:
• *relaxation therapies*: which encourage slow regular deep breathing
• *diaphragmatic breathing*: patients are taught to consciously expand their abdominal wall during inspiratory diaphragm descent. Outward abdominal excursion can be detected by placing one hand on the abdomen and the other on the chest. When carried out in the supine position 3 times a day for 10–20min for 6–8 weeks, improvement can be seen in breathing pattern, blood gases and expiratory muscle strength. Clear benefit from diaphragmatic breathing on function and breathlessness has not been shown[22]
• *pursed lip breathing*: performed as nasal inspiration followed by expiratory blowing against partially closed lips, expiration taking twice as long as inspiration. Some patients adopt this instinctively. Encourage its use during periods of increased ventilation. Can lead to improvements in breathing pattern, respiratory muscle function and blood gases in patients with COPD, but improvement in breathlessness is variable.[22]

Table 4.2 Correctable causes of breathlessness

Cause	Treatment
Respiratory infection	Antibiotics Physiotherapy
COPD/asthma	Bronchodilators Corticosteroids Physiotherapy
Hypoxia	Trial of oxygen (see p.156)
Obstruction of trachea, bronchus	Corticosteroids Radiotherapy LASER Stent (see Box 4.D)
Obstruction of SVC	Corticosteroids Radiotherapy Chemotherapy (e.g. SCLC, lymphoma) Stent (see Box 4.D)
Lymphangitis carcinomatosa (see p.173)	Corticosteroids Diuretics Bronchodilators
Pleural effusion (see p.167)	Thoracocentesis Drainage and pleurodesis
Ascites (see p.127)	Diuretics Paracentesis
Pericardial effusion (see p.368)	Paracentesis Corticosteroids
Anaemia (see p.229)	Blood transfusion
Heart failure	Diuretics ACE inhibitors
Pulmonary embolism	Anticoagulation (for more information, see *PCF3*)
Respiratory muscle weakness	Assisted ventilation, e.g. in selected patients with MND/ALS (see Box 4.E, p.154)

Positioning

Some patients with COPD find breathlessness improves in positions which:
- increase abdominal pressure, improving the efficiency of the flattened diaphragm, reducing abdominal paradoxical breathing and accessory muscle use, e.g. leaning forward with arms/elbows resting on the knees or a table, or lying prone
- maximize ventilation–perfusion matching; patients with unilateral broncho-pulmonary disease, e.g. collapse, consolidation, or pleural effusion are less likely to experience a deterioration in blood gases when lying on their side with the normal lung down (this advantage is lost with a large pleural effusion).

Box 4.C Non-drug treatment of breathlessness[17]

Exploring the perception of the patient and carers
What is the meaning of the breathlessness to the patient and to the carers?

Explore anxieties, particularly fear of sudden death when breathless.

Inform the patient and carers that breathlessness in itself is not life-threatening.

State what is/is not likely to happen, e.g. 'You won't choke or suffocate to death'.

Decide on realistic goals and help the patient adjust to the progressive deterioration.

Help the patient to cope with and adjust to loss of role, abilities, etc.

Maximizing the feeling of control over breathlessness
Breathing control advice.

Relaxation techniques.

Plan of action for acute episodes:
• simple written instructions outlining a step-by-step plan
• increase confidence in coping with acute episodes.

Use of an electric fan.

Complementary therapies benefit some patients.

Maximizing functional ability
Encourage exertion to breathlessness to increase tolerance/desensitize to breathlessness and maintain fitness.

Evaluation by district nurse, occupational therapist, physiotherapist and social worker may all be necessary to identify where additional support is required.

Reduce feelings of personal and social isolation
Meet others in a similar situation.

Attendance at a day centre.

Respite admissions.

Desensitization
Exposure to greater than usual levels of breathlessness in a safe environment may increase a patient's confidence to cope with the symptom. Exercise in a supervised environment enables some patients to overcome the anxiety provoked by exertional breathlessness and increase their exercise tolerance.

Drug treatment
For more information, see *PCF3*.

Severe breathlessness in the last days of life:
• no patient should die with distressing breathlessness
• failure to relieve terminal breathlessness is a failure to use drug treatment correctly
• give an opioid with a sedative-anxiolytic parenterally, e.g. morphine and midazolam by CSCI, and p.r.n.[23]
• if the patient becomes agitated or confused (sometimes aggravated by a benzodiazepine), haloperidol or levomepromazine should be added (see p.430).

Box 4.D   Local techniques to restore or maintain airway patency[18]

With immediate effect
An immediately effective treatment is required when airway obstruction is life-threatening, e.g. when acute or when stenosis > 50% of lumen:
- LASER, e.g. neodymium yttrium aluminium garnet (Nd:YAG):
  ▷ coagulates and vaporizes tissue
  ▷ aids removal of endobronchial cancer via rigid bronchoscope
  ▷ often used with stenting
- airway stent:
  ▷ includes self-expanding nitinol wall-covered stents
  ▷ most effective in obstruction of the trachea
  ▷ complications include cancer ingrowth, migration, excessive granulation tissue.

Delayed effect
- brachytherapy
- cryotherapy
- photodynamic therapy.

Note: if an obstruction causes atelectasis which persists for > 4 weeks, complete re-expansion of the lung is generally considered unlikely even when the obstruction is removed.

Box 4.E   Assisted ventilation[19]

Assisted ventilation is used:
- short-term in patients with acute ventilatory failure, e.g. an exacerbation of COPD
- long-term in patients with chronic ventilatory failure, e.g. respiratory muscle weakness in MND/ALS.

Long-term assisted ventilation is generally considered when there are symptoms or signs of:
- *both* nocturnal hypoxaemia and/or hypercapnia, e.g. disturbed sleep, morning headache, poor concentration, daytime sleepiness; nocturnal oxygen desaturation or increased morning $PaCO_2$
- *and* respiratory muscle weakness, e.g. breathlessness on exertion, at rest, on lying flat (orthopnoea); reduced FVC or sniff nasal pressure.

Non-invasive and invasive ventilation improves survival in patients with MND/ALS and ventilatory failure, and its use is likely to increase. A pre-emptive discussion is recommended about what to do when the non-invasive ventilation is no longer able to compensate for the effects of disease progression, e.g. change to invasive ventilation or withdraw all assisted ventilation. This is a good example of a situation where a patient can use an Advance Decision to Refuse Treatment (ADRT) to clearly state their wishes (see p.409).

Generally, symptomatic drug treatments for breathlessness are used after appropriate corrective and non-drug treatments have been fully exploited.

Bronchodilators

Patients with lung cancer and COPD tend to report the highest levels of breathlessness. Airflow obstruction is often undiagnosed and consequently untreated. Bronchoconstriction is not always associated with wheeze, particularly in patients with a history of chronic asthma, COPD or heavy smoking. The diagnosis of asthma or COPD is mainly based on the history and examination, supported by objective tests, e.g. peak expiratory flow and the response to treatment (for more information see *PCF3*).

In palliative care, unless asthma is suspected, spirometric reversibility testing is likely to play a minor role. When airflow obstruction is suspected, evaluating the impact on symptoms of a 1–2 week trial of a bronchodilator is a more pragmatic and probably more relevant approach than a reversibility test.

Bronchodilator therapy, e.g. a β_2-adrenergic receptor stimulant $\pm$ an antimuscarinic, inhaled via a spacer or nebulizer, improves breathlessness in most cancer patients with COPD even without any changes in ventilatory indices.[24,25] Both classes of drug improve breathlessness by airway bronchodilation and/or reducing air-trapping at rest (static hyperinflation) and on exertion (dynamic hyperinflation). A reduction in hyperinflation probably explains why clinical benefit may be seen in patients with COPD with little or no change in the FEV_1.

Morphine

Generally, opioids are more beneficial in patients who are breathless at rest than in those who are breathless only on exertion. Even with maximal exertion, breathlessness generally recovers within a few minutes, much quicker than the time it takes to locate, administer and obtain benefit from an opioid. Thus, non-drug measures are of primary importance in managing breathlessness on exertion.

Morphine and other opioids reduce the ventilatory response to hypercapnia, hypoxia and exercise, thereby decreasing respiratory effort and breathlessness. Improvement is seen at doses that do *not* cause respiratory depression.[26–31] In opioid-naïve patients:
- start with small doses of morphine, e.g. 2.5–5mg PO p.r.n.; larger doses may be poorly tolerated
- if $\geqslant 2$ doses/24h are needed, prescribe morphine regularly and titrate the dose according to response, duration of effect and undesirable effects
- relatively small doses may suffice, e.g. 20–60mg/24h.[26,27,29,30,32–35]

In patients already taking morphine for pain and with:
- severe breathlessness ($\geqslant 7/10$), a dose that is 100% or more of the q4h analgesic dose may be needed
- moderate breathlessness (4–6/10), a dose equivalent to 50–100% of the q4h analgesic dose may suffice
- mild breathlessness ($\leqslant 3/10$), a dose equivalent to 25–50% of the q4h analgesic dose may suffice.

However, as with pain, individual titration is required for optimal benefit. In some patients, morphine by CSCI is better tolerated and provides greater relief, possibly by avoiding the peaks (with undesirable effects) and troughs (with loss of effect) of oral medication. If using an alternative opioid to morphine, adopt the same approach as above. The use of oral transmucosal fentanyl (Actiq®) has been reported in a small case series.[36]

Nebulized morphine

A systematic review supports the use of opioids for the relief of breathlessness by the oral and parenteral routes, but *not* by nebulizer.[37]

Apart from an RCT, the use of nebulized morphine should be discouraged.[37–43] Potential adverse events include:
- the release of histamine from mast cells by the morphine → bronchoconstriction
- unexpected respiratory depression (as reported in a patient already receiving oral morphine; an additional 4mg via a nebulizer caused serious respiratory depression necessitating artificial ventilation for several hours).[44]

Anxiolytics

Unlike opioids, anxiolytics probably do not have a specific anti-breathlessness effect.[45] Nonetheless, there is an association between breathlessness and anxiety, and reducing anxiety may help a patient to cope better with their breathlessness (see p.187). Non-drug approaches to managing anxiety ± panic attacks should be considered before using drugs (see p.189). Panic attacks generally settle within minutes, much quicker than the time it takes to administer and benefit from an anxiolytic. If a patient is severely disabled by their anxiety or panic, consider if a pathological anxiety, panic or depression disorder exists, which requires more specific therapy, e.g. an antidepressant.

If the patient is very anxious, diazepam can be given, e.g. 2–10mg stat, 5–20mg at bedtime, 2–5mg p.r.n. Reduce the dose if the patient becomes drowsy as a result of drug accumulation. Some centres use lorazepam SL b.d. and p.r.n. Midazolam with an opioid is of particular benefit in relieving terminal breathlessness (see p.426).[23]

Buspirone which acts predominantly via serotonin $5HT_{1A}$-receptors is free of sedative or respiratory depressant effects.[46] It is as effective as diazepam in the relief of generalized anxiety but not panic disorder.[47] Buspirone may be a useful alternative to a benzodiazepine when sedation or the risk of ventilatory depression is unacceptable, but trial results in COPD are conflicting. However, the effect of buspirone is not immediate; its anxiolytic effect is seen only after 2–4 weeks.[48–50] This is too slow for most breathless patients with end-stage disease. If used for more stable patients:
- start with 5mg t.d.s.
- if necessary, titrate up to 10–20mg t.d.s.

Antipsychotics have an anxiolytic but not a specific antipanic effect. They are helpful in patients who are anxious and delirious. Haloperidol is the antipsychotic of choice and is without significant respiratory depressant effects.

A cannabinoid, e.g. nabilone 100–250microgram b.d.–q.d.s., is used at some centres in patients with severe breathlessness at risk of developing hypercapnic respiratory failure if given opioids or benzodiazepines. With higher doses, most patients complain of drowsiness and/or dysphoria; hypotension and tachycardia may also be limiting factors.[51]

Oxygen

Oxygen therapy helps to correct most common causes of arterial hypoxaemia (Table 4.3). However, breathlessness is a complicated sensation which does not only relate to oxygen tension. Thus, there is great variation in the response to oxygen; and this cannot be reliably predicted by the level of oxygen saturation at rest, the degree of desaturation on exercise or by the degree of improvement in oxygen saturation.[52–54]

Table 4.3 Common causes of arterial hypoxaemia[55]

	Example	Arterial O_2 level increases with oxygen	Arterial CO_2 level
Alveolar hypoventilation	Respiratory depression Severe COPD Respiratory muscle weakness	Yes	Inevitably increases as ventilation falls; CO_2 level will not respond to oxygen therapy
Diffusion impairment	Lung oedema or fibrosis	Yes	Normal or low due to hypoxia $\rightarrow$ reflex increase in ventilation
Right-to-left shunt	Lung consolidation or atelectasis	No or minimal	May be increased in extremis, e.g. exhaustion in near fatal asthma
Ventilation–perfusion mismatch	Asthma COPD	Yes	

In patients with cancer, oxygen is generally better than air in severely hypoxic patients (SaO_2 < 90%).[53,56] With lesser degrees of hypoxia/normoxia there is no difference in the benefit achieved with oxygen or piped air delivered by nasal prongs.[57]

In patients with COPD, there also seems little difference in benefit between oxygen and compressed air when used p.r.n., e.g. to recover from exercise.[58–60] Even for the minority of patients who could distinguish oxygen from compressed air, there is only 80sec improvement in the time to subjective recovery with oxygen compared with air; about 3.5min vs. 5min.[61]

These findings suggest that the sensation of airflow $\pm$ a cooling effect may be the main determinants of benefit for many patients.[62–66] Breathless patients should be encouraged to test the benefit of a cool draught (open window or fan) before being offered oxygen.

It has been recommended that they should have a formal evaluation, e.g. shuttle walk test,[52] before being offered oxygen. As a minimum, for those breathless at rest, a trial of oxygen therapy should be given via nasal prongs for 10–15min, with pre- and post-evaluations.[52,59,67,68]

A pulse oximeter will help identify patients who are severely hypoxic and for whom it is reasonable to give sufficient oxygen to achieve an SaO_2 > 90%. If benefit is obtained, review again after a longer period of use, e.g. 48h. If the patient has persisted in using the oxygen and has found it useful, it can be continued but, if the patient has any doubts about its benefit, it should be discontinued.

National guidelines on the use of oxygen in acutely ill patients are available.[69] *PCF3* contains advice about:

- prescribing oxygen (Table 4.4).
- long-term/continuous use in patients with COPD, cystic fibrosis, interstitial lung disease, etc.
- in-flight oxygen provision.

Table 4.4 Oxygen therapy in brief

Treatment schedule	Oxygen concentration	Condition
Short-term/ intermittent	High (60%)	Pneumonia, pulmonary embolus, fibrosing alveolitis, acute asthma
Short-term/ intermittent	Low (28%)	Ventilatory failure due to COPD, and other causes. Also cancer, interstitial lung disease, CHF
Long-term/ continuous Ambulatory	Individually titrated, generally low (28%)	Severe disabling breathlessness due to cancer and other progressive life-threatening diseases; also in patients with COPD, cystic fibrosis, interstitial lung disease, pulmonary hypertension, etc. meeting certain criteria

Helium-oxygen mixtures
Helium 79%-oxygen 21% mixture (Heliox®) is less dense and viscous than air.[70] It reduces resistance in the airway when flow is turbulent, and its use helps to reduce the respiratory work required when there is high ventilatory demand or upper airway obstruction.[71–73] It can be used as a temporary measure in patients breathless at rest while more definitive therapy is arranged. A high concentration/non-rebreathing mask must be used for optimal benefit, and the patient's voice will be squeaky.

A mixture containing a higher concentration of oxygen is now available (Heliox28®; helium 72%-oxygen 28%). This improves exercise capacity, SaO_2 and breathlessness in patients with lung cancer[74] and COPD.[75] The reduction in expiratory airflow resistance may benefit COPD patients by reducing the work of breathing and degree of hyperinflation. However, this approach is limited by its expense (each cylinder lasts only 2–3h), and the practical difficulties of transporting a large gas cylinder.

CHEYNE-STOKES RESPIRATION

Cheyne-Stokes respiration is an eponymous term use to describe recurrent central apnoea alternating with a crescendo–diminuendo pattern of tidal volume. Nocturnal Cheyne-Stokes respiration is present in 30–50% of patients with severe stable congestive heart failure (CHF) and may contribute to symptoms such as orthopnoea, paroxysmal nocturnal breathlessness, insomnia, difficulty falling asleep and excessive daytime sleepiness.[76] Physiological changes associated with Cheyne-Stokes respiration, e.g. in heart rate, blood pressure and sympathetic nervous system activity, may be detrimental in heart failure, and cause further deterioration. Cheyne-Stokes respiration is associated with a poorer prognosis, particularly when present during the day.[77,78]

Cheyne-Stokes respiration is also seen after strokes and in sporadic cases of brain stem degeneration or injury.[79-81] In advanced cancer, it is mostly seen in moribund patients.

Physiology
The key mechanism is the fluctuation of $PaCO_2$ levels above and below the apnoeic threshold.[82]

In patients with heart failure, the reduced cardiac output leads to increased sympathetic nervous system activity. Pulmonary congestion may also increase pulmonary vagal afferent traffic. The result is hyperventilation and lower than expected $PaCO_2$ levels when awake and asleep. Relatively small increases in ventilation then reduce $PaCO_2$ levels below a threshold which triggers apnoea. The $PaCO_2$ subsequently increases and stimulates the chemoreceptors causing hyperventilation.

Hypoxaemia develops during the episodes of apnoea increasing the chemoreceptor sensitivity to CO_2 and facilitates arousal from sleep. Both enhance the hyperventilation which subsequently leads to a fall in $PaCO_2$ and the cycle is repeated.

The episodes of apnoea are also associated with diastolic dysfunction, increased sympathetic nervous system activity and a greater risk of arrhythmia.

Diagnosis
Observation of an apnoea in an at-risk patient is suggestive. Diagnostic criteria require each of the following to be present:[83]
- excessive daytime sleepiness or frequent nocturnal arousals/awakenings
- polysomnography showing >5 central apnoeas/hypopnoeas per hour of sleep (polysomnography also helps to differentiate between central and obstructive apnoea which can co-exist in patients with CHF)
- $PaCO_2$ <5.9kPa.

Management
Congestive heart failure (CHF)
- treat the underlying heart failure
- consider nocturnal continuous positive airway pressure (CPAP):[82,84]
  ▷ has other beneficial effects in heart failure, benefit may take 1–3 months
  ▷ improves symptoms
  ▷ improves co-existent obstructive sleep apnoea
- administer nocturnal oxygen 2–4L/min:[82,85]
  ▷ reduces hypoxaemia, number of arousals and improves sleep
  ▷ reduces total duration of Cheyne-Stokes respiration
  ▷ may not improve symptoms
  ▷ no effect on fluctuations in heart rate and blood pressure
- theophylline:[86]
  ▷ reduces total duration of Cheyne-Stokes respiration
  ▷ no effect on cardiac function
  ▷ limited data compared with CPAP and oxygen.

About 40% of patients respond to CPAP or oxygen. Those with more severe Cheyne-Stokes respiration are less likely to respond to either treatment.

Moribund patients
No specific treatment is necessary.

COUGH

Coughing helps clear the central airways of foreign matter, secretions or pus and should generally be encouraged. It is pathological when:
- ineffective
- it adversely affects sleep, rest, eating, or social activities
- it causes other symptoms such as muscle strain, rib fracture, vomiting, syncope, headache, or urinary incontinence.

Cough effectiveness is reduced by factors which:
- decrease expiratory pressure and airflow, i.e. respiratory or abdominal muscle weakness
- increase mucus tenacity, i.e. reduce the water content of secretions
- decrease mucociliary function, e.g. smoking, infection.

In patients with cancer, the prevalence of cough is 50–80%, and is highest in patients with lung cancer.[87] An acute cough is defined as one lasting <3 weeks, a chronic cough >8 weeks.[88]

Pathogenesis
Cough is caused by mechanical and/or chemical stimulation of:
- rapidly adapting myelinated stretch ('irritant') and C-fibre receptors in the airway
- other structures innervated by the vagi, trigeminal and phrenic nerves.

Afferent input terminates in the nucleus tractus solitarius within the brain stem (Figure 4.4). Input from higher centres allows cough to be voluntarily induced or suppressed.[17,89,90]

Acid and non-acid reflux can cause cough via a vagally-mediated bronchoconstrictor reflex or by macro- or micro-aspiration into the airways. Typical symptoms of reflux are often absent and may occur predominantly during the day when upright.

Cough is a typical feature of asthma. Cough can also occur in both cough-variant asthma and in eosinophilic bronchitis. In these conditions there is a lack of variable airflow obstruction, plus eosinophilic inflammation in the latter, and a positive response to a therapeutic trial of corticosteroids.[88]

In COPD, cough is caused by inflammation and/or the need to eliminate large volumes of bronchial secretions. Because ciliary clearance of mucus is slow in COPD, coughing helps to clear secretions even if it seems non-productive.

ACE inhibitors cause a dry cough in $<10\%$ of patients either immediately or after weeks/months of use. Inhibition of angiotensin-converting enzyme prevents inactivation of inflammatory mediators which accumulate and increase the sensitivity of the cough reflex. Confirmation of the diagnosis is by resolution of the cough within 4 weeks of discontinuing the ACE inhibitor. In many patients, the severity and frequency of the cough is reduced by aspirin.[91]

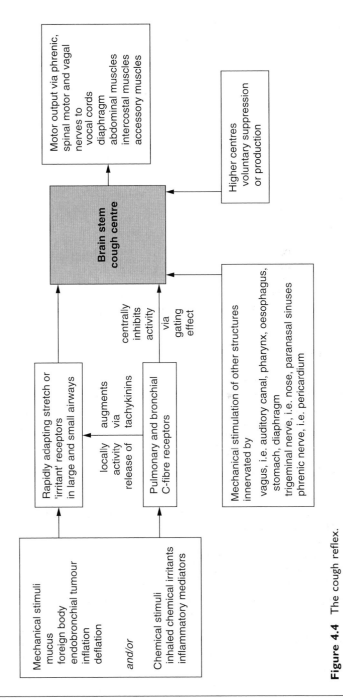

Figure 4.4 The cough reflex.

Evaluation

The commonest cause of acute cough is respiratory tract infection (Box 4.F). In advanced cancer, chronic cough is most likely caused by endobronchial tumour within the central airways.

Box 4.F   Causes of cough in patients with cancer

Cardiopulmonary
Post-nasal drip
Smoking
Asthma
COPD
Heart failure
Chest infection
Tumour
   endobronchial
      airway infiltration, distortion,
      obstruction
   lung parenchyma
      airway distortion, obstruction
      lymphangitis carcinomatosis
   mediastinum
   pleura, pericardium
   pleural effusion
Tracheo-oesophageal fistula
Vocal cord paralysis

Oesophageal
Gastro-oesophageal reflux

Aspiration
Gastro-oesophageal reflux
Bulbar muscle weakness
Neuromuscular inco-ordination

Treatment
Chemotherapy, e.g.
   bleomycin, methotrexate,
   cyclophosphamide
Radiotherapy, dose-related
   pneumonitis in 5–15% (early onset)
   fibrosis (late onset, >6 months)
ACE inhibitors
Nitrofurantoin
β-Blockers

Is the cough wet or dry?

A wet cough generally serves a physiological purpose and expectoration should be encouraged. A dry cough serves no purpose and should be suppressed. A wet cough distressing a dying patient who is too weak to expectorate should also be suppressed with antitussives.[17]

Is the cough caused by the cancer?

It is generally obvious when the cough is caused by the cancer. Associated features such as episodic wheezing (asthma) or heartburn (gastro-oesophageal reflux) suggest an alternative cause.[92] Appropriate investigations may include:

- chest radiograph
- sputum culture
- induced sputum to detect airway eosinophilia
- spirometry (pre- and post-bronchodilator)
- laryngoscopy
- bronchoscopy
- CT scan of the thorax.

Common causes, alone or in combination, include:

- post-nasal drip syndrome
- asthma
- gastro-oesophageal reflux
- COPD.

Can the cancer be modified?
Radiotherapy (teletherapy or endobronchial brachytherapy) improves cough in 50–60% of patients.[93] Other options may include chemotherapy, hormone therapy or surgery.[94] If in doubt, seek advice from an oncologist.

Can the impact of the cancer be modified?
For example, by draining a pleural effusion.

Management
Correct the correctable
Ideally, antitussive therapy should be specific, i.e. directed at the underlying cause or the presumed mechanism responsible for cough (Table 4.5).[95]

When cause-specific treatment is not possible or is inappropriate, non-specific treatment with an antitussive is generally indicated.[96] A protussive (expectorant) may be of benefit, making the sputum less tenacious and easier to expectorate. Nebulized saline is generally the protussive of choice, but sometimes an irritant mucolytic (e.g. guaifenesin) or a chemical mucolytic (e.g. carbocisteine) may be preferable (Figure 4.5).

Wet cough
Non-drug treatment
- advise how to cough efficiently; it is impossible to cough effectively lying on your back
- physiotherapy
- steam inhalations.

A forced expiration (a huff) from a low–medium lung volume:
- is effective in clearing secretions
- is better tolerated than the assisted cough manoeuvre (involves compressing the lower thorax and abdomen with the hands)
- requires less effort for the patient
- can be augmented by postural drainage.[97]

Drug treatment
For more information, see *PCF3*.

Avoid antitussives (cough suppressants) if possible, although these may be necessary to ensure sleep at night and to prevent exhaustion during the day. If used, the aim is to make expectoration more effective and less tiring. There is a wide range of protussives (expectorants). In practice, it is best to limit choice to a few preferred drugs:
- nebulized 0.9% saline, 2.5mL q.d.s., p.r.n. and before physiotherapy (this is generally sufficient)
- an irritant mucolytic, which produces a greater volume but less tenacious secretions, e.g. guaifenesin, ipecacuanha or squill
- a chemical mucolytic, which reduces the viscosity of secretions, e.g. carbocisteine 750mg t.d.s.

Cough efficacy in patients with cystic fibrosis or bronchiectasis is increased by nebulized:
- hypertonic saline (commonly 6–7%, range 3–12%)
- amiloride[98]
- terbutaline after physiotherapy.[99]

Table 4.5   Correctable causes of cough

Cause	Treatment
Smoking	Stop smoking; median time to improvement is 4 weeks
Post-nasal drip	
allergic rhinitis	Nasal corticosteroid $\pm$ sodium cromoglicate
	Antihistamine; second-generation antihistamines are non-sedating but are less drying than the older sedative antimuscarinic antihistamines
perennial and post-infection rhinitis	Antihistamine $\pm$ decongestant
vasomotor rhinitis	Nasal ipratropium bromide
bacterial sinusitis	Antibiotic $\pm$ decongestant $\pm$ nasal corticosteroid (acute) $\pm$ antihistamine (chronic)
Asthma	Bronchodilators $\pm$ corticosteroids
Gastro-oesophageal reflux	Avoid coffee, smoking or drugs which decrease lower oesophageal sphincter tone
	Prokinetic agent, increases oesophageal sphincter tone
	PPI to reduce gastric acid
COPD	Stop smoking
	Bronchodilators, e.g. ipratropium bromide
	Corticosteroids?
ACE inhibitor	Discontinue the ACE inhibitor; if not possible, substitute an angiotensin-II receptor antagonist, e.g. losartan
	Alternatively, consider:
	aspirin 600mg each morning; anti-platelet doses, e.g. 75–150mg each morning, are ineffective[91]
	nifedipine; acts via an inhibitory effect on PG synthesis
	theophylline
	baclofen
	sodium cromoglicate by inhaler

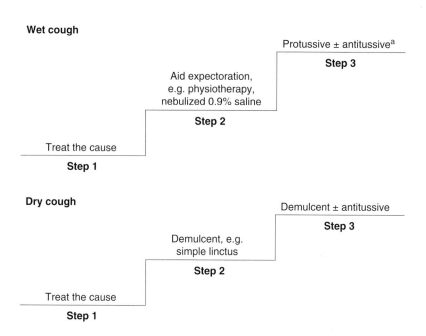

Wet cough

Protussive ± antitussive[a]

Step 3

Aid expectoration,
e.g. physiotherapy,
nebulized 0.9% saline

Step 2

Treat the cause

Step 1

Dry cough

Demulcent ± antitussive

Step 3

Demulcent, e.g.
simple linctus

Step 2

Treat the cause

Step 1

Figure 4.5 Treatment ladders for cough.

a. a protussive makes coughing more effective and less distressing; an antitussive reduces the intensity and frequency of coughing.

Dry cough
Drug treatment
For more information, see *PCF3*.

If a locally soothing demulcent (e.g. simple linctus BP 5mL t.d.s.–q.d.s.) is inadequate, consider a centrally-acting opioid antitussive, e.g.:
• codeine linctus 15–30mg (5–10mL) t.d.s.–q.d.s.

If codeine is not effective, switch to morphine:
• start with 5–10mg q.d.s.–q4h (but 2.5–5mg q.d.s.–q4h if not switching from codeine)
• if necessary, increase the dose until the cough is relieved or until undesirable effects prevent further escalation.

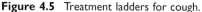

If a patient is already receiving a strong opioid for pain relief it is nonsense to prescribe codeine or a second strong opioid for cough suppression.

Opioid antitussives act centrally by facilitating serotoninergic mechanisms which inhibit the release of glutamate, an excitatory amino acid from the afferent fibres originating in the airways. Calcium channels are also involved; calcium-channel blockers and opioids both close calcium channels and in animals have a synergistic antitussive effect.[100]

If opioid antitussives are unsatisfactory, other possible treatments include:
- nebulized local anaesthetics, e.g. 5mL of either 2% lidocaine or 0.25% bupivacaine t.d.s.–q.d.s
- sodium cromoglicate 10mg inhaled q.d.s. improves cough in patients with lung cancer within 36–48h[101]
- baclofen 10mg PO t.d.s. or 20mg PO once daily has an antitussive effect in healthy volunteers and in patients with ACE inhibitor cough; 2–4 weeks of treatment is required to attain maximum effect[102,103]
- gabapentin 100mg PO b.d. up to 800mg PO b.d. is reported to have an antitussive effect in idiopathic chronic cough[104]
- diazepam in usual doses, e.g. 5mg PO once daily/at bedtime is reported to have an effect in intractable cough associated with lung metastases.[105]

Baclofen, diazepam and gabapentin are all GABA agonists, which suggests this inhibitory neurotransmitter has a role in inhibiting cough.

Non-UK options include:
- levodropropizine 75mg PO t.d.s. is as effective as dihydrocodeine 10mg PO t.d.s. in patients with lung cancer and causes less drowsiness[106]
- benzonatate 100mg PO t.d.s.; if necessary, increase to 200mg t.d.s.[107]

BRONCHORRHOEA

Bronchorrhoea is defined as the production of >100mL of sputum/24h. It sometimes occurs as a late feature in bronchiolo-alveolar cell cancer. In this uncommon form of lung cancer, the tumour cells 'coat' the bronchiolar surfaces and cause mucosal inflammation. This results in the production of massive amounts of mucus in the affected areas.

Management
Correct the correctable
When possible and appropriate, treat the underlying cancer. Response to a tyrosine kinase inhibitor (e.g. erlotinib, gefitinib) may be more impressive compared with conventional chemotherapy. Reduced mucus production can occur within hours–days and probably relates to inhibition of the epidermal growth factor receptor.[108–110]

Drug treatment
For more information, see PCF3.

The inflammatory response in the bronchioles is said to be reduced by:
- PO, IV or inhaled corticosteroids[111]
- nebulized furosemide 20mg q.d.s.
- nebulized indometacin 25mg in 2mL q8h–q4h (pH corrected to 7.4 with sodium bicarbonate); this may work even if corticosteroids fail[112]
- macrolide antibiotics, e.g. clarithromycin, erythromycin.[113,114]

Anecdotal reports suggest that an antisecretory drug, e.g. octreotide, hyoscine butylbromide or glycopyrronium, may also be of benefit.[115]

PLEURAL EFFUSION

A small amount of fluid (20–30mL) is present in the pleural space for lubrication. It is produced by capillaries and is removed by lymphatics in the parietal interstitium and pleura at a rate of 100–200mL/24h. These lymphatics ultimately drain into the mediastinal lymph nodes.

A pleural effusion forms as a result of excess production and/or reduced resorption of fluid. In malignant pleural effusion there is:
- obstruction of lymphatic transport in the pleura or regional lymph nodes by cancer cells
- cytokine production, e.g. VEGF by mesothelial and cancer cells which promote:
  ▷ effusion formation by increasing capillary permeability
  ▷ local cancer growth by enhancing angiogenesis.

Effusions may be classified as exudates or transudates (Table 4.6). Exudates develop when permeability of the pleural surface and/or capillaries is increased; transudates when there is altered hydrostatic forces favouring pleural fluid accumulation. Over 95% of malignant pleural effusions are exudates. Haemorrhagic malignant pleural effusions generally result from invasion of blood vessels or cancer-related angiogenesis.

Table 4.6 Classification of pleural effusions

	Exudate	Transudate
Distinguishing features		
Protein content	>35g/L	<25g/L
Pleural fluid:serum protein ratio	>0.5	<0.5
Pleural fluid LDH	>2/3 of upper limit of normal serum concentration	<2/3 of upper limit of normal serum concentration
Pleural fluid:serum LDH ratio	>0.6	<0.6
pH	<7.3	>7.3
RBC count	>100,000mm^3	<100,000mm^3
WBC count	>1,000mm^3	<1,000mm^3
Glucose	Low (infection) Very low (<3.3mmol/L in cancer and other causes of exudate)	Similar to plasma glucose
Common causes		
	Cancer lymphangitis carcinomatosa pleural infiltration lymphatic obstruction venous obstruction Pneumonia	Cirrhosis Hypo-albuminaemia LVF Peritoneal dialysis

Pleural effusions cause breathlessness as a result of:
- restricted movement of the chest wall and diaphragm
- lung compression, causing ventilation–perfusion mismatch
- hypoxia.

There may also be associated cough and chest pain.

Almost 50% of patients with advanced cancer develop a pleural effusion. Most will be in patients with cancer of the lung, breast or ovary, or lymphoma. Median survival for patients with malignant pleural effusion ranges from 3–12 months and is dependent upon the type of cancer and the response to anticancer therapies.

Evaluation

Clinical examination will detect an effusion >500mL. Useful investigations include:
- *chest radiograph*: detects an effusion >200mL
- *ultrasound*: helpful when there is difficulty in distinguishing pleural fluid from solid tumour or collapse of the lung
- *cytological, microbiological and biochemical examination*: carried out if there is diagnostic uncertainty; it can help to identify the effusion as an exudate or transudate (Table 4.6).

When serum protein is normal, pleural protein levels of <25g/L suggest a transudate and >35g/L an exudate. When the pleural protein concentration falls between 25–35g/L or when serum protein is abnormal, a more accurate approach is to take the pleural fluid to serum protein and LDH ratios into account (Table 4.6).[116]

Management

Advice should be sought from the local thoracic cancer multiprofessional team. Treatment depends on the severity of symptoms, the patient's performance status/prognosis and likelihood of the cancer responding to chemotherapy. Symptomatic pleural effusions should be drained (Table 4.7). Small asymptomatic effusions are best just monitored.

Correct the correctable

Guidelines: Therapeutic thoracocentesis, p.170.

Consider other common causes of pleural effusion, e.g. pneumonia, pulmonary embolism, heart failure, and treat appropriately. Give specific anticancer treatment if available.

Can the impact of the cancer be modified?
Thoracocentesis
Large symptomatic effusions should generally be removed by chest tube drainage (see below). However, the effusion may be removed by aspiration (thoracocentesis) in patients:
- with a poor prognosis
- who decline chest tube drainage
- who have failed chest tube drainage and medical pleurodesis.

Generally, no more than 1–1.5L of fluid should be removed at any one time, and the procedure discontinued if it causes cough or chest pain.[117] It can be undertaken in the hospice setting (see p.170).[119]

Chest tube drainage
Chest tube drainage and medical pleurodesis is preferred over simple aspiration because it offers better long-term control (Table 4.7). Small bore (10–14Fr) catheters are increasingly used. They are as effective as the traditional large bore intercostal

Table 4.7   Thoracocentesis vs. chest tube drainage and pleurodesis[117,118]

Thoracocentesis	Chest tube drainage and pleurodesis
Preferred option when poor prognosis (<4 weeks)	Preferred option when prognosis longer (>4 weeks)
Differences	
Relatively straightforward for operator and patient	Greater operator experience required and greater inconvenience to patient
Can be carried out as an outpatient	Requires inpatient admission for chest tube insertion or thoracoscopy
	Tube may kink or block
Repeat treatments likely because only 1–1.5L removed short time to recurrence (50% within 4 days; 97% within 4 weeks)	Long-term control likely chest tube + sclerosant >50% thoracoscopy + talc poudrage 90%
May paradoxically worsen ventilation–perfusion mismatch and increase hypoxia	Rapid drainage may lead to re-expansion pulmonary oedema
	Sclerosants may cause chest pain and fever
Similarities	
Both may lead to pneumothorax, haemothorax, empyema, fluid loculation, making further intervention difficult	
Cancer seeding in the chest wall	

tubes (24–32Fr), and are better tolerated.[117] Ultrasound guidance for the insertion of a drain for fluid is strongly advised by the National Patient Safety Agency.[120]

Drainage of a large pleural effusion should be at a controlled rate, i.e. about 500mL/h to avoid re-expansion pulmonary oedema. Removal of more than 1–1.5L at one time should be avoided. Drainage should be discontinued if the patient develops chest pain, persistent cough or vasovagal symptoms.[117]

Medical pleurodesis
Medical pleurodesis can proceed as soon as the lung has re-expanded, irrespective of the amount of pleural fluid draining/24h. It involves the instillation of an irritant substance into the pleural cavity to induce inflammation and activation of the coagulation system in order to produce fibrin. This leads to adhesion of the pleural layers, thereby obliterating the pleural space. In animal models, the concurrent use of corticosteroids reduces the likelihood of success by reducing the inflammatory response.[117] Success is increased by:
• removal of effusion to allow the lung to fully re-expand
• good dispersal of the irritant substance.

Guidelines: Therapeutic thoracocentesis

Ideally, thoracocentesis should be undertaken where there are radiological facilities to confirm the presence of pleural fluid, and to guide aspiration. However, if there is a high degree of clinical confidence that substantial pleural fluid is present, thoracocentesis can be undertaken in a hospice setting in breathless patients for whom a journey to hospital would be excessively arduous.

Indications for thoracocentesis

Pleural effusions are generally managed with tube drainage followed by pleurodesis. However, removal of the effusion by aspiration (thoracocentesis) may still be indicated in symptomatic patients:

- with a poor prognosis, e.g. <4 weeks
- who decline chest tube drainage
- who have failed chest tube drainage and medical pleurodesis and who are unsuitable for, or decline, repeated pleurodesis or indwelling pleural catheter drainage.

Radiological confirmation

Using clinical examination alone to diagnose a pleural effusion can be misleading, particularly in patients with advanced cancer. Ideally, thoracocentesis should be undertaken where there are radiological facilities to:

- identify the pleural effusion on a chest radiograph
- if necessary, use ultrasound to confirm the presence of fluid and exclude solid lung or thickened pleura
- guide the aspiration; generally with ultrasound scan.

When radiological facilities are not available

1 The patient should be in a comfortable position, leaning slightly forward with arms elevated and folded, resting on a pillow positioned on an adjustable bed table.

2 Identify the point of maximum dullness to percussion:
- *either* in the mid-axillary line (as for pleural drainage) where the 'safe triangle' for insertion is outlined by the lateral border of the pectoralis major, the anterior border of latissimus dorsi and a line drawn horizontal to the level of the nipple (4th intercostal space)
- *or* on the posterior chest wall medial to the angle of the scapula; this may be an easier approach but there is more risk of puncturing an intercostal artery because posteriorly this lies in the centre of the intercostal space and not under the lip of the rib above as it does more laterally. It is thus important to *ensure the point of insertion is immediately above a rib.*

3 Under aseptic technique:
- *at a point immediately above a rib*, infiltrate the skin with a small amount of 1% lidocaine using a 5mL syringe and a 25G needle (orange) and leave for 2–3 minutes
- switch to a 21G needle (green) and, perpendicular to the skin, progress the needle inwards, stopping every few millimetres to aspirate before infiltrating with 1% lidocaine to ensure you have not punctured a blood vessel or reached the pleural space

continued

- continue until pleural fluid is aspirated; then withdraw the needle
- if pleural fluid is not aspirated, the procedure should be abandoned, and not attempted again unless the presence of a pleural effusion is confirmed by imaging
- insert a 18G (green) IV cannula on the end of a 10mL syringe applying a small amount of suction. As soon as pleural fluid is aspirated, stop and advance only the cannula over the needle. Once the cannula is fully inserted, remove the needle
- attach a 3-way tap to the cannula and aspirate the effusion using a 30–50mL syringe; removing as little as 500mL of fluid may provide relief
- although more has occasionally been aspirated by some practitioners without problem (as much as 5L), generally no more than 1–1.5L of fluid should be removed at any one time
- discontinue if the patient develops chest pain, cough or an increase in breathlessness
- if there is difficulty aspirating fluid, do not continue; possibilities include solid lung, thickened pleura or loculated effusion. Seek advice from the thoracic oncology multiprofessional team.

4 Monitor the patient for at least 1 hour (respiratory rate and possibly oxygen saturation). If the patient becomes more breathless, consider a pneumothorax and obtain a chest radiograph.

5 Benefit may be short-lived as the effusions will re-accumulate (50% in <4 days, most in <4 weeks).

6 The procedure can be repeated as long as beneficial.

Suction is occasionally required to achieve complete lung re-expansion. A gradual increase in pressure up to -20cm H_2O should be applied using a high volume, low pressure system. Persistent incomplete lung re-expansion may relate to trapped lung, caused by:

- a thick visceral peel
- pleural loculations
- proximal large airway obstruction
- a persistent pneumothorax.

Patients with persistent incomplete lung re-expansion should be considered for thoracoscopy (see below). However, if thoracoscopy is not considered appropriate, medical pleurodesis can still be attempted as favourable responses have been seen in patients with only partial re-expansion.[117]

Undesirable effects of sclerosants include chest pain and fever. Adult respiratory distress syndrome is a rare (<1%) complication following talc administration. This may relate to the size of talc particles used. The risk is reduced by the use of graded talc which has had the smaller particles removed.[121] Pain should be managed by:

- premedication with a systemic opioid ± benzodiazepine 10min before the pleurodesis, to achieve a level of sedation which does not interfere with the patient's ability to communicate or co-operate, together with
- the instillation into the pleural space of lidocaine solution (3mg/kg; up to a maximum of 250mg, i.e. 25mL of lidocaine 1%) just before the sclerosant.[117,122]

Talc 2–5g instilled via a chest tube as a suspension ('slurry') is cheap, widely available and a more effective sclerosant than doxycycline, tetracycline or bleomycin.[123,124]

The tube is clamped for 1h and it is not necessary to rotate the patient if the lung has re-expanded.[117,124] The tube should be removed within 12–72h if the lung remains fully expanded and fluid drainage is <250mL/24h. When there is persistent drainage of >250mL, repeat pleurodesis with an alternative substance should be considered.[117]

In patients with mesothelioma, prophylactic radiotherapy should be given to the thoracoscopy/chest tube insertion site to reduce the likelihood of seeding and local recurrence.[117]

Loculated effusions
The drainage of a loculated effusion may be helped by intrapleural streptokinase 250,000units b.d. or urokinase 100,000units once daily in 30–100mL of 0.9% saline. These degrade fibrin and thereby disrupt adhesions. Improvement is generally seen within 3 days and allows medical pleurodesis to be attempted. Some patients become pyrexial after streptokinase but not after urokinase which is not antigenic. Haemorrhagic complications have not been reported.[118,125,126]

Thoracoscopy
Video-assisted thoracoscopy under sedation or general anaesthesia should be considered for patients with a reasonable prognosis and:
• suspected but unproven malignant pleural effusion
• persistent incomplete lung re-expansion despite drainage
• a loculated effusion
• recurrent effusion following medical pleurodesis.

Thoracoscopy allows biopsies to be taken which have a high diagnostic yield and adhesions and loculations to be broken down. This can be followed by talc instillation with an atomiser (poudrage), which prevents recurrence of effusion in >90% of patients. Overall, talc is equally effective whether administered as a poudrage or a slurry. However, poudrage appears superior for patients with lung or breast cancer. On the other hand, compared with chest tube drainage, there is a slightly higher mortality and complication rate following thoracoscopy.[18]

Indwelling tunnelled pleural catheters and pleuroperitoneal shunts
Indwelling tunnelled pleural catheters and pleuroperitoneal shunts can be considered for recurrent pleural effusions or when the lung fails to re-inflate (trapped lung) making pleurodesis unlikely to succeed.

Indwelling tunnelled pleural catheters (e.g. Pleurx®) help to keep hospital admissions to a minimum which may be important when prognosis is limited.[117] They are inserted under local anaesthesia and patients and carers instructed on how to drain off small amounts at regular intervals using vacuum bottles. The irritant effect of the tube may contribute to a 'spontaneous' pleurodesis which is observed in 1/2–3/4 of patients after 1–2 months, allowing their removal.[18,127] Complications include blockage, displacement, loculations, empyema, cellulitis, cancer seeding along the catheter tract and pneumothorax.

A pleuroperitoneal shunt consists of a valved chamber with fenestrated pleural and peritoneal catheters attached at either end. It is sited at thoracoscopy or mini-thoracotomy. A pressure gradient allows pleural fluid to drain into the peritoneal cavity, and this can be augmented by manual compression of the pump chamber.[117] Although effective, 1/4 of shunts become occluded within a median of 10 weeks.[124]

Pleurectomy
Although effective, pleurectomy is associated with mortality rates of ≥10% and should be reserved for a carefully selected group of patients who have failed other treatment options. A parietal pleurectomy undertaken by thoracoscopy is a safer alternative.[117]

LYMPHANGITIS CARCINOMATOSA

Lymphangitis carcinomatosa is a term used to describe the diffuse infiltration of lymphatics of the lungs by cancer cells. Clinically it is characterized by increasing breathlessness and cough ± pleuritic chest pain and central cyanosis. Prognosis is poor with a median survival of 3 months from presentation; only 10% survive longer than 10 months.[128]

Physiology

Lymphatic channels in the lungs follow the bronchi, the pulmonary arterial and venous system and form an extensive network in the pleura. These become distended with cancer cells causing lymph stasis which in turn stimulates fibrosis and smooth muscle proliferation.

Evaluation

Chest radiographs

These are generally abnormal but not always diagnostic. Abnormalities reflecting lymphatics permeated with cancer cells, fibrous tissue or oedema include:

- small nodular opacities, 1–5mm with hazy border
- a diffuse reticular pattern
- a combination of the above (reticulonodular)
- Kerley A lines <1mm thick, straight >2cm, pointing towards hilum and not touching the pleura
- Kerley B lines <1mm thick, straight <2cm, perpendicular to and touching the pleura (reflects peripheral septal thickening)
- irregular thickening of interlobular septal lines associated with cancer cells, fibrous tissue or oedema.[129]

Hilar lymphadenopathy and/or pleural effusions may also be present.

CT

High resolution CT increases diagnostic accuracy.[130]

Pulmonary function tests

These show a restrictive ventilatory disturbance, i.e. vital capacity, residual volume, total lung capacity, diffusing capacity for carbon monoxide and pulmonary compliance all reduced. Tidal volume is also reduced and the respiratory rate increases. Reduced compliance increases the work of breathing. Hypoxia is common because of impaired gas exchange due to interstitial oedema secondary to impaired lymphatic drainage.[131]

Management

Correct the correctable

Can the cancer be modified?

Chemotherapy or hormone therapy in responsive cancers improves survival by 6–30 months.[128] Corticosteroids may have an anticancer effect in some cancers, e.g. breast, lymphoma, prostate, occasionally leading to a dramatic response.

Can the impact of the cancer be modified?

Corticosteroids, e.g. dexamethasone 4–8mg PO once daily, may improve the breathlessness with an objective improvement in lung function. Give initially on a trial basis for 1 week. Theoretically, diuretics may reduce alveolar membrane congestion. Furosemide 20–40mg PO stat is used at some centres on presentation; if benefit is seen ≤4h, it is continued each morning indefinitely.

Drug treatment

For more information, see *PCF3*.

PO morphine should be considered to relieve breathlessness, and oxygen to correct moderate–severe hypoxia (see p.156). Benzodiazepines may help reduce concurrent anxiety (see p.187).

HICCUP

Hiccup is a pathological (involuntary) reflex characterized by sudden, (generally) unilateral repetitive contraction of the diaphragm. This causes sudden inspiration and abrupt closure of the glottis, producing the characteristic sound.

Although generally transient, lasting just minutes or a few hours, hiccup can be more persistent, and can then result in disturbed sleep, exhaustion, and increased debility. Occasionally, hiccup can be so intractable as to make the subject suicidal.

Causes

Hiccup has many possible causes, including:[132]

- gastric distension
- gastro-oesophageal reflux
- gastritis
- cholecystitis
- diaphragmatic irritation
- phrenic nerve irritation
- tympanic membrane irritation
- metabolic:
  ▷ uraemia
  ▷ hypokalaemia
  ▷ hypocalcaemia
  ▷ hyperglycaemia
  ▷ hypocapnia
- toxicity:
  ▷ fever, infection
- brain tumour, stroke, infection, demyelination
- psychological, e.g. related to stress or excitement.

Of these, gastric distension ± gastro-oesophageal reflux probably account for most cases.

Many drugs have been implicated as a cause of hiccup, including:[132,133]

- alcohol
- benzodiazepines (notably with PR midazolam in children)[134]
- corticosteroids (particularly when IV dexamethasone is given with cisplatin chemotherapy)[135]
- methyldopa
- opioids.[136]

Midazolam has also been reported as a cure for persistent hiccup (see below). The mechanism underlying opioid-related hiccup could be delayed gastric emptying, exacerbating gastric distension ± gastro-oesophageal reflux, or secondary to spasm of the sphincter of Oddi and distension of the common bile duct.

Evaluation and explanation
Generally, proceed on the basis that measures to reduce gastric distension (see below) are likely to lead to relief. If such measures do not work, consider an alternative cause, e.g.:
- biochemical abnormalities
- direct irritation of the diaphragm by, for example, subphrenic metastases; try baclofen (see below) or
- peripheral or central neural lesion; try gabapentin (see below).

If this fails, a thorough diagnostic evaluation may be necessary, which may include imaging of the upper abdomen/thorax or brain as appropriate.

Management
Prevent the preventable
Advise the patient to consider adopting the equivalent of a 'small stomach' or post-gastrectomy approach to eating and drinking, i.e. 'small and often', separating the main food from the main fluid intake.

Non-drug treatment
Pharyngeal stimulation
This may be worth considering for occasional hiccup. Pharyngeal stimulation triggers a 'gating' mechanism which inhibits the hiccup reflex. Most of the 'folk' remedies for hiccup involve pharyngeal stimulation (Box 4.G). Medical variations include:
- nebulized 0.9% saline (2mL over 5min)[137]
- forceful tongue traction sufficient to induce a gag reflex
- a nasogastric tube inserted as far as the oropharynx and oscillated (Figure 4.6).[138]

Box 4.G   Some traditional 'folk' remedies for hiccup

Direct stimulation of the pharynx
Rapidly ingest two heaped teaspoons of granulated sugar or two glasses of liqueur.
Swallow dry bread or crushed ice.

Indirect stimulation of the pharynx (via hyperextension of the neck)
Drink from the wrong side of a cup (or sitting 'doubled up' and drinking water).
A cold key dropped inside the back of the person's shirt or blouse.[140]

Massage of the junction between hard and soft palate with a cotton bob is also an effective gating mechanism.[139]

Counter-irritation of the diaphragm
- leaning forward
- pull knees up to the chest.

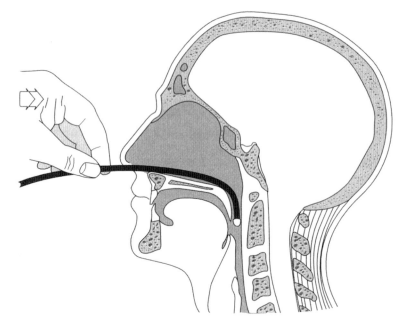

Figure 4.6 Pharyngeal stimulation to stop hiccup. A nasal catheter is inserted 8–12cm so that it is opposite the second cervical vertebra. Jerky to-and-fro movements lead to the immediate cessation of hiccup. Afferent innervation = vagus and glossopharyngeal nerves. Reproduced with permission from Salem *et al.*[138]

Elevation of PaCO$_2$
This inhibits processing of the hiccup reflex in the brain stem:
- breath holding
- rebreathing from a paper bag.

Drug treatment
For more information, see *PCF3*.

Only chlorpromazine and haloperidol are licensed for the treatment of hiccup. However, chlorpromazine has many undesirable effects, and is not recommended as a first-line or second-line drug (Table 4.8). Consideration of the underlying pathophysiology suggests that simeticone with metoclopramide should generally be considered as first choice drug treatment for troublesome hiccup in advanced cancer.

Table 4.8 Drug treatment of hiccup

Class of drug	Drug	Acute relief	Maintenance regimen
Reduce gastric distension ± gastro-oesophageal reflux			
Antiflatulent (carminative)	Peppermint water[a,b]	10mL	10–20mL b.d.
Antiflatulent (defoaming agent)	Simeticone, e.g. in Asilone®	10mL	10mL q.d.s.
Prokinetic	Metoclopramide[a,c]	10mg	10mg t.d.s.–q.d.s.
PPI	Lansoprazole	30mg	30mg each morning
Muscle relaxant (all of these also have central suppressant effects)			
GABA agonist	Baclofen	5mg PO	5–20mg t.d.s., occasionally more[141,142]
Calcium-channel blocker	Nifedipine	10mg PO/SL	10–20mg t.d.s., occasionally more[143,144]
Benzodiazepine	Midazolam	2mg IV, followed by 1–2mg increments every 3–5min	10–60mg/24h by CSCI if patient in last days of life[145]
Central suppression of the hiccup reflex			
Dopamine antagonist	Metoclopramide	As above	As above
	Haloperidol	5–10mg PO or IV if no response	1.5–3mg at bedtime[146,147]
	Chlorpromazine	10–25mg PO or IV if no response	25–50mg t.d.s.
	Methylphenidate	5mg PO	5–10mg b.d.[148]
GABA agonist	Baclofen	As above	As above
Anti-epileptic	Sodium valproate	200–500mg PO	15mg/kg/24h in divided doses[149]
	Gabapentin	'Burst gabapentin', e.g. 400mg t.d.s. for 3 days, then 400mg once daily for 3 days, then stop; repeat if necessary[d,150]	Repeat burst gabapentin, if necessary[15,151,152]

a. facilitates belching by relaxing the lower oesophageal sphincter; an old-fashioned remedy, but can cause gastro-oesophageal reflux
b. peppermint water and metoclopramide should not be used concurrently because of their opposing actions on the gastro-oesophageal sphincter
c. tightens the lower oesophageal sphincter and hastens gastric emptying
d. a smaller dose advisable in elderly frail patients and those with renal impairment, e.g. start with 100mg t.d.s.

1 American Thoracic Society (1999) Dyspnea, mechanisms, assessment and management: a consensus statement. *American Journal of Respiratory and Critical Care Medicine.* **159**: 321–340.

2 Tanaka K et al. (2002) Prevalence and screening of dyspnea interfering with daily life activities in ambulatory patients with advanced lung cancer. *Journal of Pain and Symptom Management.* **23**: 484–489.

3 O'Driscoll M et al. (1999) The experience of breathlessness in lung cancer. *European Journal of Cancer Care.* **8**: 37–43.

4 Henoch I et al. (2008) Dyspnea experience and management strategies in patients with lung cancer. *Psychooncology.* **17**: 709–715.

5 Davis C (1997) Breathlessness, cough, and other respiratory problems. *British Medical Journal.* **315**: 931–934.

6 Wilcock A et al. (2008) Symptoms limiting activity in cancer patients with breathlessness on exertion: ask about muscle fatigue. *Thorax.* **63**: 91–92.

7 Solano J et al. (2006) A comparison of symptom prevalence in far advanced cancer, AIDS, heart disease, chronic obstructive pulmonary disease and renal disease. *Journal of Pain and Symptom Management.* **31**: 58–69.

8 Reuben DB and Mor V (1986) Dyspnoea in terminally ill cancer patients. *Chest.* **89**: 234–236.

9 Reuben DB et al. (1988) Clinical symptoms and length of survival in patients with terminal cancer. *Archives of Internal Medicine.* **148**: 1586–1591.

10 Bianchi A et al. (1995) Central control of breathing in mammals: neuronal circuitry, membrane properties, and neurotransmitters. *Physiological Reviews.* **75**: 1–45.

11 O'Donnell DE et al. (2007) Pathophysiology of dyspnea in chronic obstructive pulmonary disease: a roundtable. *Proceedings of the American Thoracic Society.* **4**: 145–168.

12 Dudgeon D and Lertzman M (1999) Dyspnea in the advanced cancer patient. *Journal of Pain and Symptom Management.* **16**: 212–219.

13 Travers J et al. (2008) Mechanisms of exertional dyspnea in patients with cancer. *Journal of Applied Physiology.* **104**: 57–66.

14 Bruera E et al. (2000) The frequency and correlates of dyspnea in patients with advanced cancer. *Journal of Pain and Symptom Management.* **19**: 357–362.

15 Dudgeon DJ et al. (2001) Physiological changes and clinical correlations of dyspnea in cancer outpatients. *Journal of Pain and Symptom Management.* **21**: 373–379.

16 Corner J and O'Driscoll M (1999) Development of a breathless assessment guide for use in palliative care. *Palliative Medicine.* **13**: 375–384.

17 Wilcock A (1998) The management of respiratory symptoms. In: C Faull et al. (eds) *The Handbook of Palliative Care.* Blackwell Scientific, London, pp. 157–176.

18 Gasper WJ et al. (2007) Palliation of thoracic malignancies. *Surgical Oncology.*

19 Radunovic A et al. (2007) Clinical care of patients with amyotrophic lateral sclerosis. *Lancet Neurology.* **6**: 913–925.

20 Thompson E et al. (2005) Non-invasive interventions for improving well-being and quality of life in patients with lung cancer–a systematic review of the evidence. *Lung Cancer.* **50**: 163–176.

21 Zhao I and Yates P (2008) Non-pharmacological interventions for breathlessness management in patients with lung cancer: a systematic review. *Palliative Medicine.* **22**: 693–701.

22 Breslin E (1995) Breathing retraining in chronic obstructive pulmonary disease. *Journal of Cardiopulmonary Rehabilitation.* **15**: 25–33.

23 Navigante AH et al. (2006) Midazolam as adjunct therapy to morphine in the alleviation of severe dyspnea perception in patients with advanced cancer. *Journal of Pain and Symptom Management.* **31**: 38–47.

24 Congleton J and Muers MF (1995) The incidence of airflow obstruction in bronchial carcinoma, its relation to breathlessness, and response to bronchodilator therapy. *Respiratory Medicine.* **89**: 291–296.

25 Janssens J-P et al. (2000) Management of dyspnea in severe chronic obstructive pulmonary disease. *Journal of Pain and Symptom Management.* **19**: 378–392.

26 Bruera E et al. (1990) Effects of morphine on the dyspnea of terminal cancer patients. *Journal of Pain and Symptom Management.* **5**: 341–344.

27 Bruera E et al. (1993) Subcutaneous morphine for dyspnoea in cancer patients. *Annals of Internal Medicine.* **119**: 906–907.

28 Mazzocato C et al. (1999) The effects of morphine on dyspnoea and ventilatory function in elderly patients with advanced cancer: A randomized double-blind controlled trial. *Annals of Oncology.* **10**: 1511–1514.

29 Abernethy AP et al. (2003) Randomised, double blind, placebo controlled crossover trial of sustained release morphine for the management of refractory dyspnoea. *British Medical Journal.* **327**: 523–528.

30 Allen S et al. (2005) Low dose diamorphine reduces breathlessness without causing a fall in oxygen saturation in elderly patients with end-stage idiopathic pulmonary fibrosis. *Palliative Medicine.* **19**: 128–130.

31 Clemens KE et al. (2008) Is there a higher risk of respiratory depression in opioid-naive palliative care patients during symptomatic therapy of dyspnea with strong opioids? *Journal of Palliative Medicine.* **11**: 204–216.

32 Cohen M et al. (1991) Continuous intravenous infusion of morphine for sever dyspnoea. *Southern Medical Journal.* **84**: 229–234.

33 Boyd K and Kelly M (1997) Oral morphine as symptomatic treatment of dyspnoea in patients with advanced cancer. *Palliative Medicine.* **11**: 277–281.

34 Poole PJ et al. (1998) The effect of sustained-release morphine on breathlessness and quality of life in severe chronic obstructive pulmonary disease. *American Journal of Respiratory and Critical Care Medicine.* **157**: 1877–1880.

35 Allard P et al. (1999) How effective are supplementary doses of opioids for dyspnea in terminally ill cancer patients? A randomized continuous sequential clinical trial. *Journal of Pain and Symptom Management.* **17**: 256–265.

36 Gauna AA et al. (2008) Oral transmucosal fentanyl citrate for dyspnea in terminally ill patients: an observational case series. *Journal of Palliative Medicine.* **11**: 643–648.

37 Jennings A et al. (2002) A systematic review of the use of opioids in the management of dyspnoea. *Thorax.* **57**: 939–944.

38 Davis C (1999) Nebulized opioids should not be prescribed outside a clinical trial. *American Journal of Hospice and Palliative Care.* **16**: 543.

39 Foral PA et al. (2004) Nebulized opioids use in COPD. *Chest.* **125**: 691–694.

40 Brown SJ et al. (2005) Nebulized morphine for relief of dyspnea due to chronic lung disease. *The Annals of Pharmacotherapy.* **39**: 1088–1092.

41 Bruera E et al. (2005) Nebulized versus subcutaneous morphine for patients with cancer dyspnea: a preliminary study. *Journal of Pain and Symptom Management.* **29**: 613–618.

42 Bruera E et al. (2006) Can we really say that nebulized morphine works? [author's response]. *Journal of Pain and Symptom Management.* **32**: 102–103.

43 Lasheen W et al. (2006) Can we really say that nebulized morphine works? *Journal of Pain and Symptom Management.* **32**: 101–102; author reply 102–103.

44 Lang E and Jedeikin R (1998) Acute respiratory depression as a complication of nebulised morphine. *Canadian Journal of Anaesthesia.* **45**: 60–62.

45 Harrison T et al. (2004) A comparison or oral lorazepam and placebo in relieving breathlessness associated with cancer (meeting abstract). *Palliative Medicine.* **18**: 305–306.

46 Rapoport D et al. (1991) Differing effects of the anxiolytic agents buspirone and diazepam on control of breathing. *Clinical Pharmacology and Therapeutics.* **49**: 394–401.

47 Smoller J et al. (1996) Panic anxiety, dyspnea, and respiratory disease. Theoretical and clinical considerations. *American Journal of Respiratory and Critical Care Medicine.* **54**: 6–17.

48 Argyopoulou P et al. (1993) Buspirone effect on breathlessness and exercise performance in patients with chronic obstructive pulmonary disease. *Respiration.* **60**: 216–220.

49 Singh N et al. (1993) Effects of buspirone on anxiety levels and exercise tolerance in patients with chronic airflow obstruction and mild anxiety. *Chest.* **103**: 800–804.

50 Datta A et al. (1994) Palliation of breathlessness in patients with COAD and anxiety without provoking sedation or respiratory depression. *Progress in Palliative Care.* **2**: 11.

51 Ahmedzai S (1997) Palliation of respiratory symptoms. In: D Doyle et al. (eds) *Oxford Textbook of Palliative Medicine* (2e). Oxford University Press, Oxford, pp. 583–616.

52 Booth S et al. (2004) The use of oxygen in the palliation of breathlessness. A report of the expert working group of the scientific committee of the association of palliative medicine. *Respiratory Medicine.* **98**: 66–77.

53 Bruera E et al. (2003) A randomized controlled trial of supplemental oxygen versus air in cancer patients with dyspnea. *Palliative Medicine.* **17**: 659–663.

54 Philip J et al. (2006) A randomized, double-blind, crossover trial of the effect of oxygen on dyspnea in patients with advanced cancer. *Journal of Pain and Symptom Management.* **32**: 541–550.

55 Ward J (2006) Oxygen delivery and demand. *Surgery (Oxford).* **24**: 354–360.

56 Vit J-P et al. (2006) The analgesic effect of low dose focal irradiation in a mouse model of bone cancer is associated with spinal changes in neuro-mediators of nociception. *Pain.* **120**: 188–201.

57 Uronis HE et al. (2008) Oxygen for relief of dyspnoea in mildly- or non-hypoxaemic patients with cancer: a systematic review and meta-analysis. *British Journal of Cancer.* **98**: 294–299.

58 Eaton T et al. (2006) Short-burst oxygen therapy for COPD patients: a 6-month randomised, controlled study. *The European Respiratory Journal.* **27**: 697–704.

59 Roberts CM (2004) Short burst oxygen therapy for relief of breathlessness in COPD. *Thorax.* **59**: 638–640.

60 O'Neill B et al. (2006) Short-burst oxygen therapy in chronic obstructive pulmonary disease. *Respiratory Medicine.* **100**: 1129–1138.

61 Quantrill SJ et al. (2007) Short burst oxygen therapy after activities of daily living in the home in chronic obstructive pulmonary disease. *Thorax.* **62**: 702–705.

62 Schwartzstein R et al. (1987) Cold facial stimulation reduces breathlessness induced in normal subjects. *American Review of Respiratory Disease.* **136**: 58–61.

63 Burgess K and Whitelaw W (1988) Effects of nasal cold receptors on pattern of breathing. *Journal of Applied Physiology.* **64**: 371–376.

64 Freedman S (1988) Cold facial stimulation reduces breathlessness induced in normal subjects. *American Review of Respiratory Diseases.* **137**: 492–493.

65 Kerr D (1989) A bedside fan for terminal dyspnea. *American Journal of Hospice Care.* **89**: 22.

66 Liss H and Grant B (1988) The effect of nasal flow on breathlessness in patients with chronic obstructive pulmonary disease. *American Review of Respiratory Disease.* **137**: 1285–1288.

67 Royal College of Physicians of London (1999) *Domiciliary Oxygen Therapy Services: Clinical Guidelines and Advice for Prescribers.* Royal College of Physicians, London.

68 Bradley J *et al.* (2005) Short-term ambulatory oxygen for chronic obstructive pulmonary disease. *Cochrane Database of Systematic Reviews.* **4**: CD004356.

69 O'Driscoll BR *et al.* (2008) Guideline for emergency oxygen use in adult patients. Thorax. Suppl VI: vi1–vi73. Available from: www.brit-thoracic.org.uk

70 Boorstein J *et al.* (1989) Using helium-oxygen mixtures in the emergency management of acute upper airway obstruction. *Annals of Emergency Medicine.* **18**: 688–690.

71 Lu T-S *et al.* (1976) Helium-oxygen in treatment of upper airway obstruction. *Anesthesiology.* **45**: 678–680.

72 Rudow M *et al.* (1986) Helium-oxygen mixtures in airway obstruction due to thyroid carcinoma. *Canadian Anaesthesiology Society Journal.* **33**: 498–501.

73 Khanlou H and Eiger G (2001) Safety and efficacy of heliox as a treatment for upper airway obstruction due to radiation-induced laryngeal dysfunction. *Heart and Lung.* **30**: 146–147.

74 Ahmedzai SH *et al.* (2004) A double-blind, randomised, controlled Phase II trial of Heliox28 gas mixture in lung cancer patients with dyspnoea on exertion. *British Journal of Cancer.* **90**: 366–371.

75 Laude EA *et al.* (2006) The effect of helium and oxygen on exercise performance in chronic obstructive pulmonary disease: a randomized crossover trial. *American Journal of Respiratory and Critical Care Medicine.* **173**: 865–870.

76 Quaranta A *et al.* (1997) Cheyne-Stokes respiration during sleep in congestive heart failure. *Chest.* **111**: 467–473.

77 Andreas S *et al.* (1996) Cheyne-Stokes respiration and prognosis in congestive heart failure. *American Journal of Cardiology.* **78**: 1260–1264.

78 Brack T *et al.* (2007) Daytime Cheyne-Stokes respiration in ambulatory patients with severe congestive heart failure is associated with increased mortality. *Chest.*

79 Escribano M *et al.* (1990) A case of dirhythmic breathing. *Chest.* **97**: 1018–1020.

80 Lalonde R and Botez M (1991) Death from bulbar involvement in Friedreich's ataxia. *Medical Hypotheses.* **36**: 250–252.

81 Nachtmann A *et al.* (1995) Cheyne-Stokes respiration in ischemic stroke. *Neurology.* **45**: 820–821.

82 Lorenzi-Filho G *et al.* (2005) Cheyne-Stokes respiration in patients with congestive heart failure: causes and consequences. *Clinics.* **60**: 333–344.

83 Banno K and Kryger MH (2007) Sleep apnea: clinical investigations in humans. *Sleep Medicine.* **8**: 400–426.

84 Naughton M (1998) Pathophysiology and treatment of Cheyne-Stokes respiration. *Thorax.* **53**: 514–518.

85 Andreas S *et al.* (1996) Improvement of exercise capacity with treatment of Cheyne-Stokes respiration in patients with congestive heart failure. *Journal of the American College of Cardiology.* **27**: 1486–1490.

86 Javaheri S *et al.* (1996) Effect of theophylline on sleep-disordered breathing in heart failure. *The New England Journal of Medicine.* **335**: 562–567.

87 Meurs M and Round C (1993) Palliation of symptoms in non-small cell lung cancer: a study by the Yorkshire Regional Cancer Organisation thoracic group. *Thorax.* **48**: 339–343.

88 Morice AH *et al.* (2006) BTS Guidelines. Recommendations for the management of cough in adults. *Thorax.* **61 Suppl 1**: i1–24.

89 Widdicombe J (1995) Neurophysiology of the cough reflex. *European Respiratory Journal.* **8**: 1193–1202.

90 Fuller R and Jackson D (1990) Physiology and treatment of cough. *Thorax.* **45**: 425–430.

91 Tenenbaum A *et al.* (2000) Intermediate but not low doses of aspirin can suppress angiotensin-converting enzyme inhibitor-induced cough. *American Journal of Hypertension.* **13**: 776–782.

92 Mello C *et al.* (1996) Predictive values of the character, timing, and complications of chronic cough in diagnosing its cause. *Archives of Internal Medicine.* **156**: 997–1003.

93 Awan A and Weichselbaum R (1990) Palliative radiotherapy. *Haematology/Oncology Clinics of North America.* **4**: 1169–1181.

94 Kvale PA (2006) Chronic cough due to lung tumors: ACCP evidence-based clinical practice guidelines. *Chest.* **129**: 147S–153S.

95 McGarvey LP and Morice AH (2006) Clinical cough and its mechanisms. *Respiratory Physiology & Neurobiology.* **152**: 363–371.

96 Homsi J *et al.* (2001) Important drugs for cough in advanced cancer. *Supportive Care in Cancer.* **9**: 565–574.

97 Irwin R *et al.* (1993) Appropriate use of antitussives and protussives. A practical review. *Drugs.* **46**: 80–91.

98 App E *et al.* (1990) Acute and long-term amiloride inhalation in cystic fibrosis lung disease: a rational approach to cystic fibrosis therapy. *American Review of Respiratory Disease.* **141**: 605–612.

99 Irwin RS et al. (1998) Managing cough as a defense mechanism and as a symptom. A consensus panel report of the American College of Chest Physicians. Chest. 114 (suppl): 133s–181s.

100 Kamei J (1995) Recent advances in neuropharmacology of the centrally acting antitussive drugs. Methods and Findings: Experimental and Clinical Pharmacology. 17: 193–205.

101 Moroni M et al. (1996) Inhaled sodium cromoglycate to treat cough in advanced lung cancer patients. British Journal of Cancer. 74: 309–311.

102 Dicpinigaitis PV (2006) Current and future peripherally-acting antitussives. Respiratory Physiology & Neurobiology. 152: 356–362.

103 Dicpinigaitis P et al. (1998) Inhibition of capsaicin-induced cough by the gamma-aminobutyric acid agonist baclofen. Journal of Clinical Pharmacology. 38: 364–367.

104 Mintz S and Lee JK (2006) Gabapentin in the treatment of intractable idiopathic chronic cough: case reports. The American Journal of Medicine. 119: e13–15.

105 Estfan B and Walsh D (2008) The cough from hell: diazepam for intractable cough in a patient with renal cell carcinoma. Journal of Pain and Symptom Management. 36: 553–558.

106 Luporini G et al. (1998) Efficacy and safety of levodropropizine and dihydrocodeine on nonproductive cough in primary and metastatic lung cancer. European Respiratory Journal. 12: 97–101.

107 Doona M and Walsh D (1997) Benzonatate for opioid-resistant cough in advanced cancer. Palliative Medicine. 16: 212–219.

108 Kitazaki T et al. (2005) Novel effects of gefitinib on mucin production in bronchioloalveolar carcinoma; two case reports. Lung Cancer. 49: 125–128.

109 Milton DT et al. (2005) Prompt control of bronchorrhea in patients with bronchioloalveolar carcinoma treated with gefitinib (Iressa). Support Care Cancer. 13: 70–72.

110 Thotathil Z and Long J (2007) Erlotinib effective against refractory bronchorrhea from advanced non-small cell lung cancer. Journal of Thoracic Oncology. 2: 881–882.

111 Nakajima T et al. (2002) Treatment of bronchorrhea by corticosteroids in a case of bronchioloalveolar carcinoma producing CA19-9. Internal Medicine. 41: 225–228.

112 Tamaoki J et al. (2000) Inhaled indomethacin in bronchorroea in bronchioloalveolar carcinoma: role of cyclooxygenase. Chest. 117: 1213–1214.

113 Suga T et al. (1994) Bronchioloalveolar carcinoma with bronchorrhoea treated with erythromycin. The European Respiratory Journal. 7: 2249–2251.

114 Hiratsuka T et al. (1998) Severe bronchorrhoea accompanying alveolar cell carcinoma: treatment with clarithromycin and inhaled beclomethasone. Nihon Kokyuki Gakkai Zasshi. 36: 482–487.

115 Hudson E et al. (2006) Successful treatment of bronchorrhea with octreotide in a patient with adenocarcinoma of the lung. Journal of Pain and Symptom Management. 32: 200–202.

116 Maskell NA and Butland RJ (2003) BTS guidelines for the investigation of a unilateral pleural effusion in adults. Thorax. 58 Suppl 2: ii8–17.

117 Antunes G et al. (2003) BTS guidelines for the management of malignant pleural effusions. Thorax. 58 Suppl 2: ii29–38.

118 Stretton F et al. (1999) Malignant pleural effusions. European Journal of Palliative Care. 6: 5–9.

119 Abbas SQ (2007) Pleural effusion aspiration in a small hospice setting. Journal of Pain and Symptom Management. 34: 114–115.

120 National Patient Safety Agency (2008) Rapid response report. NPSA/2008/RRR003. Available from: www.npsa.nhs.uk

121 Janssen JP et al. (2007) Safety of pleurodesis with talc poudrage in malignant pleural effusion: a prospective cohort study. Lancet. 369: 1535–1539.

122 Sherman S et al. (1988) Optimum anaesthesia with intrapleural lidocaine during chemical pleurodesis with tetracycline. Chest. 93: 533–536.

123 Shaw P and Agarwal R (2004) Pleurodesis for malignant pleural effusions. Cochrane Database of Systematic Reviews. CD002916.

124 Tan C et al. (2006) The evidence on the effectiveness of management for malignant pleural effusion: a systematic review. European Journal of Cardio-thoracic Surgery. 29: 829–838.

125 Erasmus J and Patz E (1999) Treatmet of malignant pleural effusions. Current Opinion in Pulmonary Medicine. 5: 250–255.

126 Davies C et al. (1999) Intrapleural streptokinase in the management of malignant multiloculated pleural effusions. Chest. 115: 729–733.

127 Warren WH et al. (2008) Identification of clinical factors predicting Pleurx catheter removal in patients treated for malignant pleural effusion. European Journal of Cardio-thoracic Surgery. 33: 89–94.

128 Bruce D et al. (1996) Lymphangitis carcinomatosa: a literature review. Journal of the Royal College of Surgeons (Edinburgh). 41: 7–13.

129 Trapnell D (1964) Radiological appearances of lymphangitis carcinomatosa. Thorax. 19: 251–260.

130 Stein M et al. (1987) Pulmonary lymphangitic spread of carcinoma: appearance on CT scans. Radiology. 162: 371–375.

131 Emirgil C (1964) Effect of metastatic carcinoma to the lung on pulmonary function in man. *American Journal of Medicine*. **36**: 382–394.

132 National electronic Library for Health (2008) NHS Clinical Knowledge Summary: Hiccups - Management. Available from: http://www.cks.library.nhs.uk/hiccups/management/quick_answers/scenario_hiccups/view_full_scenario

133 Giudice M (2007) Drugs may cause hiccups in rare cases. *Canadian Pharmacists Journal*. **140**: 124–126.

134 Marhofer P et al. (1999) Incidence and therapy of midazolam induced hiccups in paediatric anaesthesia. *Paediatric Anaesthesia*. **9**: 295–298.

135 Liaw CC et al. (2005) Cisplatin-related hiccups: male predominance, induction by dexamethasone, and protection against nausea and vomiting. *Journal of Pain and Symptom Management*. **30**: 359–366.

136 Lauterbach E (1999) Hiccup and apparent myoclonus after hydrocodone: Review of the opiate-related hiccup and myoclonus literature. *Clinical Neuropharmacology*. **22**: 87–92.

137 De-Ruysscher D et al. (1996) Treatment of intractable hiccup in a terminal cancer patient with nebulized saline. *Palliative Medicine*. **10**: 166–167.

138 Salem MR et al. (1967) Treatment of hiccups by pharyngeal stimulation in anesthetized and conscious subjects. *Journal of the American Medical Association*. **202**: 126–130.

139 Goldsmith A (1983) A treatment for hiccups. *Journal of the American Medical Association*. **249**: 1566.

140 Lamphier TA (1977) Methods of management of persistent hiccup (singultus). *Maryland State Medical Journal*. **November**: 80–81.

141 Ramirez FC and Graham DY (1992) Treatment of intractable hiccup with baclofen: results of a double-blind randomized, controlled, crossover study. *American Journal of Gastroenterology*. **87**: 1789–1791.

142 Guelaud C et al. (1995) Baclofen therapy for chronic hiccup. *European Respiratory Journal*. **8**: 235–237.

143 Lipps DC et al. (1990) Nifedipine for intractable hiccups. *Neurology*. **40**: 531–532.

144 Brigham B and Bolin T (1992) High dose nifedipine and fludrocortisone for intractable hiccups. *Medical Journal of Australia*. **157**: 70.

145 Wilcock A and Twycross R (1996) Case report: midazolam for intractable hiccup. *Journal of Pain and Symptom Management*. **12**: 59–61.

146 Scarnati RA (1979) Intractable hiccup (singultus): report of case. *Journal of the American Osteopathic Association*. **79**: 127–129.

147 Ives TJ et al. (1985) Treatment of intractable hiccups with intramuscular haloperidol. *American Journal of Psychiatry*. **142**: 1368–1369.

148 Marechal R et al. (2003) Successful treatment of intractable hiccup with methylphenidate in a lung cancer patient. *Support Care Cancer*. **11**: 126–128.

149 Jacobson P et al. (1981) Treatment of intractable hiccups with valproic acid. *Neurology*. **31**: 1458–1460.

150 Moretti R et al. (2004) Gabapentin as a drug therapy of intractable hiccup because of vascular lesion: a three-year follow up. *Neurologist*. **10**: 102–106.

151 Schuchmann JA and Browne BA (2007) Persistent hiccups during rehabilitation hospitalization: three case reports and review of the literature. *American Journal of Physical Medicine & Rehabilitation*. **86**: 1013–1018.

152 Tegeler ML and Baumrucker SJ (2008) Gabapentin for intractable hiccups in palliative care. *The American Journal of Hospice & Palliative Care*. **25**: 52–54.

5: PSYCHOLOGICAL SYMPTOMS

Patients with cancer experience psychological as well as physical symptoms. The results of a survey at a major cancer centre in the USA illustrate this (Table 5.1). Problems are also common among patients' relatives.

Table 5.1 Common symptoms in cancer patients[1]

Physical	%	Psychological	%
Lack of energy	73	Worrying	72
Pain	63	Feeling sad	67
Drowsiness	60	Feeling nervous	62
Dry mouth	55	Difficulty sleeping	53
Nausea	45	Feeling irritable	47
Anorexia	45	Difficulty concentrating	40

Psychological problems are often overlooked by doctors and nurses. This is partly because of selective attention to physical problems.[2] About 10% of patients with advanced cancer have an identifiable psychiatric illness. Open questions such as 'How are you feeling?' and 'How are you coping?' frequently facilitate the expression of negative emotion.[3]

Some psychological problems can be prevented by:
- good staff–patient communication, giving information according to individual need. Unfortunately, staff do not always give as much information as patients and families want, even when asked directly
- good staff–patient relationships, with continuity of care
- allowing patients to have some control over the management of their illness.

RESPONSES TO LOSS

Many of the psychological problems seen in advanced cancer relate to actual or anticipated loss (Table 5.2). Similar psychological responses occur with major losses of any kind, e.g. redundancy, divorce, amputation, bereavement, as well as the anticipated loss of one's own life. These responses do not necessarily occur in sequence. Several may occur together and some may not occur at all. Oscillations in the patient's feelings are common. In cancer patients, more marked responses are often seen:

- at or shortly after the time of diagnosis
- at the time of the first recurrence
- as death approaches.

Table 5.2 Psychological responses to loss[4]

Phase	Symptom	Typical duration
Disruption	Disbelief Denial Shock/numbness Despair	Days → weeks
Dysphoria	Anxiety Insomnia Anger Guilt Sadness Poor concentration Activities disrupted	Weeks → months
Adaptation	Dysphoria diminishes Implications confronted New goals established Hope refocused and restored Activities resumed	Months

Denial

Denial is a common defence mechanism. It signifies an ability to obliterate or minimize threat by ignoring it.[5] However, it may be associated with physiological and other non-verbal evidence of anxiety. Occasionally, because a patient is unable to accept that he is dying, he deludes himself into believing that there is a plot to kill him or that the treatment is the cause of his deterioration. However, such paranoid states are more likely to be caused by brain tumours, biochemical disturbances or corticosteroids. There is no one right way of responding and adjusting to a poor prognosis. The doctor's task is to help the patient adjust in the best way possible, given that particular patient's family, cultural and spiritual background. Many people have a combination of inner resources and good support from their family and others which enables them to cope without prolonged and disabling distress.

Even so, most patients and relatives continue to make use of denial to a varying extent. Patients experience conflict between the wish to know the truth and the wish to avoid anxiety, and denial is one way of coping with this. Professional intervention may be needed when denial persists and interferes with:
- the acceptance of treatment
- planning for the future
- interpersonal relationships.

FAMILY PROBLEMS

Cancer always changes family psychodynamics, either for better or for worse. Within families, there is a conflict between the wish to confide and to receive emotional and practical support on the one hand and the wish to protect loved ones from distress on the other, particularly children or frail parents. A conspiracy of silence (collusion) is a source of tension. It blocks discussion of the future and preparation for parting. If it is not resolved, the bereaved often experience much regret.[6]

OTHER PROBLEMS

Cancer-related
These include for example, impact on sexual function, difficulty in accepting a colostomy, paraplegia, or the effects of cerebral secondaries.

Treatment-related
For example, undesirable drug effects such as hair loss. Patients may want to share in decisions about when to stop treatment aimed at prolonging life. Fear of death may make some want to go on even when undesirable effects are severe and the chance of improvement is minimal. Others may wish to opt for a shorter life with better quality at a time when doctors are advocating more aggressive measures.

Concurrent
For example, a bereavement or a pre-existing psychiatric illness.

ANGER

'A person loses their temper when the emotional demands of the situation exceed their emotional resources.'

'Anger is an emotional response to the perception of an overwhelming threat.'

Anger is an uncomfortable dynamic emotion which ranges from a mild sense of irritation to uncontrollable rage. Anger is generally transient but may be chronic. Anger can:
- increase vigour/energy
- facilitate the expression of negative feelings

- disrupt relationships (temporarily or permanently)
- induce impulsive action
- help a person defend himself physically and psychologically
- instigate aggression.

If anger is unjustifiably displaced or projected onto the family or staff, it tends to alienate. Anger can also interfere with the acceptance of limitations, and may stop a patient from making positive adjustments to physical disability. If anger is suppressed, the patient may become withdrawn, unco-operative and possibly depressed.

Causes

Anger is a common response to the losses associated with advanced cancer and bereavement. However, there are many specific causes which need to be identified (Box 5.A).

Box 5.A   Selected causes of anger

Personality trait
Delay in diagnosis
Manner in which the patient was told the diagnosis
Part of an adjustment reaction to diagnosis and prognosis
Delay in treatment
Uncommunicative doctors
Failed treatment
Feeling of unfairness about illness
Feeling let down by God
Frustration because of the limitations imposed by progressive illness
Depression

Management

Anger is a normal response to bad news and may be directed at the doctor as the bearer of the bad news. It is important to:
- listen carefully to what is being expressed
- avoid defensiveness
- validate the patient's feelings, e.g. 'Given what you're having to cope with, you've every right to be angry'
- remember that a period of silence can be therapeutic
- clarify the cause(s) of anger, e.g. 'Are you able to tell me exactly what's making you so angry?
- consider whether anger is part of a clinical depression; if this seems probable, treat accordingly (see p.194)
- if anger becomes chronic, consider obtaining help from a counsellor, psycho-therapist, psychiatrist or chaplain/spiritual adviser
- support staff involved, and maintain team unity.

With time, in most patients, anger resolves to a variable extent. On the other hand, it may not; some patients die angry.[7]

ANXIETY

Anxiety is an unpleasant emotion with which everybody is familiar. Anxiety can be acute (transient) or chronic (persistent) and varies in intensity. Many cancer patients sleep badly, have frightening dreams or are reluctant to be left alone at night, and sometimes during the day as well; these all suggest heightened anxiety.

At some stage, about 10% of palliative care patients suffer from generalized anxiety disorder or panic disorder, accompanied by various physical symptoms (Box 5.B). Such patients experience greater distress from physical symptoms, social concerns and existential issues.[8,9]

Box 5.B Symptoms of anxiety[10,11]

Psychological
Apprehension
Cannot distract self or be distracted
Depersonalization
Derealization
Catastrophic thoughts
Indecisiveness
Intrusive thoughts of death
Irritability
Persistently tense, unable to relax
Poor concentration
Worry

May be associated with low morale or depressive illness

Physical
Nervous system
    headache, tremor, fatigue, dizziness, paraesthesia, panic attacks, leg weakness
Gastro-intestinal
    nausea, dry mouth, dysphagia, anorexia, indigestion, diarrhoea
Cardiovascular
    palpitations, chest pain
Respiratory
    hyperventilation, yawning, sighing,
Genito-urinary
    frequency or urgency of micturition, impotence
Skin
    rash, sweating

Causes
There are many causes of anxiety in advanced cancer (Box 5.C).

Evaluation
An expectation that cancer patients are bound to be anxious is a common obstacle to evaluation and treatment. Evaluation is primarily through careful listening and questioning. In addition, the family may well be able to provide useful background information.

Investigate the cause of any biochemical or neuro-endocrine abnormality. Other investigations are sometimes indicated, e.g. cardiac monitoring in patients suspected of having an arrhythmia. Review medication; for example, has the patient recently started a corticosteroid or an SSRI?

Box 5.C Causes of heightened anxiety[12]

Situational
Adjustment reaction
Fear of hospital, chemotherapy,
    radiotherapy
Worry about family and finances
Withdrawal of active treatment

Psychological
Thoughts about the past, e.g.
    wasted opportunities
    guilt
Thoughts about the future, e.g.
    fear of pain
    fear of mental impairment
    fear of loss of independence
Thoughts about after death

Psychiatric
Adjustment disorder with anxiety
Panic disorder
Generalized anxiety disorder
Post-traumatic stress disorder
Depression
Psychosis
Delirium

Uncontrolled symptoms
Insomnia
Breathlessness
Nausea
Severe pain
Weakness

Physical disorders
Brain tumour
Cardiac arrhythmias
Hyperadrenalism
Hyperthyroidism
Hypoglycaemia

Drugs
Drug-induced hallucinations, e.g.
    benzodiazepines
    opioids
Antidepressants, e.g.
    SSRIs
Anti-epileptics, e.g.
    carbamazepine
Antimicrobials, e.g.
    aciclovir
    cephalosporins
    isoniazid
    ofloxacin
Antipsychotics (akathisia, see p.396)
Bronchodilators, e.g.
    β_2-agonists
    theophyllines
Corticosteroids
Thyroxine

Drug withdrawal
Alcohol
Antidepressants
Benzodiazepines

Management
Correct the correctable
Management depends on the cause:
• relieve pain and other distressing symptoms
• facilitate the airing and sharing of worries and fears; 'a trouble shared is a trouble halved'[13]
• correct misconceptions
• develop a strategy for coping with uncertainty.[14]

Non-drug treatment
There are many psychological approaches to anxiety but these are beyond the scope of this book (Box 5.D). They are also used in chronic pain management, particularly when anxiety is a concurrent feature. In practice their use depends on the availability of an appropriate therapist, e.g. psychologist, music therapist, hypnotherapist.

Box 5.D Psychological methods for managing anxiety and/or pain

Anxiety management training	Art therapy
CBT	Biofeedback
Brief therapy	Hypnotherapy
Music therapy	

Relaxation therapy is often provided by an occupational therapist or physiotherapist. CBT and psychotherapy are generally provided over several months. The duration and goals of treatment may need to be adjusted in the palliative care setting.[15,16]

Drug treatment
For more information, see *PCF3*.

The following should be used together with psychological support:
- benzodiazepines, e.g.:
  ▷ lorazepam 1–2mg PO b.d.–t.d.s.
  ▷ diazepam 2–20mg PO at bedtime and 2–5mg p.r.n.
- antidepressants:
  ▷ particularly if anxiety-depression (see p.194)
  ▷ if persistent panic attacks (see below)
- antipsychotics:
  ▷ if the patient is psychotic, e.g. has paranoid ideas or is hallucinating
  ▷ if the anxiety is a feature of an agitated delirium
  ▷ if the situation is made worse by benzodiazepines.

PANIC DISORDER

Panic is an episodic pathological failure of the protective 'fight or flight' response to a major threat, in which all structure and reality checks are lost. In the dying, an overwhelming sense of doom or absolute despair often supervenes. Panic is associated with various autonomic symptoms (Box 5.E). It is physiologically demanding and cannot be maintained indefinitely. Panic is therefore episodic but attacks may occur in clusters.

Physiology
Serotonin (5HT) plays a central role in panic disorder.[18] Supporting evidence for this comes from the clinical efficacy of SSRIs.[19] It is unclear whether there is a deficit in the synthesis and/or neurotransmission of serotonin. Serotonin may improve anxiety (and hyperventilation) by inhibiting:
- excitatory cortical inputs to the amygdala
- excitatory stimulation of the peri-aqueductal gray area, locus ceruleus and, chronically, the hypothalamo-pituitary-adrenal axis
- corticotrophin-releasing factor production and/or release
- ventilatory control abnormalities associated with low serotoninergic tone.

Panic circuitry is complex and mediated by region-specific subtypes of serotonin receptors that adapt to the effects of panic disorder and its treatment.[20,21]

Box 5.E   DSM-IV-TR criteria for panic attack and panic disorder[17]

Panic attack

A discrete period of intense fear or discomfort in which four or more of the following symptoms develop abruptly and reach a peak within 10 minutes:
• palpitations, pounding heart, or accelerated heart rate
• sweating
• trembling or shaking
• sensations of shortness of breath or smothering
• feeling of choking
• chest pain or discomfort
• nausea or abdominal distress
• feeling dizzy, unsteady, lightheaded or faint
• derealization (feelings of unreality) or depersonalization (being detached from oneself)
• fear of losing control or going crazy
• fear of dying
• paraesthesias (numbness or tingling sensations)
• chills or hot flushes.

Panic disorder

Recurrent unexpected panic attacks, and at least one of the attacks followed by 1 month or more of one or more of the following:
• persistent concern about having further attacks
• worry about the implications of the attack or its consequences, e.g. fear of death or suffocation
• a significant change in behaviour related to the attacks.

The serotoninergic system also interacts with the GABA-ergic, noradrenergic and neuropeptide systems. Impairment of the brain's inhibitory GABA-ergic system also plays a part. Elevated levels of noradrenaline (norepinephrine) within the CNS are also implicated, as is supersensitivity of parts of the sympathetic nervous system. Various neuropeptides have also been implicated, notably corticotrophin-releasing factors and cholecystokinin.[18,20]

The amygdala is instrumental in the generation of the fear response.[22] Anxiety-provoking sensory stimuli from the cardiorespiratory and GI systems or signals from the sensory cortex are relayed to the central nucleus of the amygdala (Table 5.3). This generates fear-related responses mediated by corticotrophin-releasing factor activation of:
• peri-aqueductal gray area (facilitates the panic response)
• noradrenergic cells of the locus ceruleus (further stimulating the amygdala)
• hypothalamic-pituitary-adrenal axis (increase in plasma cortisol)
• parabrachial nucleus and dorsal motor nucleus of the vagus (activating cardio-respiratory responses, i.e. hyperventilation).

Many of the areas which mediate panic are also chemosensitive to carbon dioxide and pH, and thereby influence the respiratory neurones in the medulla. Depletion of serotonin increases respiratory rate, ventilation, and ventilatory response to carbon dioxide; these are reversed by administration of a serotonin precursor.[23]

Table 5.3 Afferent pathways in panic disorder[18]

Input	Modifier	Destination
Viscerosensory		
Respiratory panicogens	Changes in pH	Amygdaloid-hippocampal
Baroreceptor stimulation	Locus ceruleus	activation
Neuropeptides		
Visuospatial-auditory-cognitive		
Visual stimuli	Hippocampus	Amygdaloid-thalamic-cortical-
Auditory stimuli	Peri-aqueductal	amygdaloid circuit activation
Catastrophic thoughts	gray area	

Hypersensitivity to carbon dioxide is present in many patients with panic disorder; this is reduced by treatment with a serotoninergic antidepressant.[21,24]

Evaluation
In cancer, panic may be:
• an exacerbation of a pre-existing anxiety disorder (in which case the onset of panic attacks may well predate the diagnosis of cancer)
• a reaction to the patient's current circumstances
• secondary to uncontrolled symptoms, e.g. breathlessness
• a feature of agitated delirium
• precipitated by medication, e.g. corticosteroids
• a form of temporal lobe epilepsy in patients with brain tumours (Box 5.F).[25]

Box 5.F Temporal lobe epilepsy

The temporal lobe is the most common site of origin for complex partial seizures.

Clinical features include:
• impaired consciousness
• hallucinations are characteristic but need not occur
  ▷ olfactory (most frequent), e.g. burning rubber
  ▷ taste, e.g. metallic
  ▷ hearing (infrequent)
  ▷ sight (infrequent)
• cognitive impairment
  ▷ *jamais-vu*, i.e. feelings of unreality which may provoke despair, panic
  ▷ *déjà-vu*, i.e. a feeling of excessive familiarity with events and environment
  ▷ intense pleasure
  ▷ intense fear or anger
• autonomic activity
  ▷ flushing
  ▷ pilo-erection ('gooseflesh')
  ▷ ill-defined abdominal sensations
• automatisms, e.g. chewing, swallowing, plucking.

Patients with breathlessness are at increased risk of panic attacks associated with exacerbations of their breathlessness. A common feature is the persistent fear about the attacks and their consequences, e.g. fear of suffocation and death during an attack.[26] Other features include:

- episodes of breathlessness occurring at rest
- poor relationship of breathlessness to exertion
- rapid fluctuations of breathlessness within minutes
- breathlessness associated with certain social situations
- previous/concurrent panic or generalized anxiety disorder.

Some patients with end-stage MND/ALS appear fearful at times but are unable to vocalize their feelings. As many such patients have incipient respiratory failure, it is probable that the non-verbally expressed fear reflects episodes of panic.

Management
Correct the correctable
If panic is a manifestation of temporal lobe epilepsy, anti-epileptics should be introduced or adjusted.

Non-drug treatment
With all breathless patients, enquire specifically about panic attacks because open discussion is the key to successful management. Panic often responds to a calming presence and encouraging the hyperventilating patient to breathe more slowly and deeply. Patients should also be taught about optimal breathing techniques, respiratory control and relaxation.[26] These are most commonly provided by a physiotherapist or, in a breathlessness clinic, by a specialist nurse.[8,27]

With panic attacks not associated with breathlessness, it is important to explore possible reasons for the attacks. In physically healthy people, panic may relate to chronic existential anxiety. In contrast, in cancer patients there is an obvious precipitating cause, namely the fear of impending death, disintegration and annihilation. Often such fears are only thinly disguised and empathic discussion can help by bringing them into the open.

Where panic disorder is diagnosed, CBT is the treatment of choice.[28] It is as effective as an antidepressant but does not cause undesirable effects.[29] However, it is of limited availability and it may take 4–8 weeks to see improvement compared with 2–4 weeks with an SSRI, and a few days with a benzodiazepine.[30] In patients with a prognosis of just weeks, the goals and duration of CBT will need to be altered. This could reduce its effectiveness.[31]

Some centres offer solution-focused brief therapy.[32] This is a modified form of CBT, developed specifically with physically ill patients in mind.[33,34]

Drug treatment
For more information, see *PCF3*.

In patients with a short prognosis, the drug of choice is a benzodiazepine with a long halflife and which needs to be given only once daily or b.d., such as diazepam or clonazepam.[35] With short-acting drugs, such as alprazolam, there is significant risk of break-through (rebound) anxiety.[36] Diazepam and clonazepam are generally best taken at bedtime, when they double as a night sedative. If episodes of rebound anxiety continue to occur, additional smaller doses can be given in the morning, or both morning and early evening.

Maintenance treatment is with either a benzodiazepine or an SSRI, or both.[35,37] In breathless patients with a short prognosis, a benzodiazepine is likely to remain the treatment of choice.

When starting an SSRI, it is best to continue the benzodiazepine for a few weeks to prevent an initial exacerbation of anxiety. To reduce the likelihood of initial nausea, the starting dose of the SSRI should be low, e.g. sertraline 25mg once daily. If necessary, the dose is titrated upwards at intervals of 1–2 weeks to 50–200mg once daily.[19,30]

For patients with a prognosis of 2–3 months, initial treatment with an SSRI is preferable.[28,38] Although the addition of a benzodiazepine produces a more rapid response, after 3 weeks the response rate is no greater than treatment with an SSRI alone.[39]

Imipramine, a TCA, is sometimes recommended as the second-line antidepressant treatment.[28] However, antimuscarinic effects may limit dose escalation,[30] and mirtazapine with its sedative and specific serotoninergic effects is probably a better alternative.[40,41]

Patients who take benzodiazepines for prolonged periods develop physical dependence, and thus the possibility of a discontinuation (withdrawal) syndrome should medication be stopped abruptly. This is characterized by anxiety, irritability, insomnia, poor concentration, headaches, palpitations and breathlessness. Discontinuation syndromes are less marked if the dose is tapered over 4–8 weeks, and with benzodiazepines with a long halflife.[42] If PO medication becomes difficult, consider switching to midazolam by CSCI.[43]

For some patients in whom symptoms of palpitation, sweating or tremor predominate, propranolol 20mg PO stat ± 20–40mg P.O. b.d.–t.d.s. may be helpful. However, it is not as effective as a benzodiazepine.[44]

An antipsychotic such as haloperidol is indicated if there are concurrent psychotic symptoms such as delusions or hallucinations.

ADJUSTMENT DISORDER

An adjustment disorder is a state of distress and emotional disturbance which impairs normal social and occupational function. It may be precipitated by any stressful event, e.g. bad news, pain or approaching death. To fulfil the diagnostic criteria, the distressed state must develop <3 months after the trigger event.

Symptoms of an adjustment disorder include anxiety, low mood, inability to cope and behavioural changes which are not severe or persistent enough to meet the diagnostic criteria for major psychiatric disorders but are beyond those of a normal stress reaction.[17,45] An adjustment disorder occurs in up to 1/3 of palliative care patients.[46] It may be difficult to differentiate between a normal and abnormal response to a distressing event.[47]

Risk factors for adjustment disorder include:
- lack of information
- lack of social support
- partner's level of distress
- other unresolved issues
- passive or avoidant coping styles.[11]

Adjustment disorder should be differentiated from post-traumatic stress disorder. This occurs as a delayed response to a stressful event and is associated with nightmares, reliving of the stressful event and avoidance of reminiscent activities.

Adjustment disorder should be evaluated and managed in the same way as anxiety. Benzodiazepines should be reserved for more severe cases; treatment with an antidepressant is not recommended.[45]

DEPRESSION

A depressive illness (major depression) occurs in some 5–10% of patients with advanced cancer.[48–50] Another 10–15% will have some depressive symptoms, often as part of an adjustment disorder or because of a loss of morale associated, for example, with unremitting distressing symptoms.

Loss of morale is sometimes called 'demoralization syndrome'. Its cardinal features are helplessness, feelings of inadequacy, meaninglessness and hopelessness. It differs from a depressive illness, and does not need or respond to antidepressants.[51,52]

It is important to identify depression particularly because conventional treatment achieves a good response in about 80% of cases. Untreated depression:
- intensifies other symptoms
- leads to social withdrawal
- prevents the patient from completing 'unfinished business'.

Depression may be undiagnosed because:
- low mood is ignored by doctors and nurses because it is considered 'understandable' or 'reactive'
- the patient may be feeling better when seen by the doctor compared with earlier in the day (diurnal variation)
- social skills mask the depressed mood (smiling depression)
- the depression is expressed through physical symptoms, e.g. pain (somatization)
- the depression is masked by concurrent symptoms of anxiety
- the depression manifests as a worsening of a personality trait, e.g. attention-seeking.

On the other hand, depression may be over-diagnosed if all patients who are sad and sometimes cry are said to have a depressive illness.

Clinical features
For major depression, at least five of the following symptoms must be present, including one or both of the first two. In addition, symptoms must be present most of the day, on most days, for at least 2 weeks:
- depressed mood
- markedly diminished interest or pleasure in almost all activities
- significant weight loss or gain
- insomnia or hypersomnia
- psychomotor agitation or retardation
- impaired concentration (indecisiveness)
- fatigue (lack of energy)
- feelings of worthlessness (or guilt)
- suicidal ideas.[53]

Causes

Many psychosocial and physiological factors predispose to depression (Box 5.G). Medication is also a cause (Table 5.4). There is also a relationship between the site and nature of an organic brain disorder and the subsequent development of depression (Box 5.H).

Box 5.G   Risk factors for depression

Psychosocial
Past history of depression
Conspiracy of silence
Inability to express emotions
Lack of supportive relationship
Loss of independence (greater risk in men)
Mutilation
Obsessional personality
Recent bereavement
Threat of death

Physiological
Unrelieved pain
Paraneoplastic[a]
Biochemical
  hypercalcaemia
  hypokalaemia
Endocrine
  hypercortisolism[b]
  hyperparathyroidism
  hypoparathyroidism
  hyperprolactinaemia
Vitamin deficiency
  folate
  nicotinic acid (Pellagra)
  thiamine (B_1)
Brain
  stroke
  head injury
  brain tumour
  epilepsy
  parkinsonism
  multiple sclerosis

---

a. incidence higher in cancer of the pancreas[54,55]
b. nearly 50% become depressed; more likely when caused by pituitary impairment.

Table 5.4   Drugs commonly associated with depression[56]

Drug class	Example
Antihypertensive	Clonidine, methyldopa, nifedipine, propanolol
Anti-arrhythmic	Digoxin, procainamide
Antiparkinsonian	Amantidine, L-dopa
Antipsychotic	Chlorpromazine (but not levomepromazine)
Cytotoxics	Interferons, vincristine
H_2-receptor antagonist	Ranitidine
Hormonal agent	Corticosteroids, oral contraceptives
Anti-epileptic	Carbamazepine, vigabatrin
Antiretroviral	Efavirenz, nevirapine

Box 5.H   Organic brain disorders and depression

Epilepsy
Higher suicide rate, particularly with temporal lobe epilepsy.

Brain tumours
Depression more common with supratemporal tumours and with frontal and temporal lobe tumours.[57]

Cerebrovascular accident (CVA) and head injury
Location of lesion relevant for the first 6 months; psychosocial factors more relevant later. Greater risk with left-sided lesion, particularly left anterior brain.[58] Positive emission tomography (PET) shows that the brain serotonin concentration is lower after a left-sided CVA than after a right-sided CVA.[59]

Parkinson's disease
Left-sided Parkinson's disease (i.e. right brain) is associated with more depression (the opposite of post-stroke depression).[60] Responds well to antidepressants.

Multiple sclerosis
Up to 1/3 become depressed and cognitively impaired; a similar proportion are relatively euphoric.[61] There is a higher than expected incidence of depression in the year before diagnosis,[62] and a greater likelihood of a past history of bipolar depression.

MND/ALS
Less depression than in multiple sclerosis.[63]

Evaluation
Diagnosing depression is difficult in the presence of a debilitating physical illness.

Some patients are seemingly depressed but in reality are simply close to death with no residual energy and a corresponding loss of pleasure in life.[64] In more robust patients, it is necessary to differentiate between:
- an adjustment reaction, i.e. sadness provoked by the change in personal circumstances
- loss of morale because of unrelieved severe pain or other distressing symptoms, anxiety, insomnia, and a sense of desolation
- depression (Figure 5.1 and Table 5.5).

Evaluation is difficult because the somatic symptoms of depression overlap with the symptoms of cancer:
- anorexia
- weight loss
- constipation
- sleep disturbance
- loss of libido.

Proxies, including close relatives, cannot reliably be used to determine a person's emotional state. The essential first step is to ask all new patients directly about their mood, e.g. 'How has your mood been recently?' If the answer suggests that their mood is lower than normal, ask more directly, 'Are you depressed?'.

In palliative care patients in the USA, this single question is reported to identify 100% of the patients with depression.[65] In contrast, in the UK, the figure is nearer 50%,[66] indicating a major cultural difference.

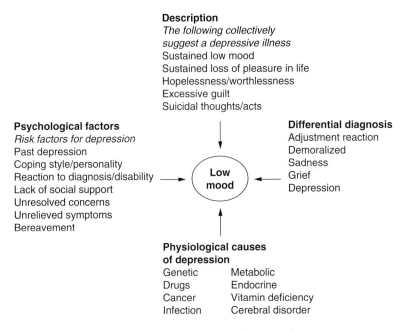

Description
The following collectively suggest a depressive illness
Sustained low mood
Sustained loss of pleasure in life
Hopelessness/worthlessness
Excessive guilt
Suicidal thoughts/acts

Psychological factors
Risk factors for depression
Past depression
Coping style/personality
Reaction to diagnosis/disability
Lack of social support
Unresolved concerns
Unrelieved symptoms
Bereavement

Low mood

Differential diagnosis
Adjustment reaction
Demoralized
Sadness
Grief
Depression

Physiological causes of depression
Genetic   Metabolic
Drugs   Endocrine
Cancer   Vitamin deficiency
Infection   Cerebral disorder

Figure 5.1 The four dimensions of evaluation of low mood.

Table 5.5 Distinguishing a depressive illness from sadness and loss of morale[70]

Features of all three conditions	Features more typical of depression
Loss of interest	Loss of all emotion and pleasure in life
Decreased concentration	Social withdrawal
Tearfulness	Not distractable (but with diurnal variation)
Anxiety	Irritability
Decreased sleep	Physical anxiety (sweating, tremor, panic attacks)
Tiredness	Hopelessness and worthlessness (particularly
Anorexia	with regard to family and friends)
Suicidal ideas	Excessive guilt
	Intractable pain
	Requests for euthanasia
	Suicide attempts

In general practice, asking two general mood-related questions, followed by a 'help' question, identified about 80% of all depressed patients, with few false positives:[67]

'During the past month, have you often been bothered by feeling down, depressed or hopeless?'

'During the past month, have you often been bothered by little interest or pleasure in doing things?'

'Is this something with which you would like help?'.

These screening questions were asked in writing, and the answer to the third was limited to 'no', 'yes, but not today', and 'yes'. However, in patients with advanced cancer, a positive answer to the second question may well be misleading because of general debility.

When there is doubt, a decision can be delayed for, say, 2 weeks. During this time, with the general support given by the palliative care service, morale may rise and adjustment reactions worked through. Sometimes it may help to use a validated screening tool, e.g. the Edinburgh Depression Scale.[68,69] However, this is unlikely to clarify the situation in cases which are not clearcut. A psychiatric consultation should be requested when doubt persists.

Explanation
The nature of the explanation will vary according to the patient's physical and psychological state. Patients are often helped by being told that depression is not shameful. For example:

'It seems to me that you've developed a depressive illness ... Being physically ill is hard work and emotionally exhausting. Ongoing stress reduces certain chemicals in the brain and this results in depression ... Antidepressants are tablets which help the brain replenish these chemicals.'

Management
Guidelines: Management of depression, p.199.

In patients who have had depression in the past, ask them what helped before and consider together whether such measures might help again.

Non-drug treatment
When a patient presents with severe depression, a combination of antidepressants and individual CBT should be considered.[71] The goals of CBT need to be tailored to the patient's prognosis and ability to participate.

Attendance at a palliative care day centre is helpful for patients who are isolated at home because of weakness and/or other debilitating symptoms. A day centre provides:
• social interaction
• psychological support
• medical supervision.

Drug treatment
For more information, see *PCF3*.

TCAs have been largely superseded as the drugs of choice for depression by the newer antidepressants, e.g. SSRIs and mirtazapine. Undesirable effects can still be troublesome. Nausea and anxiety are common reasons for discontinuing an SSRI.[72]

Guidelines: Management of depression

Sadness and tears alone, even if associated with transient suicidal thoughts, do not justify the diagnosis of depression or the prescription of an antidepressant. Patients may have an adjustment reaction and/or become demoralized. These do not respond to antidepressants, but may improve with psychosocial support and time.

Evaluation

1 Screening: about 5–10% of patients with advanced cancer develop a major depression. Cases will be missed unless specific enquiry is made of all patients:

'What has your mood been like lately?... Are you depressed?'
'Have you had serious depression before? Are things like that now?'

2 Assessment interview: if depression is suspected, explore the patient's mood more fully by encouraging the patient to talk further with appropriate prompts. Symptoms overlap with those of cancer (e.g. loss of weight, lack of energy, fatigue) making diagnosis more difficult. However, the following are suggestive of clinical depression:
- sustained low mood (most of every day for several weeks) ⎫ core symptoms
- sustained loss of pleasure/interest in life (anhedonia) ⎭
- withdrawal from family and friends
- insomnia or hypersomnia
- psychomotor agitation or retardation
- impaired concentration (indecisiveness)
- feelings of worthlessness (or excessive guilt)
- indecisiveness or diminished ability to concentrate
- persistent suicidal ideas, and requests for euthanasia.

3 If in doubt whether the patient is suffering from depression, an adjustment reaction or sadness, review after 1–2 weeks and/or obtain the help of a psychologist/psychiatrist.

4 Medical causes of depression: depression may be the consequence of:
- a medical condition, e.g. hypercalcaemia, cerebral metastases
- a reaction to severe uncontrolled physical symptoms
- drugs, e.g. cytotoxics, benzodiazepines, antipsychotics, corticosteroids, antihypertensives.

Management

5 Correct the correctable: treat medical causes, particularly severe pain and other distressing symptoms.

6 Non-drug treatment:
- explanation and assurance that symptoms can be treated
- depressed patients often benefit from the ambience of a Palliative Care Day Centre
- specific psychological treatments (via a clinical psychologist, etc.)
- other psychosocial professionals, e.g. chaplain and creative therapists, have a therapeutic role but avoid overwhelming the patient with simultaneous multiple referrals.

continued

7 Drug treatment:
- if the patient is expected to live for >4 weeks, prescribe an antidepressant
- the initial and continuing doses of antidepressants are generally lower in debilitated patients compared with the physically fit
- all antidepressants can cause withdrawal symptoms if stopped abruptly; generally withdraw gradually over 2–3 weeks
- except for MAOIs, when switching from one antidepressant class to another, overlap the withdrawal of the old antidepressant with the gradual introduction of the new antidepressant over 2–3 weeks.

PCF preferred antidepressants

First-line antidepressants
Psychostimulant, e.g. methylphenidate
Particularly if prognosis <2–3 months:
- start with 2.5–5mg b.d. (on waking/breakfast time and noon/lunchtime)
- if necessary, increase by daily increments of 2.5mg b.d. to 20mg b.d.
- occasionally higher doses are necessary, e.g. 30mg b.d. or 20mg t.d.s.

SSRI, e.g. sertraline
Particularly if prognosis >2–3 months, and if associated anxiety:
- no antimuscarinic effects, but may cause an initial increase in anxiety
- if necessary, prescribe diazepam at bedtime
- start with 50mg each morning, preferably p.c.
- if no improvement after 2 weeks, increase dose by 50mg every 2–4 weeks
- maximum dose 200mg each morning.
- low likelihood of a withdrawal (discontinuation) syndrome.
If no response at all after 4 weeks, switch to a second-line antidepressant; but if partial response, wait a further 2 weeks.

Second-line antidepressants
Mirtazapine
A good choice for patients with anxiety/agitation:
- starting dose 15mg at bedtime
- if little or no improvement after 2 weeks, increase to 30mg at bedtime
- concurrent H_1-receptor antagonism leads to sedation but this decreases at the higher dose because of noradrenergic effects.
- fewer undesirable effects than TCAs.
If no response after 4 weeks, switch to a TCA or seek advice from a psychiatrist.

Tricyclic antidepressant, e.g. amitriptyline or imipramine
- start with 10–25mg at bedtime
- if tolerated, after 3–7 days increase to 25–50mg at bedtime
- if limited improvement, increase dose by 25mg every 4 weeks to 75–150mg at bedtime
- undesirable effects may limit dose escalation, e.g. dry mouth, sedation.
If no response after 8 weeks, seek advice from a psychiatrist.

Antidepressants take time to work. Latencies of 1–2 weeks for SSRIs and 2–3 weeks for TCAs are too optimistic for most patients, particularly with slow dose escalation.[73] The *median* response time in older patients is 2–3 months.[74]

Thus, because of the rapid onset of action (days rather than weeks), a psychostimulant, e.g. methylphenidate, should be considered in a severely retarded patient with a prognosis of <2–3 months.[75–77] Psychostimulants are possibly of greater benefit in medically ill patients than in the physically healthy.[78]

Psychostimulants are used at some centres for other purposes:
- troublesome opioid-induced drowsiness
- restoring a normal day and night rhythm of waking and sleeping.[79]

THE WITHDRAWN PATIENT

Some patients seem to be psychologically inaccessible. Although this may not be detrimental to the patient, there are times when the patient's facial expression and behaviour suggests considerable underlying psychological distress.

Causes
These fall into several categories (Box 5.1). Sometimes there may be several concurrent causal factors.

Box 5.1 Differential diagnosis of the withdrawn patient[80]

Personality

Pathological
Brain tumour
Cerebrovascular disease
Secondary mental disorders (see p.204)
Concurrent illness, e.g. hypothyroidism

Pharmacological
Oversedation
Tardive dyskinesia

Psychological
Anger
Collusion   } 'no point in talking about my feelings'
Distrust
Fear   'too painful'
Guilt   } 'too embarrassed'
Shame

Psychiatric
Depression   } 'no point in talking about my feelings'
Paranoia   } 'too dangerous'

Management

Management depends on the cause. If a psychological cause seems likely, try to find a 'window' in the patient's protective shell in order to help him acknowledge the problem and to begin to move forward to a healthier/more comfortable frame of mind. Good communication skills are essential to achieve this:

- acknowledge *your* difficulty, e.g. 'We seem to be finding it difficult to get into conversation'
- offer the patient an invitation which he can accept or reject, e.g. 'Are you able to tell me why you find it difficult to talk to me about things?'
- if the patient then gives a clue as to the reason for the reticence, this should be gently but firmly followed up, e.g. 'Can you tell me exactly what's troubling you?'
- it is important to establish the frequency and intensity of any mood disturbance in case the patient is psychiatrically ill rather than just psychologically disturbed
- ask for specialist help if you feel you are getting nowhere.

THE DIFFICULT PATIENT

It is not possible to be equally positive towards all patients. Some patients we find difficult. It is important to remember that the problem is primarily ours and not the patient's, although it could be a joint problem. Thus it is better to say, 'I find Mrs Brown difficult to look after' and not, 'Mrs Brown is difficult'.

Causes

There are many reasons why a patient may be difficult to care for (Box 5.J). The difficulties elicit feelings of impotence and inadequacy in us; we feel we have failed and we have come to the end of our therapeutic resources.

Box 5.J Reasons why patients can be difficult to care for

Patients or relatives perceived as
Unpleasant
Seductive
Ungrateful
Critical
Antagonistic
Demanding
Manipulative
Overdependent

Transference and countertransference

Patient's behaviour
Withdrawn
Psychologically volatile, angry
Depressed

Patient's symptoms
Gross disfigurement
Malodour
Poor response to symptom management
Somatization

Management

- acknowledge your difficulty with the rest of the team
- explore possible reasons why the patient seems difficult
- consider transference and countertransference reactions, i.e. negative feelings evoked by behaviour or personality traits in the patient because of your past experiences

---

(transference), or your personality evoking negative feelings in the patient (counter-transference). Both parties sense the negative 'vibes' and react to them
- agree on a management plan with the rest of the team and record it in the notes, including short-term goals and time to be spent with the patient and family. Accept that some problems cannot be solved.

INSOMNIA

Insomnia is difficulty in falling or staying asleep, leading to impaired daytime functioning. Some patients catnap during the day so much that they do not sleep well at night. If this is the case, it is important to determine whether being awake during the night is a problem for the patient or only for the family or carers.[81]

Causes
If the patient is not sleeping well at night, the situation needs to be evaluated; there may be a correctable cause (Box 5.K).

Box 5.K Causes of wakeful nights	

Physiological
Dementia with reversal of normal
  sleep-wake cycle
Normal old age
Sleep during day
  long siesta
  catnaps
  sedative drugs
Wakeful stimuli
  light
  noise
  urinary frequency
 	
Psychological
Anxiety (see p.187)
Depression (see p.194)
Fear of dying in the night
 	
Sleep disorders
Sleep apnoea
	Unrelieved symptoms
	Breathlessness
	Diarrhoea
	Incontinence
	Pain
	Pruritus
	Restless legs
	Vomiting
	
	Drugs
	Alcohol (may cause rebound
	  wakefulness)
	β-Blockers (bad dreams)
	Caffeine
	Corticosteroids
	Diuretics
	Sympathomimetics
	Withdrawal of night sedative

Management
Correct the correctable
- relieve disturbing symptoms
- if night pain, consider increasing the bedtime dose of morphine from double to treble the daytime q4h dose or supplement bedtime m/r morphine with ordinary morphine tablets or solution; in practice this is rarely necessary.

Non-drug treatment
- rise at the same time each day regardless of the amount of sleep the previous night
- increase daytime activity and reduce or stop daytime naps
- facilitate expression of anxieties and fears
- change mattress/bed if not comfortable
- avoid stimulants in the evening, e.g. alcohol, caffeine, smoking
- avoid mentally demanding tasks, e.g. studying, for 1–2h before bedtime
- do not use the bedroom for work or TV
- reduce light and noise at bedtime *and*
- institute a routine before bedtime e.g. hot drink, warm bath, reading
- soothing music or relaxation therapy/tape
- massage, e.g. of hands or feet
- if not asleep within 15–20min, leave the bedroom and go back to bed only when feeling sleepy
- CBT, particularly if there are dysfunctional beliefs about sleep and the insomnia is chronic; in practice, this is rarely necessary.[82]

Drug treatment
For more information, see *PCF3*.

Modify the drug regimen:
- corticosteroids, give as a single morning dose
- anxiolytics, if receiving diazepam in the daytime, convert to a single dose at bedtime
- diuretics, give as a single dose each morning.

Night sedatives (hypnotics):
Because of the risk of dependence, night sedatives should be used only when insomnia is severe, disabling or causing the patient extreme distress. Night sedatives can cause cognitive impairment and falls in the elderly; prescribe with caution,[83] e.g. half the normal starting dose.[81] Good choices include:
- temazepam 10–40mg at bedtime, occasionally more
- trazodone 25–100mg at bedtime, occasionally more.

Other drugs:
- if the patient is depressed or wakes early (see p.194), prescribe an antidepressant with sedative properties, e.g. amitriptyline, mirtazapine
- if sleep is disturbed by unpleasant dreams, and if specific discussion does not lead to a resolution, it may be necessary to prescribe haloperidol 1.5–5mg at bedtime.

SECONDARY MENTAL DISORDERS

These are mental disorders which are secondary to a general medical condition or related to chemical substances (drugs, alcohol), or both (Box 5.L). Causes include:
- biochemical derangement
- organ failure
- brain tumours
- paraneoplastic syndromes.

All types of secondary mental disorders are seen in patients with advanced cancer.

Box 5.L   Secondary mental disorders

Delirium	Personality disorder
Dementia	Intoxication
Amnestic disorder	Withdrawal state
Anxiety disorder	Psychosis
Mood disorder	

Delirium (synonyms: acute brain syndrome, acute confusion), dementia (synonym: chronic brain syndrome) and amnestic disorder are all characterized by cognitive impairment. The word confusion is often used of all three conditions. Note that:
- sometimes dementia is compounded by delirium
- dementia is not generally associated with drowsiness
- some patients with cancer appear to develop dementia rapidly and this may cause difficulty in diagnosis (Box 5.M).

Box 5.M   Comparison of global cognitive impairment disorders

Delirium		**Dementia**
Acute		Chronic
Often remitting and reversible		Usually progressive and irreversible
Disturbed consciousness		Consciousness intact
Reduced attention		Brain damage
(information not taken in)		*(information not retained)*
+	Impaired short-term memory	+
+	Disorientation	+
+	Living in the past	+
+	Misinterpretations	+
++	Hallucinations	+
+	Delusions	+
Speech rambling and incoherent	Speech stereotyped and limited	
Often diurnal variation	Constant (in later stages)	
Often aware and anxious	Unaware and unconcerned (in later stages)	

Patients with cognitive impairment disorders (confusion) have identifiable cognitive defects if tested formally using, e.g. the Mini-Mental State Examination.

Caution! Patients manifesting the following are sometimes misdiagnosed as confused:
- not taking in what is said:
  - ▷ deaf
  - ▷ anxious
  - ▷ too ill to concentrate
- muddled speech:
  - ▷ poor concentration
  - ▷ nominal dysphasia
- non-convulsive status epilepticus (see p.283).

It is also important to identify hypnagogic (going to sleep) and hypnopompic (waking up) hallucinations as these are normal phenomena, although possibly more common in ill patients receiving sedative drugs.

Dementia

Dementia is a generic term used to describe a chronic syndrome characterized by:
- progressive loss of intellectual function
- decreasing ability to carry out activities of daily living
- behavioural disturbances.

Dementia is usually caused by Alzheimer's disease, cerebral atherosclerosis or Lewy body disease.[84,85] Behavioural disturbances include:
- agitation, restlessness, wandering
- shadowing, physical aggression
- inappropriate sexual activity
- culturally inappropriate behaviours
- hoarding
- cursing, screaming
- sleep disorders.

Structured systematically applied behaviour management is the mainstay of treatment for the neuropsychiatric and behavioural features of dementia.[86,87] Cholinesterase inhibitors are sometimes prescribed to slow the rate of deterioration of cognition, or to help in the management of non-cognitive symptoms and/or behavioural disturbances when other interventions have failed.[88,89]

Antipsychotics are associated with an increase in cerebrovascular events in elderly patients with dementia and mortality.[90] They should be used only as a last resort, i.e. when behavioural interventions fail (Box 5.N).

Box 5.N   Drugs for behavioural problems in elderly patients with dementia

With violent or dangerous patients, use haloperidol IM, SC or PO to control the acute crisis.

If the patient has chronic psychotic symptoms (delusions or hallucinations) or marked behavioural fluctuation, consider prescribing an atypical antipsychotic despite the associated risk.[a]

For other behavioural disturbances unresponsive to non-drug measures, use trazodone first but switch to an atypical antipsychotic if trazodone is unsatisfactory.

Review after 2–3 months: if possible reduce the dose of the psychotropic medication.

---

a. if the patient has visual hallucinations, consider a cholinesterase inhibitor (refer to psychogeriatrician).

DELIRIUM

Delirium is the term commonly used for acute brain failure (acute confusion) associated with a general medical condition. The global cerebral dysfunction of delirium is characterized by concurrent disturbances of consciousness and cognition.

Disturbances in consciousness may manifest as reduced clarity of awareness and/or impaired ability to focus, shift or sustain attention. Change in cognition may present as memory impairment, disorientation, language disturbance or perceptual disturbances, e.g. hallucinations. Other associated features may include alterations in psychomotor behaviour, emotion, and the sleep–wake cycle.[17,91,92]

Delirium typically fluctuates in intensity, and there may well be lucid intervals; it commonly recurs or worsens as daylight fades. Delirium occurs at some stage in up to 3/4 of palliative care patients.[93,94]

Psychopathogenesis
Everybody is at risk of delirium. However, the risk varies from person to person depending on their vulnerability both physically and psychologically (Box 5.O) Thus, it is useful to think in terms of a 'delirium threshold' (cf. pain threshold).[92] The risk

---

Box 5.O   Risk factors for delirium

Deliriant threshold lowered	Precipitating factors for delirium	
Extremes of age	Change of environment	Biochemical disturbance
Dementia	Unfamiliar excessive	hypercalcaemia
Learning disability	stimuli	hyponatraemia
Visual impairment	too hot	Drug-induced
Previous episode	too cold	opioids
of delirium	wet bed	antimuscarinics
Alcohol abuse	crumbs in bed	corticosteroids
Depression	creased sheets	chemotherapy, e.g.
Reduced activities	General deterioration	cisplatin
of daily living	fatigue	5-FU, ifosfamide,
	Uncontrolled symptoms	methotrexate
	anxiety	immunomodulators, e.g.
	depression	interferon,
	pain	interleukin
	faecal impaction	Withdrawal state
	urinary retention	alcohol
	infection	nicotine
	dehydration	psychotropics
	hypoxia	Thiamine deficiency
	Brain tumour or	Organ failure
	secondaries	brain
	Paraneoplastic syndromes	hepatic
		renal
		respiratory

---

factors are generally synergistic rather than additive. To a certain extent, the occurrence of lucid intervals reflects normal biological diurnal rhythms, and the impact of fatigue towards the end of the day, and primitive fears associated with dangers in darkness.

Clinical features

The clinical features of delirium are numerous (Box 5.P). The disordered level of arousal and cognition is typically of acute onset (hours–days) and is generally accompanied by evidence of the underlying causal condition.[95]

Box 5.P   Clinical features of delirium

Prodromal symptoms (restlessness, anxiety, sleep disturbance and irritability)
Fluctuating course
Disorganized thinking and incoherent speech
Reduced attention (easily distractible)
   perseveration (inability to shift attention onto a new subject)
   memory impairment (cannot register new material)
   disorientation for time, place or person
Increased or decreased psychomotor activity
   altered arousal
   motor abnormalities (tremor, asterixis, myoclonus, purposeless overactivity, altered tone and reflexes)
   disturbance of the sleep–wake cycle
Affective symptoms (emotional lability, sadness, anger, euphoria, fear)
Agitation ± noisy aggressive behaviour
Altered perceptions
   misinterpretations
   hallucinations (predominantly visual and tactile rather than auditory)
   illusions
   psychosis and delusions (poorly formed)
Cortical abnormalities (dysgraphia, constructional apraxia, dysnomic aphasia)
EEG abnormalities (global slowing of activity)

Delirium can be classified as:
- hyperactive (agitated), characterized by hallucinations and delusions
- hypo-active (lethargic), characterized by confusion and sedation
- mixed, alternating features of both agitation and lethargy.

Hyperactive delirium may be associated with overactivity of the autonomic nervous system, e.g. facial flushing, dilated pupils, injected conjunctivae, tachycardia, sweating.[96]

Identifying early signs of delirium in patients at risk allows appropriate treatment to be started sooner rather than later, thereby preventing a crisis. Inability to write one's name and address correctly or to draw a clock face correctly may be as sensitive an indicator of early delirium as some of the more lengthy and intrusive tests.[97,98]

Evaluation

Delirium is present in most moribund patients, and will almost always have multiple causes.[95]

Investigation will depend upon the patient's overall condition, and the aims of care. If the patient is not close to death, consider:

- FBC
- plasma electrolytes, calcium and glucose
- blood, urine, sputum cultures
- SaO_2
- brain CT or MRI.

Management

Treat sooner rather than later, before symptoms are marked, persistent and are causing distress to the patient and/or family.

Correct the correctable

Even when the prognosis is thought to be days rather than weeks, delirium may be reversible because of the presence of one or more prominent correctable causal factors. Underlying causes should be considered and, if appropriate, specifically treated (see Box 5.O).[99,100] For example:

- relieve bladder retention and/or disimpact the rectum
- prescribe antibacterials for infection (if appropriate)
- give oxygen if cyanosed
- reduce opioid and psychotropic medication (if feasible)
- prescribe dexamethasone 8–16mg each morning if brain tumour
- if nicotine withdrawal is suspected, encourage smoking or apply a medicinal nicotine patch, e.g. Nicotinell®:
  - ▷ if smoking <20cigarettes/day, prescribe the '20' patch (releasing 14mg/24h nicotine)
  - ▷ if smoking 20+ cigarettes/day, prescribe the '30' patch (releasing 21mg/24h nicotine)[42,101]
- if alcohol withdrawal is suspected, consider offering an alcoholic beverage or prescribing a benzodiazepine (see p.389).

In >1/2 of patients with advanced cancer and delirium the cause may not be identified.[102]

Non-drug treatment

An attempt should be made to help the patient to express their distress. Hallucinations, nightmares and misinterpretations often reflect the patient's fears and anxieties. Their content should be explored with the patient.[103]

Clear explanation about the cause and fluctuations in mental state should be provided for the family. They should be assured that the patient is not 'losing their mind', and advised not to be too forceful if and when they contradict the patient.[104] In addition staff should:

- keep calm and avoid confrontation
- respond to the patient's comments
- clarify perceptions, and validate those which are accurate
- explain what is happening and why
- state what can be done to help
- repeat important and helpful information

- when indicated, recommend some tablets or an injection 'to help settle things down so that you can relax and rest for a few hours'
- stress to both the patient and the family that delirium is not madness, and that they can expect lucid intervals
- continue to treat the patient with courtesy and respect
- restraints should never be used
- bed rails should be avoided, they can be dangerous
- patient should be allowed to walk about accompanied
- allay fear and suspicion, and reduce misinterpretations by:
  - ▷ use of night light
  - ▷ not changing the position of the patient's bed
  - ▷ explaining every procedure and event in detail
  - ▷ the presence of a family member or close friend
  - ▷ limiting the number of staff caring for a patient.

In severe delirium, the doctor should acknowledge and accept the patient's distress, e.g. 'I can see that you are very upset', and invite the patient to return to his room and/or bed so that they can discuss things further. The presence of a close relative or friend, continuity of professional carers and a single room to minimize external visual and auditory stimulation may all help to provide a safe environment.[105]

Drug treatment

For more information, see *PCF3*.

Where it is not possible to treat the underlying cause, or in addition, consider an antipsychotic, e.g.:

- haloperidol 1.5/1mg PO/SC q1h p.r.n., and at bedtime; if necessary, increase to 3/2.5mg q1h p.r.n., and 5mg at bedtime
- olanzapine 2.5mg PO stat and at bedtime; if necessary, increase to 5–10mg
- risperidone 500microgram PO b.d.; if necessary, increase by 500microgram b.d. every other day to a maximum of 3mg/day.

Note: even with doses of haloperidol ≤5mg/24h, akathisia (psychomotor restlessness) may occur. This could be misinterpreted as a worsening of an agitated delirium, and lead to the inappropriate administration of even more haloperidol. Compared with haloperidol, the incidence of extrapyramidal effects is lower with olanzapine and risperidone (both atypical antipsychotics).[106]

In patients with AIDS, the effective dose of haloperidol is generally lower than in other patients.[107,108] Benzodiazepines alone often worsen delirium.[107,109] The exception to this rule is delirium associated with alcohol withdrawal for which benzodiazepines are the drug of choice.[110,111]

Levomepromazine 12.5–25mg PO/SC stat, and at bedtime, may be used instead if a period of sedation is required in an agitated delirious patient (see p.430). Alternatively, a benzodiazepine can be added to the haloperidol, e.g. haloperidol 5mg with diazepam or midazolam 10mg.

If the patient is already receiving regular psychotropic medication, a relatively high dose may be needed. Thus, if already receiving lorazepam 1mg t.d.s., a stat dose of diazepam 20mg would not be excessive (lorazepam 1mg = diazepam 5mg).

On rare occasions with an agitated patient who is a danger either to others or themselves, it is necessary to give an injection against their wishes. Forcing a patient to have an injection is an assault which must be justifiable on the grounds of necessity, and clearly in the patient's best interests.[112] It is a treatment of last resort; a step taken only after discussion within the caring team.

The doctor should stay until the patient begins to settle down. It may be necessary for a nurse to stay longer to discourage the patient from getting up and wandering about. A doctor should remain easily contactable in case further measures are necessary. In any case, the ward should be contacted after 1–2h to review the situation and to prescribe ongoing medication.

Occasionally, a dying patient becomes severely agitated despite the above measures. It is occasionally necessary to deeply sedate a patient as the only way to contain the situation, i.e. give sedation sufficient to diminish the level of consciousness (see p.430).[113]

1 Portenoy R et al. (1994) The memorial symptom assessment scale: an instrument for the evaluation of symptom prevalence, characteristics and distress. European Journal of Cancer. **30A**: 1326–1336.

2 Heaven C and Maguire P (1997) Disclosure of concerns by hospice patients and their identification by nurses. Palliative Medicine. **11**: 283–290.

3 LeFevre P et al. (1999) Screening for psychiatric illness in the palliative care inpatient setting: a comparison between the Hospital Anxiety and Depression Scale and the General Health Questionnaire-12. Palliative Medicine. **13**: 399–407.

4 Massie M and Holland J (1989) Overview of normal reactions and prevalence of psychiatric disorders. In: J Holland and J Rowland (eds) Handbook of Psychooncology. Oxford University Press, Oxford, pp. 273–282.

5 Vos MS and de Haes JC (2007) Denial in cancer patients, an explorative review. Psychooncology. **16**: 12–25.

6 Kramer BJ et al. (2006) Family conflict at the end of life: lessons learned in a model program for vulnerable older adults. Journal of Palliative Medicine. **9**: 791–801.

7 Philip J et al. (2007) Anger in palliative care: a clinical approach. Internal Medicine Journal. **37**: 49–55.

8 Periyakoil VS et al. (2005) Panic, anxiety, and chronic dyspnea. Journal of Palliative Medicine. **8**: 453–459.

9 Wilson KG et al. (2007) Depression and anxiety disorders in palliative cancer care. Journal of Pain and Symptom Management. **33**: 118–129.

10 Faulkner A and Maguire P (1994) Talking to Cancer Patients and their Relatives. Oxford Medical Publications, Oxford.

11 MacLeod S (2007) The Psychiatry of Palliative Medicine – the Dying Mind. Radcliffe Publishing, Oxford, pp. 5–6.

12 House A and Stark D (2002) Anxiety in medical patients. British Medical Journal. **325**: 207–209.

13 Maguire P and Pitceathly C (2003) Improving the psychological care of cancer patients and their relatives. The role of specialist nurses. Journal of Psychosomatic Research. **55**: 469–474.

14 Twycross R (2003) Introducing Palliative Care (4e). Radcliffe Medical Press, Oxford, pp. 28–30.

15 Roth AJ and Massie MJ Anxiety and its management in advanced cancer. Current Opinion in Supportive and Palliative Care. **1**: 50–56.

16 Bray D and Groves K (2007) A tailor-made psychological approach to palliative care. European Journal of Palliative Care. **14**: 141–143.

17 APA (American Psychiatric Association) (2000) Diagnostic and Statistical Manual of Mental Disorders. (Text revision). (4e). American Psychiatric Association, New York.

18 Hood S and Nutt D (2000) Panic disorder. Central Nervous System. **2**: 7–10.

19 Boyer W (1995) Serotonin uptake inhibitors are superior to imipramine and alprazolam in alleviating panic attacks: A meta-analysis. International Clinics of Psychopharmacology. **10**: 45–49.

20 Adgyropoulos SV and Nutt DJ (2003) Ch 11: Neuropchemical aspects of anxiety. In: DJ Nutt and JC Ballenger (eds) Anxiety Disorders. Blackwell Publishing, Oxford.

21 Maron E and Shlik J (2006) Serotonin function in panic disorder: important, but why? Neuropsychopharmacology. **31**: 1–11.

22 Kent J et al. (1998) Clinical utility of the selective serotonin reuptake inhibitors in the spectrum of anxiety. Biological Psychiatry. **44**: 812–824.

23 Bianchi A et al. (1995) Central control of breathing in mammals: neuronal circuitry, membrane properties, and neurotransmitters. Physiological Reviews. **75**: 1–45.

24 Griez E and Perna G (2003) Ch 14: Respiration and anxiety. In: DJ Nutt and JC Ballenger (eds) Anxiety Disorders. Blackwell Publishing, Oxford.

25 Thompson SA et al. (2000) Partial seizures presenting as panic attacks. British Medical Journal. **321**: 1002–1003.

26 Smoller J et al. (1996) Panic anxiety, dyspnea, and respiratory disease. Theoretical and clinical considerations. American Journal of Respiratory and Critical Care Medicine. **54**: 6–17.

27 Bredin M et al. (1999) Multicentre randomized controlled trial of nursing intervention for breathlessness in patients with lung cancer. British Medical Journal. **318**: 901–904.

28 McIntosh A et al. (2004) *Clinical Guidelines and Evidence Review for Panic Disorder and Generalised Anxiety Disorder.* NICE Sheffield: University of Sheffield/London: National Collaborating Centre for Primary Care.

29 Mitte K (2005) A meta-analysis of the efficacy of psycho- and pharmacotherapy in panic disorder with and without agoraphobia. *Journal of Affective Disorders.* **88**: 27–45.

30 Katon WJ (2006) Clinical practice. Panic disorder. *The New England Journal of Medicine.* **354**: 2360–2367.

31 Roth AJ and Massie MJ (2007) Anxiety and its management in advanced cancer. *Current Opinion in Supportive & Palliative Care.* **1**: 50–56.

32 Iveson C (2002) Solution-focused brief therapy. *Advances in Psychiatric Treatment.* **8**: 149–156.

33 Moorey S et al. (1994) Adjuvant psychosocial therapy for patients with cancer: outcome at 1 year. *Psychooncology.* **3**: 39–46.

34 Moorey S et al. (1998) A comparison of adjuvant psychological therapy and supportive counselling in patients with cancer. *Psychooncology.* **7**: 218–228.

35 Marshall J (1997) Panic disorder: a treatment update. *Journal of Clinical Psychiatry.* **58**: 36–42.

36 Herman J et al. (1987) The alprazolam to clonazepam switch for the treatment of panic disorder. *Journal of Clinical Psychopharmacology.* **7**: 175–178.

37 Tyrer P (1989) Treating panic. *British Medical Journal.* **298**: 201.

38 Baldwin DS et al. (2005) Evidence-based guidelines for the pharmacological treatment of anxiety disorders: recommendations from the British Association for Psychopharmacology. *Journal of Psychopharmacology.* **19**: 567–596.

39 Goddard AW et al. (2001) Early coadministration of clonazepam with sertraline for panic disorder. *Archives of General Psychiatry.* **58**: 681–686.

40 Carpenter L et al. (1999) Clinical experience with mirtazapine in the treatment of panic disorder. *Annals of Clinical Psychiatry.* **11**: 81–86.

41 Berigan T and Harazin J (1999) Mirtazapine in the treatment of panic disorder. *Primary Psychiatry.* **6**: 36.

42 BNFC (2007) British National Formulary for Children. In: *British National Formulary.* BMJ Publishing Group Ltd, RPS Publishing, RCPCH Publications Ltd, London. Current BNFC available from: http://bnfc.org/bnfc/bnfc/current/.

43 Periyakoil VS (2007) Panic disorder at the end of life. *Journal of Palliative Medicine.* **10**: 483–484.

44 Noyes R, Jr. et al. (1984) Diazepam and propranolol in panic disorder and agoraphobia. *Archives of General Psychiatry.* **41**: 287–292.

45 Voltz R et al. (eds) (2004) Palliative Care in Neurology (No. 69). Oxford University Press, Oxford.

46 Akechi T et al. (2004) Major depression, adjustment disorders, and post-traumatic stress disorder in terminally ill cancer patients: associated and predictive factors. *Journal of Clinical Oncology.* **22**: 1957–1965.

47 Miller K and Massie MJ (2006) Depression and anxiety. *Cancer Journal.* **12**: 388–397.

48 Plumb MM and Holland J (1977) Comparative studies of psychological function in patients with advanced cancer–I. Self-reported depressive symptoms. *Psychosomatic Medicine.* **39**: 264–276.

49 Chochinov HM et al. (1994) Prevalence of depression in the terminally ill: effects of diagnostic criteria and symptom threshold judgments. *The American Journal of Psychiatry.* **151**: 537–540.

50 Hotopf M et al. (2002) Depression in advanced disease: a systematic review Part 1. Prevalence and case finding. *Palliative Medicine.* **16**: 81–97.

51 Kissane DW et al. (2001) Demoralization syndrome–a relevant psychiatric diagnosis for palliative care. *Journal of Palliative Care.* **17**: 12–21.

52 Clarke DM and Kissane DW (2002) Demoralization: its phenomenology and importance. *The Australian and New Zealand Journal of Psychiatry.* **36**: 733–742.

53 APA (American Psychiatric Association) (2000) Practice guideline for the treatment of patients with major depressive disorder. Available from: www.guideline.gov/summary/summary.aspx?ss=15&doc_id=2605&nbr=1831

54 Green A and Austin C (1993) Psychopathology of pancreatic cancer: a psychobiologic probe. *Psychosomatics.* **34**: 208–221.

55 Passik S and Breitbart W (1996) Depression in patients with pancreatic carcinoma. *Cancer.* **78**: 615–626.

56 Ruttley A and Reid S (2006) Depression in physical illness. *Clinical Medicine.* **6**: 533–536.

57 Hecaen H and deAjuriaguerra J (1956) *Troubles Mentaux au cours des Tumeurs Intracraniennes.* Masson, Paris.

58 Lishman W (1998) *Organic Psychiatry* (thirde). Blackwells Scientific Publication, Oxford, p. 386.

59 Mayberg H et al. (1988) PET imaging of cortical S2 serotonin receptors after stroke: lateralized changes and relationship to depression. *American Journal of Psychiatry.* **145**: 937–943.

60 Fleminger S (1991) Left-sided Parkinson's disease is associated with greater anxiety and depression. *Psychological Medicine.* **21**: 629–638.

61 Surridge D (1969) An investigation into some psychiatric aspects of multiple sclerosis. *British Journal of Psychiatry.* **115**: 749–764.

62 Whitlock F and Siskind M (1980) Depression as a major symptom of multiple sclerosis. *Journal of Neurology, Neurosurgery and Psychiatry.* **43**: 861–865.

63 Schiffer R and Babigian H (1984) Behavioral disorders in multiple sclerosis, temporal lobe epilepsy, and amyotrophic lateral sclerosis. An epidemiologica study. *Archives of Neurology.* **41**: 1067–1069.

64 Block S (2000) Assessing and managing depression in the terminally ill patient. *Annals of internal medicine.* **132**: 209–218.

65 Chochinov H et al. (1997) 'Are you depressed?' screening for depression in the terminally ill. *American Journal of Psychiatry.* **154**: 674–676.

66 Lloyd-Williams M et al. (2003) Is asking patients in palliative care, 'are you depressed?' Appropriate? Prospective study. *British Medical Journal.* **327**: 372–373.

67 Arroll B et al. (2005) Effect of the addition of a 'help' question to two screening questions on specificity for diagnosis of depression in general practice: diagnostic validity study. *British Medical Journal.* **331**: 884.

68 Lloyd-Williams M et al. (2003) Which depression screening tools should be used in palliative care? *Palliative Medicine.* **17**: 40–43.

69 Miller KE et al. (2006) Antidepressant medication use in palliative care. *The American Journal of Hospice & Palliative Care.* **23**: 127–133.

70 Casey P (1994) Depression in the dying – disorder or distress? *Progress in Palliative Care.* **2**: 1–3.

71 NICE (2007) Depression: management of depression in primary and secondary care. In: *National Clinical Practice Guideline Number 23 (amended).* National Institute for Clinical Excellence. Available from: www.nice.org.uk/CG023NICEguideline

72 Trindade E et al. (1998) Adverse effects associated with selective reuptake inhibitors and tricyclic antidepressants: a meta-analysis. *Canadian Medical Association Journal.* **17**: 1245–1252.

73 Tylee A and Walters P (2007) Onset of action of antidepressants. *British Medical Journal.* **334**: 911–912.

74 Reynolds C et al. (1998) Effects of age at onset of first lifetime episode of recurrent major depression on treatment response and illness course in elderly patients. *American Journal of Psychiatry.* **155**: 795–799.

75 Breitbart W and Mermelstein H (1992) An alternative psychostimulant for the management of depressive disorders in cancer patients. *Psychosomatics.* **33**: 352–356.

76 Emptage R and Semla T (1996) Depression in the medically ill elderly: a focus on methylphenidate. *Annals of Pharmacotherapy.* **30**: 151–157.

77 Homsi J et al. (2000) Methylphenidate (MP) in the management of depression in advanced cancer. *Supportive Care in Cancer.* **8**: 40–41.

78 Satel S and Nelson J (1989) Stimulants in the treatment of depression: A critical overview. *Journal of Clinical Psychiatry.* **50**: 241–249.

79 Dalal S and Melzack R (1998) Potentiation of opioid analgesia by psychostimulant drugs: a review. *Journal of Pain and Symptom Management.* **16**: 245–253.

80 Maguire P and Faulkner A (1993) Handling the withdrawn patient – a flow diagram. *Palliative Medicine.* **7**: 333–338.

81 CKS (2005) Insomnia (PRODIGY Guidance). In: *Clinical Knowledge Summaries Service.* Available from: http://cks.library.nhs.uk/insomnia

82 Montgomery P and Dennis J (2003) Cognitive behavioural interventions for sleep problems in adults aged 60+. *Cochrane Database of Systematic Reviews.* CD003161.

83 DTB (2004) What's wrong with prescribing hypnotics? *Drug and Therapeutics Bulletin.* **42**: 89–93.

84 APA (American Psychiatric Association) (2000) Dementia. In: *Diagnostic and Statistical Manual of Mental Disorders (Text revision)* (4e). American Psychiatric Association, New York.

85 Jones RW (2003) The dementias. *Clinical Medicine.* **3**: 404–408.

86 Howard R et al. (2001) Guidelines for the management of agitation in dementia. *International Journal of Geriatric Psychiatry.* **16**: 714–717.

87 Fossey J et al. (2006) Effect of enhanced psychosocial care on antipsychotic use in nursing home residents with severe dementia: cluster randomised trial. *British Medical Journal.* **332**: 756–761.

88 SIGN (Scottish Intercollegiate Guidelines Network) (2006) Management of patients with dementia. In: *SIGN.* Available from: http://www.sign.ac.uk/pdf/sign86.pdf

89 NICE (2007) Dementia: A NICE-SCIE Guideline on supporting people with dementia and their carers in health and social care. National Clinical Practice Guideline Number 42. National Institute for Health and Clinical Excellence. Available from: http://guidance.nice.org.uk/cg42/guidance/pdf/English

90 Wang PS et al. (2005) Risk of death in elderly users of conventional vs. atypical antipsychotic medications. *The New England Journal of Medicine.* **353**: 2335–2341.

91 Breitbart W and Passik SD (1998) Psychiatric aspects of palliative care. In: D Doyle et al. (eds) *Oxford Textbook of Palliative Medicine.* Oxford University Press, Oxford, pp. 933–956.

92 Macleod AD (2006) Delirium: the clinical concept. *Palliat Support Care.* **4**: 305–312.

93 Massie MJ and Holland JC (1987) The cancer patient with pain: psychiatric complications and their management. *The Medical Clinics of North America.* **71**: 243–258.

94 Spiller JA and Keen JC (2006) Hypoactive delirium: assessing the extent of the problem for inpatient specialist palliative care. *Palliative Medicine.* **20**: 17–23.

95 Breitbart W and Strout D (2000) Delirium in the terminally ill. *Clinics in Geriatric Medicine.* **16**: 357–372.

96 Young J and Inouye SK (2007) Delirium in older people. *British Medical Journal.* **334**: 842–846.

97 Macleod A and Whitehead L (1997) Dysgraphia and terminal delirium. *Palliative Medicine.* **11**: 127–132.

98 Shulman KI (2000) Clock-drawing: is it the ideal cognitive screening test? *International Journal of Geriatric Psychiatry.* **15**: 548–561.

99 Anonymous (2000) Practice guidelines for pharmacotherapy specialists. The ACCP Clinical Practice Affairs Committee, Subcommittee B, 1998–1999. American College of Clinical Pharmacy. *Pharmacotherapy.* **20**: 487–490.

100 Cole M (1999) Delirium: effectiveness of systematic interventions. *Dementia and Geriatric Cognitive Disorders.* **10**: 406–411.

101 Krajnik M and Zylicz Z (1995) Terminal restlessness and nicotine withdrawal. *Lancet.* **346**: 1044.

102 Bruera E *et al.* (1992) Cognitive failure in patients with terminal cancer: A prospective study. *Journal of Pain and Symptom Management.* **7**: 192–195.

103 Lodder K and Read J (2007) Psychological management in delirium. *Progress in Palliative Care.* **15**: 61–66.

104 Centeno C *et al.* (2004) Delirium in advanced cancer patients. *Palliative Medicine.* **18**: 184–194.

105 Macleod A (1997) The management of delirium in hospice practice. *European Journal of Palliative Care.* **4**: 116–120.

106 Gilbody S *et al.* (2000) Risperidone versus other atypical antipsychotic medication for schizophrenia. *The Cochrane Database of Systematic Reviews.* **3**: CD002306.

107 Breitbart W *et al.* (1996) A double-blind trial of haloperidol, chlorpromazine, and lorazepam in the treatment of delirium in hospitalized AIDS patients. *American Journal of Psychiatry.* **153**: 231–237.

108 Lonergan E *et al.* (2007) Antipsychotics for delirium. *Cochrane Database of Systematic Reviews.* CD005594.

109 Meagher DJ (2001) Delirium: optimising management. *British Medical Journal.* **322**: 144–149.

110 Lundberg J and Passik S (1997) Alcohol and cancer: a review for psycho-oncologists. *Psycho-oncology.* **6**: 253–266.

111 Chick J (1998) Review: benzodiazepines are more effective than neuroleptics in reducing delirium and seizures in alcohol withdrawal. *Evidence-Based Medicine.* **3**: 11.

112 Anonymous (2005) Mental Capacity Act 2005 s.6: Elizabeth II. Chapter 9 Reprinted May and December 2006; May 2007. Available from: www.opsi.gov.uk/acts/acts2005/50009–b.htm#5

113 de Graeff A and Dean M (2007) Palliative sedation therapy in the last weeks of life: a literature review and recommendations for standards. *Journal of Palliative Medicine.* **10**: 67–85.

6: BIOCHEMICAL SYNDROMES

HYPERCALCAEMIA

Hypercalcaemia is an *ionized* plasma calcium concentration above the upper limit of normal. In most centres, the total plasma calcium concentration is measured. This includes both protein-bound and ionized calcium. If a patient is hypo-albuminaemic, the total plasma concentration may give a false impression of normality. Thus, it is necessary to 'correct' for hypo-albuminaemia using a formula based on the *mean normal plasma albumin concentration* for that particular biochemical laboratory (Box 6.A).

Box 6.A Correcting plasma calcium concentrations

If the mean normal plasma albumin for the local laboratory is 40g/L:
Corrected calcium (mmol/L) = measured calcium + 0.022 × (40 − albumin (g/L))
e.g. measured calcium = 2.45; albumin = 32
    corrected calcium = 2.45 + 0.022 × 8 = 2.63mmol/L
    (normal range 2.12–2.65mmol/L)

Incidence

Overall, hypercalcaemia occurs in 10–20% of patients with cancer, and up to 50% of patients with breast cancer or myeloma. However, the incidence in these two conditions may fall because of the more widespread use of bisphosphonates.[1]

Hypercalcaemia is also common in cancer of the lung (squamous cell), head and neck, kidney and cervix uteri. It is uncommon in SCLC, stomach, large bowel and prostate cancers. Cancer-related hypercalcaemia is generally associated with metastatic disease and, despite treatment, survival is often < 3 months, with only 20% alive at 12 months.[2]

Pathogenesis

Any type of cancer with or without skeletal metastases may be associated with hypercalcaemia. However, more than 80% of patients with cancer-related hypercalcaemia have skeletal metastases.[3] The extent of bony disease does not correlate with the level of hypercalcaemia.[4]

Biochemical evidence of humoral mechanisms is detectable in almost all cases of hypercalcaemia in cancer (Box 6.B). In solid tumours, the most common mediator of hypercalcaemia is cancer-secreted parathyroid hormone-related protein (PTHrP).

This is *not* detected by radio-immuno-assay for parathyroid hormone (PTH). Unless there is concurrent primary hyperparathyroidism (see below), plasma PTH concentrations are low or undetectable in cancer-induced hypercalcaemia.

PTHrP stimulates osteoclastic bone resorption, and also impairs calcium excretion by the distal renal tubule. Vomiting causes sodium loss and leads to sodium-linked calcium resorption by the proximal renal tubule.[5]

Myeloma and breast cancer also produce osteoclast-activating factors (Box 6.B). Most osteoclast activating factors increase the expression of RANK-L (receptor activator of nuclear factor-κB ligand) on marrow stromal cells, rather than by acting directly on osteoclast precursors. RANK-L is a member of the tumour necrosis factor (TNF) family and is released by activated T lymphocytes. RANK-L increases osteoclast formation and osteoclast activity and thus bone resorption. Bone resorption releases growth factors (Box 6.B) which increase the production of PTHrP. This leads to a vicious cycle of osteolytic metastases and hypercalcaemia.[6] Osteoblastic activity is also suppressed in myeloma.[6]

Box 6.B Humoral factors and hypercalcaemia of malignancy[6,8]

Parathyroid hormone-related protein (PTHrP)
Most common mediator of cancer-related hypercalcaemia:
• produced by many solid cancers, e.g. lung (squamous cell), breast and kidney
• activates PTH receptors in tissue
• stimulates osteoclastic bone resorption; enhances renal tubular calcium resorption.

Osteoclast-activating factors
Increase expression of RANK-L and osteoclast formation and bone resorption:
• interleukin-6 produced by T lymphocytes, myeloma, breast cancer and uterine endometrial cancer
• macrophage inflammatory protein-1α (MIP-1α) produced by myeloma
• tumour necrosis factor-α (TNF-α) produced by breast cancer
• TNF-α and TNF-β (lymphotoxin) produced by activated T lymphocytes, myeloma.

Growth factors
Increased expression by many solid cancers, e.g.:
• transforming growth factor-α (TGF-α) produced by lung (squamous cell), head and neck, breast, and kidney cancers; it is a potent bone resorber
• TGF-β produced by normal and cancer cells; enhances production of PTHrP
• insulin-like growth factors (breast and prostate cancer).

1,25-dihydroxyvitamin D (vitamin D)
Generally plays a minor role (some lymphomas; see text).

With hypercalcaemia in lymphoma, PTHrP is responsible in some cases, and similar factors to those in myeloma are responsible in others. Some lymphomas also produce an enzyme which converts 25-hydroxyvitamin D into biologically active

1,25-dihydroxyvitamin D (1,25 DHCC). This leads to increased GI absorption and increased renal resorption of calcium, and enhanced osteoclastic bone resorption.[7]

Clinical features

The severity of the symptoms appears to relate more to the rate of increase in the plasma calcium concentration than to the actual plasma calcium concentration. Thus, chronic severe hypercalcaemia may cause few symptoms, but a rapid moderate elevation in plasma calcium concentration may cause marked symptoms. Patients with existing cognitive impairment or neurological dysfunction are likely to experience more severe symptoms (Box 6.C).[1] Severe symptoms may develop rapidly without a clearly defined prodrome.

Box 6.C   Symptoms of hypercalcaemia

Mild		**Severe**	
Patient ambulatory		*Patient increasingly incapacitated*	
Polyuria	} not constant	Nausea	} → dehydration and
Polydipsia/thirst	features	Vomiting	cardiovascular collapse
Fatigue		Ileus	
Lethargy		Delirium	
Mental dullness		Drowsiness	
Weakness		Coma	
Anorexia			
Constipation			

Occasionally there may be neurological symptoms and signs, e.g. upper motor neurone deficits, scotomata, ataxia, fits, and also severe dysphagia for food and fluid.[9] *Pain may be precipitated or exacerbated by hypercalcaemia.*[10–12] If untreated, severe hypercalcaemia >4mmol/L is generally fatal because of renal failure and cardiac arrhythmia.

Evaluation

Diagnosis is based on a high level of clinical suspicion, and confirmed by appropriate blood tests. Primary hyperparathyroidism should also be considered; this is the sole cause of hypercalcaemia in about 6% of cancer patients with hypercalcaemia and a contributory factor in 4–15% more.[13,14] Thus, some centres suggest the routine measurement of plasma PTH in patients with known cancer and hypercalcaemia, particularly if there is no evidence of bone metastases.[15] Plasma PTH concentration is low or undetectable in cancer but is raised in primary hyperparathyroidism and where the two disorders co-exist. If the cause of hypercalcaemia remains unclear, PTHrP may be measured.[1]

Management

Stop and think!
Are you justified in correcting a potentially fatal complication in a moribund patient?

The following together comprise a set of indications for the correction of hypercalcaemia:

- corrected plasma calcium concentration of >2.8mmol/L
- symptoms attributable to hypercalcaemia
- first episode or long interval since previous one
- previous good quality of life (in the patient's opinion)
- medical expectation that treatment will achieve a durable effect (based on the results of previous treatment)
- patient willing to have IV treatment and requisite blood tests.

Not all symptoms respond equally to treatment (Box 6.D). This may be because some are caused by other factors, principally the underlying disseminated disease.

Box 6.D Impact of correcting hypercalcaemia[16]

Consistent response
Polydipsia/thirst
Polyuria
Delirium
Mental dullness
Constipation

Variable response
General malaise
Fatigue
Anorexia

Fluid replacement

Some centres give IV fluid replacement routinely until oral fluid intake is adequate, e.g. 0.9% saline 2–3L/24h with potassium supplements. Other centres do so only when there are severe symptoms or renal impairment.

Saline improves hypercalcaemia by improving the glomerular filtration rate and by promoting a sodium-linked calcium diuresis. Saline alone will reduce plasma calcium concentrations by 0.2–0.4mmol/L.

Bisphosphonates

For more information, see PCF3.

IV bisphosphonates are the treatment of choice for hypercalcaemia of malignancy.[17] The choice of bisphosphonate is often dictated by local policy.

Bisphosphonates inhibit osteoclast activity and thereby inhibit bone resorption, but have no impact on the effect of PTHrP on renal tubular resorption of calcium. Bisphosphonates are generally given IV, at least initially, because of poor alimentary absorption (Table 6.1). Bisphosphonates are adsorbed onto the bone surface where they remain bound to hydroxyapatite for weeks or months. Thus, a single infusion has a prolonged duration of action on osteoclasts.

Calcitonin

Calcitonin (salmon) has a rapid calcium-lowering effect which is evident within 2h. It inhibits osteoclast activity and renal tubular resorption of calcium. It is generally given SC or IM but PR is also effective. Maximum effect is seen with 100units/24h and the effect lasts 2–3 days.

More calcitonin is less effective because of down-regulation of calcitonin receptors in osteoclasts. Relapse is delayed to 6–9 days by the concurrent use of a corticosteroid.[21]

Table 6.1 Bisphosphonates and the initial treatment of hypercalcaemia[18–20]

	Zoledronic acid	Ibandronic acid	Disodium pamidronate	Disodium clodronate
IV dose	4mg	2–6mg	30–90mg	(a) 1,500mg (b) 300–600mg once daily for 5 days
Onset of effect	<4 days	<4 days	<3 days	<2 days
Maximum effect	4–7 days	7 days	5–7 days	3–5 days
Duration of effect	4 weeks	2.5 weeks (4mg) 4 weeks (6mg)	2.5 weeks	(a) 2 weeks (b) 3 weeks
Restores normocalcaemia	90%	75%	70–75%	40–80%

The combination of calcitonin and corticosteroids long-term is not as effective as bisphosphonates. The main use of calcitonin is in combination with a bisphosphonate in order to obtain a rapid early response.

Corticosteroids

Corticosteroids are no longer recommended for cancer-related hypercalcaemia because of the poor response rate.[21] However, they are beneficial when used as an adjunct to SC calcitonin.[22]

If more effective treatments are not available, the use of prednisolone 60mg once daily or dexamethasone 8mg once daily should be considered in patients with breast cancer, renal cancer, myeloma or lymphoma.[23] Smaller doses are unlikely to be effective.

Octreotide

For more information, see *PCF3*.

Octreotide, a somatostatin analogue, has been used successfully in the treatment of hypercalcaemia associated with neuro-endocrine tumours resistant to other measures.[24]

DIABETES MELLITUS

Because of its increasing prevalence, palliative care clinicians will increasingly encounter patients with diabetes mellitus. This section provides an overview of diabetes mellitus, but limits information on its management to the last few weeks or days of life. Because regimens are individually tailored, there is no standard approach and guidance from a diabetologist is invaluable.

Diabetes mellitus comprises a group of metabolic diseases characterized by hyperglycaemia resulting from defects in insulin secretion, insulin action or both (Box 6.E).[25] It has a prevalence of 4% of the general population in the UK.[26,27]

Type 1 generally develops in children, young people and adults <40 years old, although it can occur at any age. There is a lack of insulin because of immune-mediated or

---

Box 6.E Causes of diabetes mellitus[25]

Type 1 ($<$10%)
Type 2 ($>$90%)
Diseases of the exocrine pancreas
  pancreatitis
  pancreatic cancer
  haemochromatosis
Drug-induced
  corticosteroids
  α-interferon
  octreotide
  thiazide diuretics
  thyroxine

Gestational diabetes mellitus
Infections
  cytomegalovirus
Associated genetic conditions
  Huntington's chorea
  porphyria
Genetic defects in
  β-cell function
  insulin action

---

idiopathic destruction of the β-cells in the pancreas. Generally, symptoms develop rapidly and the diagnosis is based on the presence of characteristic symptoms plus a high blood glucose concentration. It requires life-long treatment with insulin.

Type 2 generally develops in adults $>$40 years old, although it is increasingly manifesting in younger people because of obesity. The pancreas does not produce sufficient insulin for the body's needs and generally there is also marked insulin resistance, i.e. cells are not able to respond to the insulin that is produced. Symptoms tend to develop gradually, with a long delay (possibly years) before diagnosis. Treatment is based on modification of diet and weight loss, together with various glucose-lowering drugs. Some patients will require insulin. However, when an illness such as cancer leads to a reduced dietary intake and weight loss, it is often possible to reduce or discontinue insulin, and sometimes oral hypoglycaemics as well.

Some patients can exhibit features of both type 1 and type 2 diabetes, making a definite classification difficult.

The prevalence of diabetes is higher in palliative care because patients:
- are mostly older
- may be taking diabetogenic drugs, e.g. corticosteroids
- may have cancer-related metabolic changes.

Glucose intolerance is one of the first metabolic consequences of cancer, and is found in nearly 40% of non-diabetic cancer patients given an oral or IV glucose tolerance test.[28,29] For corticosteroid-induced diabetes, see p.223.

Clinical features

Diabetes may present with:
- symptomatic hyperglycaemia; polyuria, thirst, polydipsia, weight loss, blurred vision, infections, e.g. vulvovaginal candidosis, UTIs
- acute life-threatening complications, e.g. hyperosmolar non-ketotic coma, keto-acidosis
- chronic complications, e.g. retinopathy, nephropathy, peripheral neuropathy
- an incidental finding of hyperglycaemia.

Patients newly presenting with diabetes are generally symptomatic with a fasting blood glucose of $\geq$12mmol/L. However, there is wide variation in the level of blood glucose at which symptoms develop. Further, for some 'asymptomatic' patients, a retrospective realization that they were in fact symptomatic only comes after blood glucose levels are normalized.

Diagnosis

In patients with symptoms suggestive of diabetes mellitus, a diagnosis can be made on the basis of the following criteria:

- a single fasting plasma glucose of ≥7.0mmol/L (normal <5.6mmol/L) *or*
- random plasma glucose concentrations of ≥11.1mmol/L.

In patients who do not have symptoms suggestive of diabetes mellitus, diagnosis should be confirmed by repeat testing on another day.[25,30] An oral glucose tolerance test may be useful when there is diagnostic uncertainty.

Management

In palliative care, the aim of treatment is to use as simple a regimen as possible to achieve the best control possible, while minimizing the risk of:

- symptomatic hyperglycaemia
- hypoglycaemia
- hyperosmolar non-ketotic states (type 2 only)
- keto-acidosis (type 1 >type 2).

Keto-acidosis can occur in patients with type 2 diabetes in association with an intercurrent illness, e.g. sepsis or myocardial infarction, which increases secretion of counter-regulatory hormones such as glucagon.[31]

Aiming for tight glycaemic control to reduce the risk of long-term complications is generally irrelevant in palliative care; higher blood glucose levels are acceptable and reduce the likelihood of hypoglycaemia in an anorexic patient.[32] Because some patients and families will have managed their diabetes closely for many years, it is important to sensitively explain the reason for the change in goals of treatment and emphasize that this is not suboptimal care.

There is a lack of consensus for blood glucose ranges at the end of life, but aiming for a fasting or pre-meal glucose of 5–15mmol/L may be reasonable. However, because different patients will have different thresholds for symptomatic hyperglycaemia, the upper limit may be reduced to avoid symptoms.

The relative advantages and disadvantages of insulin or oral hypoglycaemics need to be considered alongside factors such as the patient's prognosis, oral nutritional intake and presence of other co-morbidities:

- *insulin*: provides rapid, effective and more predictable control; easier to titrate and has less risk of prolonged hypoglycaemia compared with some oral hypoglycaemics; better choice in patients with:
  - ▷ a short prognosis (≤3 months)
  - ▷ unwell and/or very symptomatic from hyperglycaemia
  - ▷ co-morbidity contributing to hyperglycaemia, e.g. infection
  - ▷ poor or erratic oral nutritional intake
  - ▷ contra-indications to the use of oral hypoglycaemics
- *oral hypoglycaemics*: control may take several weeks, less effective, less predictable and harder to titrate than insulin; possible treatment option in patients with:
  - ▷ a long prognosis (>3 months)
  - ▷ mild symptoms of hyperglycaemia
  - ▷ good performance status
  - ▷ good and stable oral nutritional intake.

When deciding the starting dose of insulin, the patient's build, oral intake and the blood glucose levels must be taken into account. A reasonable starting dose in an adult patient newly diagnosed with diabetes mellitus is isophane insulin 6–8units b.d. (small build) or 10–12units b.d. (normal/large build), administered before breakfast and before the evening meal. When adding insulin to oral hypoglycaemics to improve blood glucose control, 6–12units of isophane insulin or long-acting insulin once daily may suffice. Blood glucose should be monitored before each dose until the insulin dose is stable. The frequency can then be reduced and the time of testing varied to monitor control during different parts of the day.

Glucose monitoring
As a patient nears the end of life, it may be possible to reduce the frequency of blood glucose monitoring. However, because symptoms of both hypo- and hyperglycaemia may mimic those frequently present at the end of life, including agitation and delirium, regular monitoring of blood glucose remains advisable, preferably with a blood glucose fingerstick test. The precise frequency of monitoring depends on the patient's symptoms, stability of insulin requirements and imminence of death.[33] For example, once daily monitoring may be sufficient in the last days of life but, if insulin requirements are unstable, a minimum of twice daily monitoring is advisable.[34]

The monitoring of urinary glucose, using glucose oxidase test strips, is less reliable because urinary glucose concentration depends on urine output, time since the bladder was last emptied, and the renal threshold. The renal threshold has a normal range of 7–13mmol/L but may be much higher in patients with renal impairment.

In palliative care patients with a limited prognosis, measurement of glycated haemoglobin (HbA$_{1c}$) becomes irrelevant. Further, it may be inaccurate in patients with cancer who have disturbed turnover of RBCs.

Treatment in type I diabetes mellitus
For more information, see PCF3.

Insulin
Injections of insulin are an essential life-long treatment, including the last days of life. However, as the patient's dietary intake and weight decline, or in the presence of nausea or vomiting, e.g. from bowel obstruction, the insulin dose will need to be reduced in order to avoid hypoglycaemia. As part of self-management of diabetes, patients may be able to estimate their carbohydrate intake and adjust their insulin dose accordingly.

Generally, short-acting insulins (e.g. given to cover mealtimes) which produce a more rapid peak and have a greater risk of hypoglycaemia, are reduced or discontinued first. Intermediate- or long-acting insulins (e.g. given once daily or b.d. to provide background control) may also need to be reduced to maintain blood glucose in the target range. For similar reasons, patients receiving mixed insulins may need to reduce or discontinue the short-acting insulin component. However, if a patient has months or weeks to live, it would be prudent to liaise with a diabetologist before making major changes to an established insulin regimen.

Discontinuing insulin in the dying patient
A decision to stop insulin completely should generally be taken only after discussion with the patient (if still has capacity) and the family. It is generally appropriate to stop insulin injections completely when the patient has become irreversibly unconscious as

part of the dying process, and not because of hypoglycaemia or diabetic keto-acidosis, and when all other life-prolonging treatments have been stopped.[35]

If it is felt strongly that the insulin should be continued, a simple regimen of once daily long-acting, or b.d. intermediate-acting insulin can be used, with the minimum of routine monitoring, i.e. once daily.[34]

Treatment in type 2 diabetes mellitus
Non-drug treatment
Patients with advanced cancer who are newly diagnosed with diabetes mellitus are unlikely to be obese and will probably have a poor appetite. The usual lifestyle and dietary advice will not be appropriate for such patients.

Patients with existing diabetes and a poor appetite should be able to relax dietary restrictions.

Drug treatment
For more information, see PCF3.

Generally, as they lose weight and reduce their calorie intake, patients with type 2 diabetes may be able to reduce the dose of oral hypoglycaemics, or even stop them.

If a patient develops an intercurrent illness causing nausea, vomiting or very poor oral intake, oral hypoglycaemics should be stopped and the blood glucose fingerstick test monitored twice daily. If hyperglycaemia occurs this can be managed with b.d. intermediate- or long-acting insulin. Patients who are very symptomatic from their hyperglycaemia may occasionally require a sliding scale. If appropriate, oral hypoglycaemics may be restarted when the patient improves. Generally, the insulin dose is progressively phased out over a 2–4 week period as the dose of the oral hypoglycaemic is titrated upwards.

Discontinuing oral hyoglycaemics in the dying patient
Ultimately, when it becomes difficult for a dying patient to swallow, oral hypoglycaemics and routine monitoring can be stopped.[36] A blood glucose level can be checked if symptoms suggestive of hypo- or hyperglycaemia develop. Unless death is imminent, hyperglycaemia can be treated with a once daily long- or b.d. intermediate-acting insulin.

Corticosteroid-induced diabetes mellitus
Corticosteroid-induced diabetes mellitus occurs in 2% of patients.[37] It can occur with any corticosteroid and is dose-related.[38,39] It is not possible to predict which patients will develop corticosteroid-induced diabetes, when it will occur, or the likelihood of a full recovery once the corticosteroids are stopped.

Pathogenesis
Corticosteroids may cause or worsen diabetes mellitus by inducing a state of relative insulin-resistance by several mechanisms including:
- down-regulation of glucose transporter 4 (GLUT-4) in the muscle, necessitating higher insulin concentrations for glucose to be taken up into muscle
- increased gluconeogenesis
- suppressed insulin secretion.[38,39]

This leads to an exaggerated post-prandial hyperglycaemia, 1–2h after meals and, when pronounced, a persistent diabetic state.

Diagnosis

Diagnostic criteria for corticosteroid-induced diabetes are the same as for type 1 and type 2 diabetes (see p.221). However, because an early morning fasting blood glucose may sometimes be normal, measuring a random glucose may be preferable.

Management

It is advisable to monitor all non-diabetic patients who are started on corticosteroids, e.g. weekly urinalysis or random blood glucose. Duration of monitoring will depend upon the stability of the glucose readings and the duration of the corticosteroid treatment.

In patients with known diabetes who are started on corticosteroids, blood glucose fingerstick tests should be carried out once daily–b.d. and the dose of hypoglycaemic titrated accordingly.

As with type 1 and type 2 diabetes, the goal of treatment for corticosteroid-induced diabetes is to prevent symptomatic hyperglycaemia and its complications, rather than tight glycaemic control. If the patient is receiving a short course of corticosteroids and has mild, asymptomatic hyperglycaemia, a random blood glucose should be monitored daily, until the corticosteroids are stopped, and once–twice weekly thereafter. Blood glucose levels should normalize within a few days of stopping corticosteroids; if they do not, the patient may have previously unrecognized diabetes.

If it is not possible to stop the corticosteroid, the dose should be reduced as much as possible. Dietary and lifestyle advice is unlikely to be appropriate in patients with advanced cancer.

Drug therapy

Some suggest that insulin should be first-line treatment for all patients with corticosteroid-induced diabetes, particularly if they have high blood glucose levels at diagnosis.[39] If glycaemic control in a patient with established diabetes deteriorates significantly when corticosteroids are started, existing hypoglycaemic treatment should be titrated accordingly. However, the treatment regimen should take into account that the greatest rise in blood glucose is likely to occur in the *first few hours* after the dose of corticosteroid.

Oral hypoglycaemics: If a non-diabetic patient with a reasonable prognosis and oral intake develops corticosteroid-induced diabetes, a trial of a sulphonylurea should be initiated. However, in patients with a poor food intake, there may be an increased risk of night-time or early morning hypoglycaemia. Repaglinide, because of its short duration of action, may be a safer alternative.

Insulin: If a patient with pre-existing non-insulin-dependent diabetes remains hyperglycaemic despite maximal doses of an appropriate oral hypoglycaemic, insulin should be given *in addition*. The most appropriate type of insulin, and the timing of its administration, will be indicated by the pattern of glucose levels, for example when high blood glucose levels are only seen after the dose of corticosteroid, a once daily dose of isophane insulin given with the corticosteroid may suffice. Advice should be sought from a diabetologist.

If tight glycaemic control is required, an ultra-short-acting insulin, e.g. aspart or lispro, can be given immediately before a meal to prevent post-prandial hyperglycaemia.[39]

When a corticosteroid is tapered, insulin requirements decline in proportion. When stopped, there may be no further need for insulin. Blood glucose should be monitored once daily when a corticosteroid is being reduced, preferably pre-breakfast because of the risk of nocturnal hypoglycaemia;[39] a blood glucose concentration of <5mmol/L indicates the need for a reduction in insulin dose.

SYNDROME OF INAPPROPRIATE ADH SECRETION (SIADH)

Inappropriate secretion of antidiuretic hormone (ADH) occurs in 2% of patients with cancer. Three-quarters of these will occur in SCLC which has an incidence of about 10%.[40,41] The incidence is 3% in head and neck cancer.[42]

Pathogenesis
There are many causes of SIADH (Box 6.F). In cancer-related SIADH there is ectopic secretion of arginine vasopressin (ADH) or vasopressin-like peptides by the cancer.[43,44] In SCLC an elevated arginine vasopressin can be detected in about 40% of patients, but in most it is asymptomatic.

Box 6.F   Causes of SIADH

Cancer
SCLC
Head and neck
Pancreas
Prostate
Carcinoid
Lymphoma
Acute myeloid leukaemia

Treatment
After neurosurgery
Chemotherapy, e.g.
   cyclophosphamide
   vincristine
Drugs
   barbiturates
   carbamazepine
   lorazepam
   phenothiazines
   SSRIs
   TCAs

Miscellaneous
Pulmonary
   pneumonia
   tuberculosis
   lung abscess
   positive pressure ventilation
Central nervous system
   meningitis
   encephalitis
   subarachnoid haemorrhage
   cerebral thrombosis
   head injury
Psychiatric
   schizophrenia
   psychosis
Recreational drugs
   alcohol
   nicotine

Hyponatraemia with consequential intracellular cerebral oedema, possibly caused by SIADH, should be considered in all patients who develop drowsiness, confusion or seizures while taking a TCA or SSRI. Risk factors for the development of SIADH with SSRIs include older age, female gender, low body weight and concurrent use of diuretics.[45]

Clinical features

Clinical features depend on both the level and the rate of decline of the plasma sodium concentration (Box 6.G). Given time, brain cells can compensate against cerebral oedema by secreting potassium and other solutes; asymptomatic hyponatraemia therefore indicates chronic rather than acute SIADH.

Box 6.G   Clinical features of SIADH

Plasma sodium 110–120mmol/L	**Plasma sodium <110mmol/L**
Anorexia	Multifocal myoclonus
Nausea and vomiting	Drowsiness
Lassitude	Seizures
Confusion	Coma

Evaluation

Paired urine and serum samples should be obtained from the patient. Diagnosis of SIADH is based on the following criteria:
* hyponatraemia (<130mmol/L)
* low plasma osmolality (<270mosmol/L)
* urine osmolality greater than plasma osmolality (>300mosmol/L)
* urine sodium concentration:
  ▷ always >20mmol/L
  ▷ up to 80mmol/L
* normal or moderately expanded plasma volume.[46]

Urine osmolality >100mosmol/L but <300mosmol/L may be consistent with a diagnosis of SIADH if there is co-existent renal tubular dysfunction, diuretic use or reset osmostat syndrome. In such cases, a raised urine sodium concentration (>30mmol/L) is more diagnostically reliable.[47,48] In practice, a plasma sodium concentration of <120mmol/L is sufficient to make a clinical diagnosis of SIADH in the absence of:
* severe vomiting
* diuretic therapy
* hypo-adrenalism
* hypothyroidism
* severe renal failure.

Management
Treat the patient and not the biochemical results.

Correct the correctable
Successful anticancer treatment will lead to a remission of SIADH.

Non-drug treatment

Restrict fluid intake to 700–1,000mL/day or daily urine output to <500mL. Although standard treatment for SIADH, fluid restriction to this extent is an added burden for most patients struggling to cope with end-stage cancer.

Drug treatment

For more information, see *PCF3*.

Demeclocycline, a tetracycline derivative, is the drug treatment of choice, and is given in a dose of 300mg PO b.d.–q.d.s. In patients unable to take demeclocycline reliably PO, it can be given PR dispersed in 5ml of a methylcellulose carrier.[49] It acts by inducing nephrogenic diabetes insipidus, i.e. inhibits the action of ADH on renal tubules.

The effect of demeclocycline is apparent after 3–5 days, and persists for several days after stopping treatment. There is no need to restrict fluid during treatment. Undesirable effects include uraemia, particularly with higher doses. Nausea and photosensitivity also occur.

Vasopressin V_2-receptor antagonists which selectively block the action of ADH on renal tubules are being developed for PO and IV use.[50,51]

1 Stewart AF (2005) Clinical practice. Hypercalcemia associated with cancer. *The New England Journal of Medicine.* **352**: 373–379.
2 Bower M et al. (2005) Endocrine and metabolic complications of advanced cancer. In: D Doyle et al. (eds) *Oxford Textbook of Palliative Medicine* (3e). Oxford University Press, Oxford, pp. 688–690.
3 Glick J and Glover D (1998) Metabolic emergencies. In: G Murphy et al. (eds) *Clinical Oncology* (seconde). American Cancer Society, Atlanta, Georgia, pp. 609–610.
4 Mundy G (1997) Malignancy and the skeleton. *Hormone and Metabolic Research.* **29**: 120–126.
5 Strewler GJ (2000) The physiology of parathyroid hormone-related protein. *The New England Journal of Medicine.* **342**: 177–185.
6 Roodman GD (2004) Mechanisms of bone metastasis. *The New England Journal of Medicine.* **350**: 1655–1664.
7 Seymour JF et al. (1994) Calcitriol production in hypercalcemic and normocalcemic patients with non-Hodgkin lymphoma. *Annals of Internal Medicine.* **121**: 633–640.
8 Ashcroft AJ et al. (2003) Aetiology of bone disease and the role of bisphosphonates in multiple myeloma. *The Lancet Oncology.* **4**: 284–292.
9 Grieve R and Dixon P (1983) Dysphagia: a further symptom of hypercalcaemia. *British Medical Journal.* **286**: 1935–1936.
10 Parsons V et al. (1974) The effects of calcitonin on the metabolic disturbances surrounding widespread bony metastases. *Acta Endocrinologica.* **76**: 286–301.
11 Davies J et al. (1979) Effect of mithramycin on widespread painful bone metastases in cancer of the breast. *Cancer Treatment Reports.* **63**: 1835–1838.
12 Coombes R et al. (1979) Agents affecting osteolysis in patients with breast cancer. *Cancer Chemotherapy and Pharmacology.* **3**: 41–44.
13 Godsall JW et al. (1986) Nephrogenous cyclic AMP, adenylate cyclase-stimulating activity, and the humoral hypercalcemia of malignancy. *Recent Progress in Hormone Research.* **42**: 705–750.
14 Hutchesson AC et al. (1995) Survival in hypercalcaemic patients with cancer and co-existing primary hyperparathyroidism. *Postgraduate Medical Journal.* **71**: 28–31.
15 Conroy S and O'Malley B (2005) Hypercalcaemia in cancer. *British Medical Journal.* **331**: 954.
16 Ralston S et al. (1990) Cancer-associate hypercalcaemia: morbidity and mortality. *Annals of Internal Medicine.* **112**: 449–504.
17 Saunders Y et al. (2004) Systematic review of bisphosphonates for hypercalcaemia of malignancy. *Palliative Medicine.* **18**: 418–431.
18 Purohit O et al. (1995) A randomised, double-blind comparison of intravenous pamidronate and clodronate in hypercalcaemia of malignancy. *British Journal of Cancer.* **72**: 1289–1293.
19 Ralston SH et al. (1997) Dose-response study of ibandronate in the treatment of cancer-associated hypercalcaemia. *British Journal of Cancer.* **75**: 295–300.
20 Major P et al. (2001) Zoledronic acid is superior to pamidronate in the treatment of hypercalcaemia of malignancy: a pooled analysis of two randomized, controlled clinical trials. *Journal of Clinical Oncology.* **19**: 558–567.

21 Percival R et al. (1984) Role of glucocorticoids in management of malignant hypercalcaemia. British Medical Journal. 289: 287.

22 Ralston S et al. (1985) Comparison of aminohydroxypropylidene diphosphonate, mithramycin, and corticosteroids/calcitonin in treatment of cancer-associated hypercalcaemia. Lancet. ii: 907–910.

23 Mannheimer I (1965) Hypercalcaemia of breast cancer. Management with corticosteroids. Cancer. 18: 679–691.

24 Harrison M et al. (1990) Somatostatin analogue treatment for malignant hypercalcaemia. British Medical Journal. 300: 1313–1314.

25 ADA (American Diabetes Association) (2008) Diagnosis and classification of diabetes mellitus. Diabetes Care. 31 Suppl 1: S55–60.

26 National Collaborating Centre for Chronic Conditions (2008) Type 2 Diabetes: National Clinical Guideline for Management in Primary and Secondary Care (Update). London: Royal College of Physicians.

27 YHPHO PBS Diabetes Prevalence Model Phase 3. Yorkshire and Humber Public Health Observatory. Available from: www.yhpho.org.uk

28 Glicksman A and Rawson R (1956) Diabetes and altered carbohydrate metabolism in patients with cancer. Cancer. 9: 1127–1134.

29 McCoubrie R et al. (2005) Managing diabetes mellitus in patients with advanced cancer: a case note audit and guidelines. European Journal of Cancer Care (Engl). 14: 244–248.

30 WHO (1999) Definition, Diagnosis and Classification of Diabetes Mellitus and its Complications; Part 1: Diagnosis and Classification of Diabetes Mellitus. World Health Organization, Geneva.

31 Williams G (2004) Ch. 12:17. Diabetes. In: DA Warrell et al. (eds) Oxford Textbook of Medicine (5e). Oxford University Press, Oxford.

32 Usborne C and Wilding J (2003) Treating diabetes mellitus in palliative care patients. European Journal of Palliative Care. 10: 186–188.

33 Quinn K et al. (2006) Diabetes management in patients receiving palliative care. Journal of Pain and Symptom Management. 32: 275–286.

34 McCann M-A et al. (2006) Practical management of diabetes mellitus. European Journal of Palliative Care. 13: 226–229.

35 Poulson J (1997) The management of diabetes in patients with advanced cancer. Journal of Pain and Symptom Management. 13: 339–346.

36 Ford-Dunn S et al. (2006) Management of diabetes during the last days of life: attitudes of consultant diabetologists and consultant palliative care physicians in the UK. Palliative Medicine. 20: 197–203.

37 Hardy J et al. (2001) A prospective survey of the use of dexamethasone on a palliative care unit. Palliative Medicine. 15: 3–8.

38 Asudani D and Calles-Escandon J (2007) Steroid Hyperglycaemia (letter reply). Journal of Hospital Medicine. 2(4): 285–286.

39 Oyer DS et al. (2006) How to manage steroid diabetes in the patient with cancer. The Journal of Supportive Oncology. 4: 479–483.

40 van-Oosterhout A et al. (1996) Neurologic disorders in 203 consecutive patients with small cell lung cancer. Cancer. 77: 1434–1441.

41 List A et al. (1986) The syndrome of inappropriate secretion of antidiuretic hormone (SIADH) in small-cell lung cancer. Journal of Clinical Oncology. 4: 1191–1198.

42 Ferlito A et al. (1997) Syndrome of inappropriate antidiuretic hormone secretion associated with head and neck cancers. Review of the literature. Annals of Otology Rhinology and Laryngology. 106: 878–883.

43 Meinders A (1993) Hyponatraemia: SIADH or SIAD? Netherlands Journal of Medicine. 43: 1–4.

44 Sorensen J et al. (1995) Syndrome of inappropriate secretion of antidiuretic hormone (SIADH) in malignant disease. Journal of Internal Medicine. 238: 97–110.

45 Jacob S and Spinler SA (2006) Hyponatremia associated with selective serotonin-reuptake inhibitors in older adults. The Annals of Pharmacotherapy. 40: 1618–1622.

46 Burtis CA et al. (eds) (2008) Pituitary disorders. In: Tietz Fundamentals of Clinical Chemistry (6e). WB Saunders, Philadelphia, pp. 746–747.

47 Smellie WS and Heald A (2007) Hyponatraemia and hypernatraemia: pitfalls in testing. British Medical Journal. 334: 473–476.

48 Ellison DH and Berl T (2007) Clinical practice. The syndrome of inappropriate antidiuresis. The New England Journal of Medicine. 356: 2064–2072.

49 Hussain I et al. (1998) Rectal administration of demeclocycline in a patient with syndrome of inappropriate ADH secretion. International Journal of Clinical Practice. 52: 59.

50 Siragy HM (2006) Hyponatremia, fluid-electrolyte disorders, and the syndrome of inappropriate antidiuretic hormone secretion: diagnosis and treatment options. Endocrine Practice. 12: 446–457.

51 Schrier RW et al. (2006) Tolvaptan, a selective oral vasopressin V2-receptor antagonist, for hyponatremia. The New England Journal of Medicine. 355: 2099–2112.

7: HAEMATOLOGICAL SYMPTOMS

HAEMATOLOGICAL CHANGES IN CANCER

Haematological changes are common in cancer, and sometimes are the presenting feature (Table 7.1). Anaemia is the most common abnormality.

ANAEMIA OF CHRONIC DISEASE

Anaemia in adults is arbitrarily defined as a haemoglobin (Hb) concentration of <13g/dL in men and <12g/dL in women. It occurs in up to 50% of patients with solid tumours and in most patients with myeloma and lymphoma. Symptoms vary but can have a major impact on a patient's quality of life (Box 7.A). In some patients there may be more than one cause, e.g. iron deficiency as well as anaemia of chronic disease (ACD).

Hepcidin, a peptide hormone which regulates iron metabolism, is a key mediator of ACD. It is produced by the liver in response to infection and inflammation, and also by some cancers.[1] This results in:
- impaired transferrin production, resulting in reduced availability of stored iron
- shortened RBC survival.

Cytokines are also increased by infection, inflammation and cancer, and contribute to ACD by suppressing erythropoietin production, and thus erythropoiesis.[2]

Evaluation
It is important to differentiate between ACD and iron deficiency (Table 7.2). Diagnostic features of ACD are:
- normochromic-normocytic anaemia (low mean cell volume (MCV) also possible)
- low/low-normal plasma transferrin (TIBC) concentration
- low plasma iron
- high/high-normal plasma ferritin concentration (note: ferritin is also raised during the acute phase response to trauma, infection and some cancers, etc.)
- bone marrow appearance generally unremarkable; may show abnormal iron distribution

- increased marrow iron stores
- reduced iron within maturing erythroblasts.[3]

Table 7.1   Haematological changes in cancer[3]

Haematological changes	Commonly associated cancers or other disorders
RBC	
Anaemia	
ACD	All
iron deficiency	GI, cervix, uterus
megaloblastic	Stomach
sideroblastic	Myeloproliferative disorders
leuco-erythroblastic	Breast, bronchus, kidney, prostate, stomach, thyroid
micro-angiopathic haemolytic	Mucin-secreting cancers: stomach, bronchus, breast
immune haemolytic	Ovary, lymphoma
Selective red cell aplasia	Thymus, lymphoma, bronchus
Polycythaemia	Kidney, liver, posterior fossa, uterus
Secondary myelosclerosis	As for leuco-erythroblastic anaemia, also reticuloses
WBC	
Leucocytosis	All
Leukaemoid reactions	As for leuco-erythroblastic anaemia
Lymphopenia	All, reticuloses
Eosinophilia	Many
Monocytosis	All
Basophilia	Myeloproliferative disorders, mastocytosis
Platelets	
Thrombocytosis	GI, bronchus
Thrombocytopenia	As for micro-angiopathies
Acquired thrombocytopathy	Macroglobulinaemia, other paraproteinaemias
Coagulation	
Thrombophlebitis	All
DIC	Many (see p.250)
Primary activation of fibrinolysis	Prostate
Miscellaneous	
Abnormal proteins, e.g. cryoglobulins	Prostate
Foetal proteins	
α-fetoprotein	Liver
carcino-embryonic	GI
foetal Hb	Leukaemia

Box 7.A Anaemia and cancer

Main causes	**Symptoms**
ACD	Tiredness (fatigue)
Iron and folate deficiency	Lack of energy (lethargy)
Malignant infiltration of the marrow	Breathlessness
Haemolytic anaemia	Angina
Renal failure	Loss of appetite
	Loss of libido
	Low mood

Table 7.2 Iron deficiency anaemia compared with ACD

Test	Normal[a]	Iron deficiency	ACD
Blood film	Normochromic-normocytic	Hypochromic-microcytic	Normochromic-normocytic or slightly microcytic
Plasma iron (micromol/L)	9–31	Low/very low	Low
Plasma ferritin (microgram/L)	12–300	Low	High/high-normal
TIBC (micromol/L)	45–76	High/high-normal	Low/low-normal
% saturation TIBC[b]	Normal	Low	Normal

a. reference values, Nottingham University Hospitals
b. some laboratories now measure transferrin saturation instead.

Management

Treat the patient and not the laboratory results. Although tiredness and weakness can be caused by the cancer itself, if associated with anaemia they are strong indicators for a trial blood transfusion (Box 7.B).

Epoetin (recombinant human erythropoietin) has been used as an alternative to blood transfusion.[6] Erythropoietin stimulates the production of RBC. Its plasma concentration is often low in patients with cancer, particularly those receiving chemotherapy. However, RCTs show a higher rate of cancer progression and reduced survival in cancer patients receiving epoetin but not on chemotherapy.[7] Blood transfusion is the preferred option in patients with cancer, particularly those being treated with curative intent, and probably those with advanced cancer with a reasonable prognosis.[8,9]

Epoetin should generally be restricted to patients with chemotherapy-related anaemia.[10–12] In other circumstances, its use should be based on an informed risk–benefit analysis, with patient participation, taking into account factors such as cancer type and stage, degree of anaemia, life expectancy and patient preference.

Box 7.B   Non-emergency blood transfusion in palliative care

Indications
Generally the following criteria should all be met:
- symptoms attributable to anaemia, e.g. fatigue, lethargy and breathlessness on exertion, which:
  ▷ are troublesome to the patient
  ▷ limit routine activity
  ▷ are likely to be corrected by transfusion
- expectation that a blood transfusion will achieve a durable effect, e.g. at least 2 weeks
- patient willing to have a transfusion and requisite blood tests.

Contra-indications for blood transfusion
- no benefit from previous transfusion
- patient is moribund, i.e. the patient's condition is terminal
- if the transfusion can best be described as simply prolonging the patient's death
- if the main reason is a demand by the family that 'something must be done'.

Blood transfusion helps about 75% of patients in terms of wellbeing, strength and breathlessness.[4] Benefit occurs equally in patients with Hb <8g/dL and in those with Hb 8–11g/dL.[4,5]

BLEEDING

Bleeding occurs in about 20% of patients with advanced cancer. It contributes significantly to the patient's death in about 5%. External catastrophic bleeding is less common than internal occult bleeding.

Stop and think!
Are you justified in treating a potentially fatal complication in a moribund patient?

Excessive bruising and bleeding from the gums and nose or the GI tract suggests a platelet abnormality, whereas bleeding into joints or muscles suggests a deficiency of at least one coagulation factor. Check:
- FBC
- prothrombin time (PT)
- activated partial thromboplastin time (APTT).

Other helpful tests may include measurement of platelet function, and a thrombin clotting time or fibrinogen level.

In patients with cancer, an elevated PT and APTT are seen with:
- severe hepatic impairment
- phytomenadione (vitamin K_1) deficiency
- DIC (see p.250).

Thrombocytopenia
Thrombocytopenia is defined as a platelet count of $<150 \times 10^9$/L. With platelet counts of $10–20 \times 10^9$/L the risk of a major bleed is small (0.1% per day). Below

---

10×10^9/L the risk rises (2% per day) with severe bleeds occurring mostly with counts below 5×10^9/L. Treatment varies with the cause (Box 7.C). Platelet function may also be impaired without thrombocytopenia by most NSAIDs, and also in myeloma and renal failure.[13]

Box 7.C Causes of thrombocytopenia

Decreased production of platelets
Marrow replacement with cancer
Chemotherapy
Carbamazepine
Thiazide diuretics
Valproate
Excessive alcohol (recovers after abstinence for 3–5 days)

Platelet sequestration by the spleen
Increased venous pressure resulting from liver disease
Heart failure
Respiratory failure

Increased platelet destruction (immune)
Idiopathic thrombocytopenic purpura (particularly with non-Hodgkin's
    lymphoma)
After transfusion of blood products
Heparin (see p.234)

Increased platelet destruction (non-immune)
Sepsis
DIC

Correct the correctable
• modify or stop chemotherapy
• prescribe antibacterials if caused by sepsis
• review drug SPCs and stop any drug which is potentially causal.

Non-drug treatment
In a relatively well patient with a platelet count $<5 \times 10^9$/L, emergency platelet transfusions should be considered. They are not indicated if the platelet count is above 10×10^9/L and there is no bleeding. Each transfusion is generally of one adult unit. The amount by which one unit will raise the platelet count varies widely between patients, depending on the rate of platelet destruction or sequestration.

Patients for whom life-supporting treatment is appropriate and who are bleeding, have sepsis or DIC should be given platelets sufficient to maintain a count of $>50 \times 10^9$/L. If the patient has had an intracerebral haemorrhage, the platelet count should be maintained $>100 \times 10^9$/L.

In reversible renal and hepatic failure, emergency treatment with cryoprecipitate infusions 10units q12h should be considered.[14]

Further, in a relatively well patient, consider a blood transfusion to raise the haematocrit above 30%.[14]

Drug treatment

In a relatively well patient, consider corticosteroids (e.g. prednisolone 1mg/kg) or immunoglobulin infusions 1g/kg if there is auto-immune destruction of platelets

Heparin-induced thrombocytopenia (HIT)

Heparin can cause thrombocytopenia. An early (4 days) mild fall in platelet count is often seen after starting heparin therapy, particularly after surgery. This corrects spontaneously despite the continued use of heparin, and is asymptomatic.[15]

However, occasionally an immune thrombocytopenia develops associated with heparin-dependent IgG antibodies. Heparin binds to and induces a conformational change in platelet factor 4 (PF4). IgG antibodies bind to the altered PF4 and form IgG/PF4/heparin complexes. These complexes bind to the platelet surface, causing activation of the platelets and a release of pro-thrombotic microparticles. These complexes may also cause direct endothelial injury, leading to increased tissue factor expression and thrombin generation.[16]

The incidence of HIT in patients receiving low molecular weight heparin (LMWH) is estimated to be 0.5–0.8% but is higher in patients receiving unfractionated heparin.[17] HIT is less common with prophylactic regimens (low doses) than with therapeutic ones (higher doses). HIT is more common in the USA (where more bovine heparin is used) than in the UK (where more porcine heparin is used). The risk in the USA has been put at 3% for unfractionated heparin.[18]

Should HIT develop, the platelet count typically drops 5–10 days after commencing heparin. It may drop sooner if the patient has received heparin during the last 3 months and has already developed antibodies. It is rare for HIT to develop >15 days after heparin exposure.

Ideally, for patients receiving LMWH, the platelet count should be checked on the day it is started, and every 2–4 days from days 4–14. The platelet count should be checked every 1–2 days for patients receiving unfractionated heparin.

Venous or arterial thrombo-embolism will occur in 1/2 of the patients with HIT, and may be fatal (Box 7.D). Patients presenting without thrombosis are at risk of developing subsequent thrombosis if heparin is not stopped and an alternative anticoagulant started.[16]

Diagnosis and management

See *PCF3*, p.62.

Phytomenadione deficiency

Phytomenadione (vitamin K_1) is required for the synthesis of several coagulation factors (II, VII, IX, X). It is present in green vegetables and is synthesized by bacteria in the GI tract; body stores are low. Patients who are malnourished, have fat malabsorption or are receiving prolonged courses of antibacterials which sterilize the GI tract are at risk of deficiency and a rapid rise in PT and APTT. Treat with:

- phytomenadione 10mg PO once daily
- menadiol sodium phosphate 10mg PO once daily (if fat malabsorption present).

When a more rapid response is required for serious bleeding:

- phytomenadione (e.g. Konakion® MM) 10mg by slow IV injection over 15min *or*
- 4 units of fresh frozen plasma or factor concentrates or prothrombin complex concentrates (PCCs).

Box 7.D   Clinical events associated with HIT[18]

Platelet count
Thrombocytopenia.
Falling platelet count, i.e. a fall in the platelet count of ⩾50% beginning on or after day 5 of heparin use.

Venous thrombosis
DVT (mostly proximal vein); if gross swelling, arterial supply may be compromised → limb gangrene.
Pulmonary embolism.
Adrenal haemorrhagic infarction (probably secondary to adrenal vein thrombosis).
Cerebral vein or cerebral dural sinus thrombosis.

Arterial thrombosis or thrombo-embolism
Arterial thrombosis, e.g. cerebral, coronary, aorta (may cause spinal cord infarction), mesenteric, renal, limb.
Vascular graft occlusion.

Reactions at heparin injection sites
Erythematous plaques.
Skin necrosis.

Hepatic impairment

Severe liver disease leads to multiple coagulation defects:
- reduced synthesis and increased consumption of nearly all of the major coagulation factors resulting in raised PT and APTT
- hypersplenism causing thrombocytopenia
- increase in fibrin degradation products and plasmin leading to platelet dysfunction
- enhanced fibrinolysis, suggested by diffuse oozing from sites of minor trauma.

A trial of phytomenadione (vitamin K_1) should be considered, although this is unlikely to benefit most patients. Desmopressin may improve haemostasis in patients with hepatic platelet dysfunction.[19] Despite the risk of coagulation abnormalities, paradoxically the risk of venous thrombosis is often increased in patients with hepatic impairment. Thus, PCCs should be used only in emergency situations after specialist advice.

Renal impairment

Patients with renal disease may have either a bleeding or a thrombotic tendency. There is loss of natural anticoagulants in nephrotic syndrome. Patients on dialysis have a high incidence of GI and genito-urinary bleeding and subdural haematomas. In end-stage renal disease, GI bleeding due to angiodysplasia or gastritis can occur. This is treated with epoetin or blood transfusion to raise the haematocrit over 30%.

In more acute situations, consider:
- desmopressin (or cryoprecipitate infusions) to increase Von Willebrand factor levels
- dialysis (in severe impairment).

The reason for a hypercoagulable state in certain renal diseases is not understood.

SURFACE BLEEDING

Surface bleeding may be exacerbated by NSAIDs. When this is the case, change to paracetamol or to an NSAID which does not affect platelet function. Other options comprise:
- physical measures
- haemostatic drugs, e.g. tranexamic acid
- radiotherapy (Box 7.E).

The maximum dose of tranexamic acid is 2g q.d.s., although a smaller dose is often satisfactory (Box 7.E). Improvement occurs in 2–4 days. Discontinue or reduce to 500mg t.d.s. 1 week after bleeding has stopped. Restart if bleeding recurs. Parenteral use may be indicated occasionally.

Box 7.E   Management of surface bleeding

Physical
Gauze applied with pressure for 10min soaked in:
- adrenaline (epinephrine) 1mg in 1mL (1 in 1,000) or ⎫
- tranexamic acid 500mg in 5mL ⎭ use standard ampoules.

Silver nitrate sticks applied to bleeding points in the nose and mouth, and on skin nodules and fungating cancers.
Haemostatic dressings, i.e. alginate (e.g. Kaltostat®, Sorbsan®).
Diathermy.

Specialist therapy:
- cryotherapy
- LASER
- embolization.[20,21]

Drugs
Review existing medication
Discontinue aspirin and/or other platelet-impairing NSAID.
Prescribe an NSAID which does *not* impair platelet function (e.g. diclofenac, nabumetone, a non-acetylated salicylate, or a coxib), or paracetamol instead.

Topical
- sucralfate paste 2g (two 1g tablets crushed in 5mL KY jelly®)[22]
- sucralfate suspension 2g in 10mL b.d. for the mouth and rectum[23]
- tranexamic acid 5g in 50mL warm water once daily or b.d. for bleeding from cancer in the rectum, bladder or pleura (e.g. 10 ampoules of undiluted injection)[24,25]
- 1% alum solution.

Systemic
- antifibrinolytic, e.g. tranexamic acid.[26] *Do not use if DIC suspected*
- etamsylate
- desmopressin (augments platelet function).[27]

Radiotherapy
Teletherapy and brachytherapy are both used to control haemorrhage from:

skin	oesophagus	bladder	vagina.
lungs	rectum	uterus	

NOSEBLEEDS

Most nosebleeds are venous. When from the anterior nasal septum (Little's area), they can often be stopped by direct pressure, i.e. by pinching the nostrils for 10–15min. If this does not work, a silver nitrate caustic pencil applied to the bleeding point is often effective. Alternatively, the nostril can be packed for 2 days with calcium alginate rope (e.g. Kaltostat®) or with ribbon gauze soaked in adrenaline (epinephrine) solution 1mg/1mL (1 in 1,000).

If bleeding continues into the nasopharynx, the source is more posterior and may require referral to an ENT department for:
- the insertion of a Merocel® tampon for 36h with antibacterial cover or
- haemostatic packing for 3 days (risk of rebound bleeding when this is removed); if no commercial product available, soak gauze in:
  ▷ bismuth iodoform paraffin paste (BIPP) or
  ▷ 1% alum or
  ▷ 1mg/1mL (1 in 1,000) adrenaline (epinephrine)
- balloon catheter or
- cauterization under local anaesthetic
- arterial embolization if severe nosebleed from nasopharyngeal cancer.[28]

Chronic recurrent mild epistaxis is often related to nasal vestibulitis which can be treated with chlorhexidine and neomycin cream (e.g. Naseptin®) applied b.d. for 2 weeks followed by petroleum jelly (Vaseline®). If bleeding is heavy, consider checking PT and APTT, and obtain FBC to check platelets and Hb.

HAEMOPTYSIS

One third of patients with lung cancer experience haemoptysis. The incidence of acute fatal bleeds is 3%, of which some occur without warning. When death results, it is generally caused by suffocation and not exsanguination. Haemoptysis of 400mL within 3h or 600mL within 24h has a mortality of about 75%.[29]

Physiology
The lungs have two blood supplies:
- low-pressure pulmonary circulation which supplies blood for gas exchange
- high-pressure bronchial circulation which supplies blood to the structures of the respiratory tract; this is the more important in haemoptysis.

Causes
In cancer, haemoptysis may be caused by the cancer itself or by other factors:
- lung cancer; massive haemoptysis is most likely with squamous cell cancer lying centrally or causing cavitation. Generally there is necrosis of vessels within the tumour bed rather than direct tumour invasion into the pulmonary vasculature
- metastatic lung disease; particularly cancers of the breast, colorectum and kidney, and melanoma
- chest infection (acute and chronic); in haematological cancers, pulmonary haemorrhage ± haemoptysis is associated with fungal infection
- pulmonary embolus.

Pattern recognition generally helps to identify non-cancer causes, e.g. infection is associated with purulent sputum and a pulmonary embolus with pleuritic pain. These should be treated as appropriate.

Note: *coughed up blood may not originate from the lungs*. Particularly in patients with a bleeding tendency or thrombocytopenia, fresh blood can be from the nose, pharynx or lungs. Dark blood is more likely to be from the lungs.

Management
Validate the patient's concern, i.e. never say, 'Don't worry about it', but 'I'm glad you mentioned it, I imagine you must be very concerned about it'. Assure the patient that, although it is a nuisance and unpleasant, life-threatening haemoptysis is rare.

Correct the correctable
Can the cancer be modified?
Radiotherapy leads to prolonged relief in 85% of patients.[26] A palliative dose of teletherapy is generally given as 1–2 treatments, which permits retreatment if necessary. For patients with unrelieved or recurrent haemoptysis in whom further external beam radiation is not possible, other options will vary according to local availability:

- *brachytherapy (endobronchial radiation)*: a fine catheter is placed at bronchoscopy which is afterloaded for a short time with a radio-active source by remote control; can be carried out as a day case procedure and is effective in 80% of patients[30]
- *cryotherapy*: in which the tumour is cooled by a liquid nitrogen probe to $-70°$C; multiple treatments may be required; it requires rigid bronchoscopy and a general anaesthetic
- *LASER therapy*: requires bronchoscopy and a general anaesthetic.

Can other factors be modified?
Substitute a non-selective NSAID with paracetamol or an NSAID which does not impair platelet function (see Box 7.F, p.240).
Consider checking the PT, APTT and FBC.

Non-drug treatment
Massive haemoptysis is an emergency, but conventional life-saving interventions, i.e. bronchoscopy, intubation and bronchial artery embolization, are generally not appropriate in palliative care. Often there will have been several warning haemorrhages which will have prompted team discussion and a decision that the patient is 'not to be resuscitated' will have been taken. The family and patient should be brought into the discussions in an appropriate way.

If life-threatening haemoptysis seems likely, it may be sensible to have a syringe containing diamorphine/morphine and one containing midazolam 10mg drawn up and kept in a convenient safe place, or to have ampoules readily available. The dose of the opioid will depend on whether the patient is already receiving diamorphine/morphine regularly. If not, 10mg will be appropriate; otherwise use the equivalent of a q4h dose. The aim is to reduce fear, not necessarily to render the patient unconscious. If the patient is shocked and peripherally vasoconstricted, medication can be given IV or IM.

Adequate maintenance of the airway is essential. Lying on the bleeding side, if known, reduces the impact on the other lung. When the site of bleeding is unknown, the patient may benefit from being placed in a head down position with oxygen and suctioning as needed. Some patients feel safer sitting upright in a comfortable high-backed chair with the head supported, tilted forward with chin down.[31] Others feel safer reclining in bed with the head and neck well supported.

Tilting the head backwards because of boredom or exasperation may restart the bleeding. On the other hand, standing up after 1–2h, bending forward and taking deep breaths helps to dislodge clots by coughing and reduces wheezing.

A fall in blood pressure helps bleeding to stop but a subsequent rise could lead to renewed bleeding. It is important that the patient is not left alone until the situation has resolved one way or the other.

Drug treatment

For more information, see *PCF3*.

Drug treatment is often helpful for persistent mild–moderate haemoptysis:
- corticosteroid, e.g. dexamethasone 2–4mg or prednisolone 15–30mg once daily, may stop or reduce mild persistent haemoptysis, i.e. blood-streaked sputum
- antifibrinolytic, e.g. tranexamic acid 1.5g stat and 1g t.d.s.; maximum dose 2g q.d.s., with improvement in 2–4 days[26]
- haemostatic, e.g. etamsylate 500mg q.d.s.

Other options include:
- nebulized adrenaline (epinephrine) 1mg in 1mL (1 in 1,000) diluted to 5mL in 0.9% saline up to q.d.s. has been used as a short-term measure
- nebulized vasopressin 5units diluted in 1–2mL 0.9% saline up to t.d.s.[32]

HAEMATEMESIS AND MELAENA

Bleeding from the gastroduodenum, manifesting as haematemesis and/or melaena, occurs in about 5% of patients with advanced cancer.[33] Melaena is more frequent than haematemesis, and they often occur together. Patients with liver cancer or liver metastases have a much increased risk of haemorrhage.[33] NSAIDs are an added risk factor, particularly when combined with a corticosteroid.

For some, the haematemesis and/or melaena is a preterminal event, with death ensuing within days. With those who survive, a decision may be needed about a blood transfusion and endoscopy (see Box 7.B, p.232).

Causes

Haematemesis and/or melaena may be caused by the cancer itself or by other factors. Non-selective NSAIDs are an added risk factor with:
- primary cancers of the GI tract
- metastases to the GI tract
- erosive gastropathy
- peptic ulcer disease
- oesophageal varices
- liver cancer or liver metastases; may lead to portal hypertension, portal vein thrombosis or portal vein occlusion, greatly increasing the risk of haemorrhage
- oesophagitis
- Mallory-Weiss tear of lower oesophagus (most often occur *after* bouts of vomiting or retching; more common in patients with hiatus hernias).

Haematemesis associated with a Mallory-Weiss tear is generally minor, and most tears heal spontaneously.[34] However, in a patient with advanced cancer, acute variceal bleeding is likely to be a terminal event (see management of severe haemorrhage, p.243).

Management
Correct the correctable
Can the cancer be modified?
With bleeding from a gastric cancer, palliative radiotherapy should be considered unless the patient is thought to be only a few weeks from death.[34]

Can other factors be modified?
If the patient is well enough, consider oesophagogastroduodenoscopy to confirm the diagnosis and to control the bleeding:
- a discrete lesion, e.g. peptic ulcer can be treated using an injection of 1:10,000 adrenaline (epinephrine) with or without a sclerosing agent, thermocoagulation or haemostatic clips
- bleeding oesophageal varices may be banded or injected with a sclerosing agent e.g. ethanolamine oleate.[34]

Drug treatment
For more information, see *PCF3*.

As always, prevention is better than cure (Box 7.F). With a patient who is not fit for endoscopy, consider SC octreotide if the bleeding continues despite the measures suggested in the Box.[35]

Box 7.F   Strategies to prevent or limit NSAID-associated gastropathy

Prescribe paracetamol instead of an NSAID.

If an NSAID must be continued, prescribe one which:
- is less likely to cause gastric injury, e.g. nabumetone, diclofenac, ibuprofen, celecoxib
- is a pro-drug, e.g. nabumetone, or is poorly absorbed in the stomach, e.g. diclofenac, ibuprofen
- does not impair platelet function, e.g. nabumetone, diclofenac, celecoxib
- use an NSAID with the above three properties, e.g. diclofenac, nabumetone, celecoxib.

Use the smallest dose of NSAID necessary.

Consider stopping concurrent corticosteroid.

Prescribe a gastroprotective drug concurrently with NSAIDs, i.e. PPI, H_2-receptor antagonist, sucralfate, misoprostol.[36]

Tranexamic acid PO or PR (to facilitate healing).

RECTAL AND VAGINAL HAEMORRHAGE

Lower GI bleeding may be caused by the cancer itself, or other factors, e.g. diverticular disease, inflammatory bowel disease or angiodysplasia. In advanced cancer, haemorrhage from the rectum or vagina is generally associated with local cancer or radiotherapy. If related to the cancer, palliative radiotherapy should be considered unless the patient is thought to be within a few weeks of death.

Bloody diarrhoea is an acute complication of intrapelvic radiotherapy, e.g. in cancers of the cervix uteri and prostate. It is caused by inflammatory damage to the mucosa of the rectum and sigmoid colon and is self-limiting. If particularly troublesome, it can be treated with retention enemas of:

- prednisolone 20mg in 100mL (Predsol® retention enema) once daily or b.d. *or*
- prednisolone 5mg and sucralfate 3g in 15mL b.d. (made up by local pharmacy).

Bleeding associated with chronic ischaemic radiation proctocolitis does *not* benefit from prednisolone, but generally responds to:

- PO or PR tranexamic acid
- PO etamsylate
- PR sucralfate suspension (see Box 7.E, p.236).

With these treatments, bleeding generally stops in 1–2 weeks. Treatment should be continued for one more week, and then stopped.

HAEMATURIA

Haematuria in advanced cancer is generally associated with urinary tract cancer, notably bladder cancer, but may be caused by chronic radiation cystitis (Box 7.G). Radiation cystitis may develop several years after pelvic radiotherapy.[37]

Box 7.G   Causes of haemorrhagic cystitis[38]

Drugs
Tiaprofenic acid
Methenamine
Anabolic steroids
Chemotherapy
    busulfan
    cyclophosphamide
    ifosfamide
    thiotepa
Immune agents

Diseases
Cancer
Amyloidosis
Rheumatoid arthritis

Viruses e.g.
Cytomegalovirus
Herpes simplex
Influenza A

Toxins
Dyes
Insecticides
Turpentine

Radiotherapy
Bladder
Pelvis
Prostate
Rectum

Table 7.3 Bladder instillations and irrigations for haemorrhagic cystitis[37,38]

Treatment	Administration	Duration	Comment
Preferred options			
0.9% Saline	Continuous irrigation	Until urine is clear	No undesirable effects but not effective in severe cases
Sodium citrate solution 3%	Continuous irrigation	Until urine is clear	No undesirable effects but not effective in severe cases
Alum 1%	Continuous irrigation (1L costs about £24!!)	Until urine is clear	Mild undesirable effects, no anaesthesia required. Recurrence common, aluminium toxicity rare
Sucralfate suspension	Instil 5g, follow with 10mL 0.9% saline flush	Repeat up to t.d.s if no response	Use sucralfate sachets as sucralfate from the bottle is not sterile. Give oral antibacterial cover if the patient is prone to urinary tract infections
Silver nitrate 0.5–1%	Instillation, retain for 10–20min	Repeat if no response	Anaesthesia required. Often successful; short duration of response
If the above fail			
Formalin 1–3%	Instillation, retain for 20–30min	Repeat if no response	Anaesthesia required. Often successful but undesirable effects are common, e.g. risk of ureteric stenosis and obstruction if formalin refluxes into the ureters

Management
In many cases haematuria is mild, and no intervention is necessary.

Correct the correctable
Can the cancer be modified?
If the patient is well enough, consider cystoscopy for cystodiathermy and resection. This will also provide an opportunity for biopsy if it is unclear whether haematuria is due to recurrence of bladder cancer or radiation cystitis.

Can other factors be modified?
- prescribe paracetamol instead of a non-selective NSAID, or an NSAID which does not impair platelet function (see Box 7.F, p.240)
- consider checking PT, APTT and FBC
- culture urine and treat if infection is present.

Drug treatment
For more information, see *PCF3*.

If the haematuria is more marked, etamsylate generally reduces it. Tranexamic acid may be used with etamsylate (even though there is a risk of clot retention until the bleeding has completely stopped).

Other options include bladder instillations and irrigations (Table 7.3). Alum may be given as an instillation, e.g. 50mL of 1% alum instilled through a catheter and retained for 1h, repeated b.d.–q.d.s. according to response.

Daily bladder instillations of carboprost tromethamine, a PGE_1 analogue, are occasionally used. Although no anaesthesia is required, carboprost is expensive and requires close monitoring.[38,39]

Rarely, it may be necessary to consider:
- cauterization
- arterial embolization (although serious adverse events may occur).[40–42]

SEVERE HAEMORRHAGE

In a patient who is close to death, it is often appropriate to regard severe haemorrhage as a terminal event, and not to intervene with resuscitative measures. However, sometimes there is uncertainty and, if the patient's condition stabilizes, a blood transfusion after 24–48h may be indicated.

Acute haematemesis, fresh melaena, vaginal bleeding
While accepting the possibility of death and thus adopting a conservative approach, the possibility that the patient may survive must be borne in mind. This prognostic uncertainty is reflected in an ambiguous approach to management:
- a nurse or doctor should stay with the patient if death seems imminent or until things have settled down
- if the patient is distressed, give midazolam 10mg buccal/SC/IV or diazepam 10mg PR (if haematemesis) or PO (if melaena or vaginal bleeding)
- note the pulse every 30min to monitor the patient's condition; if it is steady or decreases, this suggests that bleeding has stopped
- possibly take blood for grouping and cross-matching
- if the patient survives 24h, consider a blood transfusion (see Box 7.B, p.232).

Erosion of an artery by a cancer (e.g. neck, axilla, groin)
If one or more warning haemorrhages have occurred, consider prescribing an anxiolytic prophylactically, e.g. diazepam 5–10mg PO at bedtime.

Local pressure should be applied with packing. The more superficial material can be changed if it becomes saturated with blood. A green surgical towel may make the extent of blood loss less obvious and less disturbing to the patient and family. Consider midazolam 10mg buccal/SC/IV or diazepam 10mg PR (rectal solution/suppository). A nurse or doctor should stay with the patient until the bleeding is under control.

Massive haemorrhage from the carotid artery in recurrent neck cancer is more likely after surgery and radiotherapy and results in death in minutes; the only sensible response is to stay with the patient.

VENOUS THROMBO-EMBOLISM

Venous thrombo-embolism (VTE) includes deep vein thrombosis (DVT) and pulmonary embolism (PE). There is a strong association between VTE and cancer. In elderly patients presenting with VTE, 10–20% will have a previously undiagnosed cancer, and in 25% a cancer manifests within the next 2 years.[43,44]

VTE is a common complication of cancer, occurring clinically in 4–20% of patients. Autopsy studies put the VTE rate as high as 50%. It is a common cause of death, accounting for about 10% of deaths in patients receiving chemotherapy. The risk of VTE varies widely with cancer type but, numerically, most will be observed in patients with common cancers and longer survival times, i.e. breast, colon, lung and prostate.[45]

Cancer induces a hypercoagulable state by:
- producing procoagulant factors, e.g. tissue factor, which triggers the extrinsic coagulation cascade, and procoagulant which activates factor X directly (Figure 7.1)
- releasing cytokines, which induce endothelial expression of tissue factor and inhibit the anticoagulant protein C pathway
- interacting with other cells, e.g. endothelial, WBC, platelets.[45,46]

These mechanisms promote fibrin formation and angiogenesis, and increase vascular permeability to cancer cells; all factors which play important roles in cancer growth and metastasis.

Any cause of systemic inflammation results in a hypercoaguable state. Other risk factors for VTE are shown in Box 7.H. The incidence of VTE appears to be increasing in cancer patients, possibly due to the use of anti-angiogenic drugs with vascular toxicity, e.g. thalidomide, lenolidomide.[47]

Most PE occur as a complication of DVT in the legs. The risk of PE from untreated proximal DVT is estimated to be 50%; the risk of a PE from a distal DVT is low. The mortality rate of untreated PE is 30–40%. Of those presenting with cardiogenic shock, most die within the first hour. Post-thrombotic syndrome (chronic limb pain and swelling) and chronic thrombo-embolic pulmonary hypertension may develop.[56] However, PE need not be symptomatic, it can present as a co-incidental finding on CT.

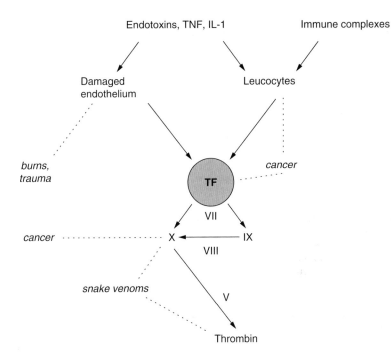

Figure 7.1 Cancer causes excessive tissue factor (TF) formation and leads to a hypercoagulable state.

Clinical features
DVT
The affected limb may be:
- swollen
- warm
- tender.

PE
The following may be seen on presentation:
- breathlessness or tachypnoea (90%)
- hypoxia (85%)
- cough (40%)
- tachycardia (30%)
- haemoptysis (10–20%)
- syncope (10–20%)
- hypotension
- cardiogenic shock
- sudden death.[57]

Pleuritic chest pain is uncommon at presentation (<10%). It tends to develop hours or days later as a result of lung infarction (66%). A DVT is detected by venous ultrasound in 30% but is not always clinically apparent.

Box 7.H Risk factors for thrombo-embolism[48–55]

Patient-related
Age ⩾40 years, particularly >60 years
Obesity
Previous thrombo-embolism
Varicose veins/chronic venous
    insufficiency

Debility
Immobility, e.g. bedbound for ⩾3 days or
    plaster immobilization of lower limbs
Major surgery within the previous
    12 weeks requiring general or regional
    anaesthesia

Co-morbidities
Chronic respiratory disease
Chronic cardiac disease
Other serious medical conditions, e.g.
    lower limb weakness, sepsis,
    inflammatory bowel disease,
    collagen disorder
Thrombophilia

Cancer (particularly if metastatic)
Bladder
Brain
Haematological
Kidney
Lung
Ovary
Pancreas
Stomach
Uterus

Treatment
Radiotherapy, e.g. to the pelvis
Hormone therapy, e.g. oral
    contraceptives, hormone
    replacement, tamoxifen,
    anastrozole, and possibly
    progestins
Chemotherapy, e.g. platinums,
    5-FU, mitomycin-C,
    thalidomide, lenalidomide
Growth factors, e.g. granulocyte
    colony stimulating factor,
    erythropoietin

Evaluation
Evaluation and management of DVT or PE depends on the patient's general condition
and the overall aims of care. For some patients, it is appropriate to confirm the
diagnosis and to treat with anticoagulants. *If the patient is close to death, no investigations
are indicated and anticoagulants are contra-indicated.*

DVT
Making a clinical diagnosis of DVT on the basis of a warm, swollen and tender limb is
unreliable. DVT can be relatively asymptomatic or mimicked by lymphatic obstruction
or external compression of the large veins by cancer or nodes in the pelvis or axilla.
A DVT is unlikely with normal D-dimer levels. Raised D-dimer levels are suggestive of
but not specific for thrombosis; *they can also be raised by cancer, infection, inflammation
or trauma.*

If the patient is well enough, investigations should be considered, e.g.:
• ultrasonography, either compression or complete duplex colour
• contrast venography, diagnostic gold standard
• CT venography, diagnostically equivalent to compression ultrasound
• MRI venography.

Compression ultrasound is good for detecting *proximal but not distal* (below knee) DVT.
If an initial scan is negative, it can be repeated after 1 week to exclude proximal
extension of an earlier undiagnosed distal DVT. Because the risk of a PE from a distal

DVT is low, it is reasonable not to treat during the interval between the first and second ultrasound examination, even with cancer patients.

Complete duplex colour ultrasonography visualizes both *distal and proximal* veins and a negative test excludes DVT.[58,59] When a distal DVT is detected, guidelines generally advocate commencing treatment with LMWH. However, the risk of a PE from a distal DVT is low; and only 3–20%[58,59] of calf vein thromboses progress to a proximal thrombosis.

Contrast venography is invasive, and venous cannulation for administration of contrast may be difficult in a swollen limb. There is a small risk of exacerbating the thrombosis. If venography is negative, DVT is excluded. The use of CT/MRI venography is likely to increase.

PE

Consideration of the history, findings on physical examination, and the presence of known risk factors will help guide the need for supporting investigations such as:

- *D-dimer levels*: methods of measurement vary in sensitivity and specificity; raised levels are suggestive of but not specific for thrombosis; they can also be raised by cancer, infection, inflammation or trauma
- *ECG*: may show non-specific tachycardia, right heart strain (e.g. S1, Q3, T3, right bundle branch block)
- *chest radiograph*: may show non-specific infiltrate or effusion (70%)
- *arterial blood gas analysis*: may show hypoxaemia.

Cardiac troponin levels can also be raised, particularly in massive acute PE.[56] However, whatever the findings, particularly in elderly inpatients with cancer, there should be a low threshold for more definitive investigations such as:

- *CT pulmonary angiography (CTPA)*: generally the current investigation of choice
- *V/Q scan*: not specific for pulmonary embolism; used less
- *pulmonary angiography*: the current gold standard but invasive
- *MRI pulmonary angiography*.[60]

Contrast-enhanced CTPA will detect almost all PE. Although the detection rate varies with technique, a negative CTPA is generally sufficient to exclude PE in patients with cancer and may identify the true alternative diagnosis.[61,62]

If a patient has a moderate–high probability of PE and no diagnosis is made on CTPA, further imaging should be considered, e.g. venous ultrasound, CT venography.[63,64] The use of contrast requires caution in patients with renal impairment and it is recommended that NSAIDs, dipyridamole or metformin are discontinued beforehand.[64]

A V/Q scan should be used only when the chest radiograph is normal and the patient has no significant cardiorespiratory disease. About 50% of patients with PE have high probability scans and no further investigations are generally necessary. However, up to 25% have low probability scans which can neither confirm nor exclude a PE, and other investigations are necessary.[61]

The use of CT or MRI pulmonary angiography together with CT or MRI leg venography are under investigation.[56]

For patients *in extremis* from a likely massive PE, bedside echocardiography and leg ultrasonography are recommended. Right ventricular enlargement/impaired function ± a positive ultrasound are indicative of PE. Further appropriate imaging can be undertaken once the patient stabilizes.[64]

Management
Prevention
Thromboprophylaxis is underused in patients with cancer.[65] It should be considered for at risk patients, which includes patients undergoing major surgery, hospitalized for any reason, or receiving thalidomide or lenolidamide together with chemotherapy or dexamethasone.[47]

Symptom relief
DVT
Bed rest is not recommended unless there is substantial pain and swelling.[56] An NSAID should be prescribed ± compression (TED stockings or Tubigrip®) ± elevation. Compression stockings ease the symptoms of venous hypertension; they also reduce the incidence of post-thrombotic syndrome.

PE
- oxygen
- SC/IV diamorphine/morphine
- anxiolytic, e.g. diazepam, midazolam.

Treatment of massive PE

Stop and think!
Are you justified in treating a potentially fatal complication in a moribund patient?

PE causing haemodynamic instability is termed massive. The resulting right ventricular failure can lead to compromised left ventricular preload, which may be fatal. Treatment of massive PE can include:[56]
- intensive support with vasopressors, oxygen and ventilation
- systemic or local (via catheter) thrombolytic therapy, e.g. tissue plasminogen activator
- catheter-based mechanical or surgical pulmonary embolectomy.

Anticoagulation
For more information, see PCF3.

Immediate treatment of DVT and PE generally comprises LMWH. In patients considered at high risk of thrombo-embolism, this should be initiated whilst awaiting imaging.

In otherwise medically fit patients, warfarin is often initiated on the same day, with LMWH continued for at least 5 days or until the INR has been in the therapeutic range (2–3) for at least 2 days. In patients with an identifiable transient risk factor, treatment duration is generally 3–6 months and there is a low risk of recurrence (<5%). About 20% of patients with no obvious risk factor will experience recurrence within 3 years; mainly due to an underlying thrombophilic disorder. Following a recurrence, life-long anticoagulation is generally recommended.

Patients with cancer are at risk of recurrent DVT/PE despite anticoagulation (about 20%) and on its cessation (up to 40%).[66] The risk of major bleeding with anticoagulation also increases in patients with metastases, immobility, renal impairment or a major bleed in the month preceding the VTE.[67] Evidence-based guidelines for patients with cancer are available,[47,68] and more specifically for those with advanced cancer from the Association for Palliative Medicine for Great Britain and Ireland (Table 7.4).[66]

Many patients find long-term LMWH acceptable, particularly if they have had previous difficulties with warfarin.[71] If patients experience recurrent VTE on the long-term decreased dose LMWH regimen, full dose LMWH can be given. The risk–benefit of

Table 7.4 Management of VTE in patients with advanced cancer[66]

Recommendation	Level of evidence[69]
Long-term LMWH is the drug of choice in the treatment of VTE in patients with cancer of any stage, performance status, or prognosis	Grade A, level Ib
Anticoagulation should be continued for at least 6 months after a first episode of VTE. However, because of the ongoing prothrombotic tendency in patients with incurable cancer, indefinite anticoagulation should be considered	Grade B, level Ib
Warfarin is not recommended for patients with extensive or metastatic disease, or poor performance status or prognosis	Grade B, level Ib
For patients considered to be at high risk of bleeding, e.g. those with extensive disease, cerebral metastases, or brain tumour, full dose LMWH for 7 days followed by a long-term decreased fixed dose should be considered, e.g. dalteparin 10,000units daily[a]	Grade B, level IIb
For patients with contra-indications to anticoagulation, an inferior vena caval filter should be considered	Grade C, level III

a. others recommend 75–80% of the initial dose.[68,70]

indefinite anticoagulation should be continually reviewed; it should be discontinued if there are bleeding complications, if the patient requests it, and generally on entering the last few days–weeks of life.

An anti-Xa level can be measured in patients who are morbidly obese (>150kg), small (<40kg) or with recurrent DVT/PE, to ensure a therapeutic level of anticoagulation.[56] However, there are limitations in the accuracy of anti-Xa monitoring.[72] Ultimately, the decision to initiate, continue, and stop anticoagulation treatment will need to be made on an individual basis, guided by the available evidence, the patient's circumstances, and their informed preferences.[66]

Thrombolytics are sometimes given in non-massive PE, e.g. in patients with:
- severe hypoxia
- massive embolic burden on imaging even without haemodynamic instability
- extensive ileofemoral venous thrombosis compromising blood supply to the leg.[56]

There are risks associated with the use of thrombolytics, particularly bleeding, and guidance should be sought.[73]

A beneficial anticancer effect of LMWH has been reported, but requires confirmation in RCTs.[74]

Non-drug treatment
IVC filters are used at some centres in cancer patients for whom anticoagulation is contra-indicated or ineffective.[75] Large scale trials are lacking, but small studies suggest that in carefully selected patients, IVC filter placement might be associated with fewer complications than anticoagulation or no intervention.[66] However, limb or

life-threatening thrombo-embolic complications can develop and there is no evidence of survival benefit.

Thrombosis in uncommon sites

Arm

Treat as for leg DVT but, if associated with a venous catheter, remove the catheter. Extensive thrombosis may require angiography-guided thrombolytic therapy.

Cerebral vein

Dehydrated patients are particularly at risk. Cerebral vein thrombosis presents with:

- non-specific symptoms or signs
- focal neurological signs ± altered level of consciousness
- symptoms and signs of raised intracranial pressure.

Because CT may remain normal despite the above clinical features, consider MRI to confirm the diagnosis.[76]

Visceral vein

The mesenteric vein is the third commonest site of thrombosis in hypercoagulable states in cancer after DVT and cerebral vein thrombosis. It presents with:

- severe abdominal pain
- extensive bowel infarction.

Priapism

This is caused by blockage of the venous drainage of the cavernosa and can occur as a result of direct tumour infiltration or DIC.

Non-bacterial endocarditis

This is characterized by cerebral embolic strokes and systemic embolization. It is most commonly associated with cancers of the lung, pancreas and prostate.[3]

Hepatic vein thrombosis (Budd-Chiari syndrome)

This manifests as a painful swollen liver and ascites and can lead to hepatic failure.

DISSEMINATED INTRAVASCULAR COAGULATION

Disseminated intravascular coagulation (DIC) is a consequence of the hypercoagulable state detectable in many cancer patients, particularly with adenocarcinoma and leukaemia. DIC results from inappropriate thrombin formation. Thrombin catalyses the activation and consumption of fibrinogen and other coagulant proteins, and the resulting fibrin thrombi consume platelets. Fibrinolysis is also activated and leads to depletion of fibrinogen. Massive haemorrhage may result. Clinical manifestations vary from asymptomatic to a fulminant haemorrhagic thrombotic state.

Causes

As well as being a paraneoplastic phenomenon, DIC occurs in other circumstances, e.g.:

- parturition
- intra-uterine death
- after surgery or trauma
- infection.

The common factor is an increased expression of tissue factor (TF) which forms a complex with coagulation factor VII, and triggers the extrinsic coagulation pathway (see Figure 7.1, p.245).

Clinical features
Acute DIC
Acute DIC is uncommon in cancer. The clinical features of acute DIC are a mixture of the manifestations of abnormal thrombosis and abnormal bleeding, and depend on the extent and site of thrombus formation and secondary thrombocytopenia.[77] In practice, it is generally the haemorrhagic features which alert the doctor to the possibility of DIC. Patients may present with organ failure and fulminant haemorrhage. In the skin, microvascular thrombosis of endarterioles and associated haemorrhage result in:
- petechiae
- purpura
- haematomas
- haemorrhagic bullae
- cyanosis of the extremities
- gangrene in areas of end circulation, i.e. digits, nose and ear lobes.

Areas of trauma tend to bleed because even small wounds cannot display normal haemostasis if there are profound deficiencies of coagulation factors and secondary concurrent activation of fibrinolytic pathways. The following are all common:
- oozing from venepuncture sites
- surgical wound bleeding
- haematuria in catheterized patients
- GI bleeding
- blood-stained secretions from endotracheal tubes.

Hypotension may also occur as a result of bradykinin release secondary to activation of the kallikrein-kinin system. This is seen in about 1/2 of patients with acute DIC. Poor tissue perfusion and acidosis prolongs the hypotension.

Chronic DIC
Although many patients with metastatic cancer have laboratory findings consistent with DIC, most remain asymptomatic. Clinical manifestations are usually thrombotic. However, a significant haemostatic stress such as surgery or an invasive procedure may result in abnormal bleeding. Thrombotic manifestations include:
- DVT
- PE
- migratory thrombophlebitis (Trousseau's syndrome), mostly in lung (adenocarcinoma), pancreas, stomach and colorectal cancers
- microvascular thrombi with micro-angiopathic haemolytic anaemia
- venous catheter thrombosis.

In DIC the most commonly clinically affected organs are:
- lungs
- kidneys
- CNS
- skin.

DIC can lead to adult respiratory distress syndrome, a common terminal event. At autopsy, microthrombi are found in most organs including the heart, pancreas, adrenals and testes.

Evaluation

Particularly in the early phase of DIC, coagulation tests may be normal or only mildly abnormal. Treatment may have to be based on clinical suspicion. Repeating coagulation tests after several hours may show significant changes. DIC is highly probable when the following features co-exist:

- thrombocytopenia, platelet count, $<150 \times 10^9$/L in 95% of cases
- decreased plasma fibrinogen concentration
- elevated plasma D-dimer concentration in 85% of cases (Figure 7.2)
- prolonged PT and/or APTT.[78]

A normal plasma fibrinogen concentration (200–250mg/100mL) is also suspicious because fibrinogen levels are usually raised in cancer (e.g. 450–500mg/100mL) unless there is extensive liver disease. Infection and cancer both may be associated with an increased platelet count which may also mask an evolving thrombocytopenia.

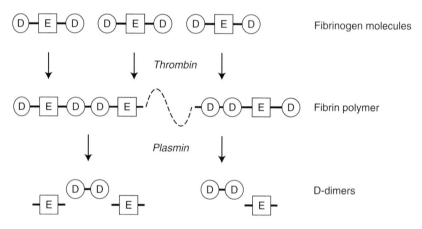

Figure 7.2 D-dimers are created by enzymatic degradation of 'cross-linked' fibrin polymers. D-dimer concentrations cannot be elevated unless fibrin polymers are being formed. D and E are the designated nomenclature for the main domains of the fibrinogen molecule.

Management

DIC results from a triggering mechanism activating the coagulation pathways. Treatment of the underlying disorder, e.g. infection, is curative but this is not possible if caused by advanced cancer.

Acute DIC

When haemorrhagic manifestations predominate, consider:
- IV fluids
- oxygen
- blood products:
  - ▷ fresh frozen plasma (to keep PT ratio <2)
  - ▷ cryoprecipitate (if fibrinogen <1g/L despite fresh frozen plasma)[79]
  - ▷ platelet transfusions (to keep count above 50×10^9/L)[14]
- the cautious use of heparin, to try to switch off consumptive process.[72]

Tranexamic acid, an antifibrinolytic, should not be used as it increases the risk of clot formation.

Chronic DIC

Chronic DIC most commonly presents as recurrent thrombosis in both superficial and deep venous systems. It does not always respond to warfarin.[80,81] Treatment is with LMWH indefinitely, e.g. dalteparin 200units/kg SC once daily up to a maximum of 18,000units. This is as effective as standard heparin and safer in patients with cancer.[82,83] It does not require routine monitoring and a long duration of action allows once daily administration.[84]

1 Ganz T (2003) Hepcidin, a key regulator of iron metabolism and mediator of anemia of inflammation. *Blood*. **102**: 783–788.

2 Miller C et al. (1990) Decreased erythropoietin response in patients with the anemia of cancer. *New England Journal of Medicine*. **322**: 1689–1692.

3 Warrell DA et al. (eds) (2004) Oxford Textbook of Medicine: Ch. 22.40.1. *Normochromic, Normocytic Anaemia* (5e). Oxford University Press, Oxford.

4 Gleeson C and Spencer D (1995) Blood transfusion and its benefits in palliative care. *Palliative Medicine*. **9**: 307–313.

5 Monti M et al. (1996) Use of red blood cell transfusions in terminally ill cancer patients admitted to a palliative care unit. *Journal of Pain and Symptom Management*. **12**: 18–22.

6 Bohlius J et al. (2006) Erythropoietin or darbepoetin for patients with cancer. *Cochrane Database of Systematic Reviews*. **3**: CD003407.

7 Steensma DP (2007) Erythropoiesis stimulating agents. *British Medical Journal*. **334**: 648–649.

8 Drug Safety Update (2007) Recombinant human erythropoietins: new prescribing advice. Medicines and Healthcare products Regulatory Agency and Commission on Human Medicines. Available from: http://www.mhra.gov.uk/Publications/Safetyguidance/DrugSafetyUpdate/CON2033216

9 Drug Safety Update (2008) Recombinant human erythropoietins: new recommendations for treatment of anaemia in cancer. Medicines and Healthcare products Regulatory Agency and Commission on Human Medicines. Available from: http://www.mhra.gov.uk/Publications/Safetyguidance/DrugSafetyUpdate/CON023078

10 EMEA (2007) Public statement. European Medicines Agency starts review of the safety of epoetins. European Agency for the Evaluation of Medicinal Products. Available from: www.emea.europa.eu/pdfs/human/press/pus/18806807en.pdf

11 FDA (2007) Medwatch 2007 safety alert: Aranesp (darbepoetin alfa). Food and Drug Administration. Available from: http://www.fda.gov/Safety/MedWatch/SafetyInformation/SafetyAlertsforHumanMedical Products/ucm150816.htm and http://www.fda.gov/Safety/MedWatch/SafetyInformation/SafetyAlertsfor HumanMedicalProducts/ucm150817.htm

12 FDA (2007) Information for healthcare professionals. Erythropoiesis stimulating agents. Food and Drug Administration. Available from: http://www.fda.gov/Drugs/DrugSafety/PublicHealthAdvisories/ucm054721.htm

13 Weigert A and Schafer A (1998) Uraemic bleeding: Pathogenesis and therapy. *The American Journal of the Medical Sciences*. **316**: 94–104.

14 British Committee for Standards in Haematology – Blood Transfusion Task Force (2003) Guidelines for the use of platelet transfusions. *British Journal of Haematology*. **122**: 10–23.

15 Warkentin TE and Greinacher A (2004) Heparin-induced thrombocytopenia: recognition, treatment, and prevention: the seventh ACCP Conference on Antithrombotic and Thrombolytic Therapy. *Chest*. **126 (suppl)**: 311s–337s.

16 Keeling D et al. (2006) The management of heparin-induced thrombocytopenia. (Guidelines of the Haemostasis and Thrombosis Task Force of the British Committee for Standards in Haematology). *British Journal of Haematology*. **133**: 259–269.

17 Keeling D et al. (2006) The management of heparin-induced thrombocytopenia. (Guidelines of the Haemostasis and Thrombosis Task Force of the British Committee for Standards in Haematology). *British Journal of Haematology*. **133**: 260.

18 Warkentin T et al. (1995) Heparin-induced thrombocytopenia in patients treated with low molecular weight heparin or unfractionated heparin. *New England Journal of Medicine*. **332**: 1330–1335.

19 Warkentin TE (2004) Ch. 22:39. Acquired coagulation disorders. In: DA Warrell et al. (eds) *Oxford Textbook of Medicine* (5e). Oxford University Press, Oxford.

20 Broadley K et al. (1995) The role of embolization in palliative care. *Palliative Medicine*. **9**: 331–335.

21 Rankin E *et al.* (1988) Transcatheter embolisation to control severe bleeding in fungating breast cancer. *European Journal of Surgical Oncology.* **14**: 27–32.

22 Regnard C and Makin W (1992) Management of bleeding in advanced cancer: a flow diagram. *Palliative Medicine.* **6**: 74–78.

23 Kochhar R *et al.* (1988) Rectal sucralfate in radiation proctitis. *Lancet.* **332**: 400.

24 deBoer W *et al.* (1991) Tranexamic acid treatment of haemothorax in two patients with malignant mesothelioma. *Chest.* **100**: 847–848.

25 McElligott E *et al.* (1991) Tranexamic acid and rectal bleeding. *Lancet.* **337**: 431.

26 Dean A and Tuffin P (1997) Fibrinolytic inhibitors for cancer-associated bleeding problems. *Journal of Pain and Symptom Management.* **13**: 20–24.

27 Mannucci P (1997) Desmopressin (DDAVP) in the treatment of bleeding disorders: the first 20 years. *Blood.* **90**: 2515–2521.

28 Wong GK *et al.* (2007) Treatment of profuse epistaxis in patients irradiated for nasopharyngeal carcinoma. *ANZ Journal of Surgery.* **77**: 270–274.

29 Lyons H (1976) Differential diagnosis of haemoptysis and its treatment. *Basics of RD.* **5**: 1.

30 Jones D and Davies R (1990) Massive haemoptysis. *British Medical Journal.* **300**: 889–890.

31 Paton W (1990) Massive haemoptysis. *British Medical Journal.* **300**: 1270.

32 Anwar D *et al.* (2005) Aerosolized vasopressin is a safe and effective treatment for mild to moderate recurrent hemoptysis in palliative care patients. *Journal of Pain and Symptom Management.* **29**: 427–429.

33 Mercadante S *et al.* (2000) Gastrointestinal bleeding in advanced cancer patients. *Journal of Pain and Symptom Management.* **19**: 160–162.

34 Imbesi JJ and Kurtz RC (2005) A multidisciplinary approach to gastrointestinal bleeding in cancer patients. *The Journal of Supportive Oncology.* **3**: 101–110.

35 Imperiale TF and Birgisson S (1997) Somatostatin or octreotide compared with H2 antagonists and placebo in the management of acute non-variceal upper gastrointestinal haemorrhage. *Annals of internal medicine.* **127**: 1062–1071.

36 Leontiadis GI *et al.* (2007) Proton pump inhibitor therapy for peptic ulcer bleeding: Cochrane collaboration meta-analysis of randomized controlled trials. *Mayo Clinic Proceedings.* **82**: 286–296.

37 Crew JP *et al.* (2001) Radiation-induced haemorrhagic cystitis. *European Urology.* **40**: 111–123.

38 West N (1997) Prevention and treatment of hemorrhagic cystitis. *Pharmacotherapy.* **17**: 696–706.

39 Denton AS *et al.* (2002) Non-surgical interventions for late radiation cystitis in patients who have received radical radiotherapy to the pelvis. *Cochrane Database of Systematic Reviews.* CD001773.

40 Lang E *et al.* (1979) Transcatheter embolization of hypogastric branch arteries in the management of intractable bladder haemorrhage. *Journal of Urology.* **121**: 30–36.

41 Appleton D *et al.* (1988) Internal iliac artery embolisation for the control of severe bladder and prostate haemorrhage. *British Journal of Urology.* **61**: 45–47.

42 Choong SK *et al.* (2000) The management of intractable haematuria. *BJU International.* **86**: 951–959.

43 Levine M and Hirsh J (1990) The diagnosis and treatment of thrombosis in the cancer patient. *Seminars in Oncology.* **17**: 160–171.

44 Piccioli A *et al.* (1996) Cancer and venous thromboembolism. *American Heart Journal.* **132**: 850–855.

45 Linkins LA (2008) Management of venous thromboembolism in patients with cancer: role of dalteparin. *Vascular Health and Risk Management.* **4**: 279–287.

46 Buller HR *et al.* (2007) Cancer and thrombosis: from molecular mechanisms to clinical presentations. *Journal of Thrombosis and Haemostasis.* **5 Suppl** 1: 246–254.

47 Lyman GH *et al.* (2007) American Society of Clinical Oncology guideline: recommendations for venous thromboembolism prophylaxis and treatment in patients with cancer. *Journal of Clinical Oncology.* **25**: 5490–5505.

48 Blann AD and Lip GY (2006) Venous thromboembolism. *British Medical Journal.* **332**: 215–219.

49 Samama MM *et al.* (1999) A comparison of enoxaparin with placebo for the prevention of venous thromboembolism in acutely ill medical patients. Prophylaxis in Medical Patients with Enoxaparin Study Group. *The New England Journal of Medicine.* **341**: 793–800.

50 Geerts WH *et al.* (2004) Prevention of venous thromboembolism: the seventh ACCP Conference on Antithrombotic and Thrombolytic Therapy. *Chest.* **126 (suppl)**: 338s–400s.

51 De Cicco M (2004) The prothrombotic state in cancer: pathogenic mechanisms. *Critical Reviews in Oncology/Hematology.* **50**: 187–196.

52 Deitcher SR and Gomes MP (2004) The risk of venous thromboembolic disease associated with adjuvant hormone therapy for breast carcinoma: a systematic review. *Cancer.* **101**: 439–449.

53 Leizorovicz A and Mismetti P (2004) Preventing venous thromboembolism in medical patients. *Circulation.* **110**: IV13–19.

54 Leizorovicz A *et al.* (2004) Randomized, placebo-controlled trial of dalteparin for the prevention of venous thromboembolism in acutely ill medical patients. *Circulation.* **110**: 874–879.

55 Chew HK et al. (2006) Incidence of venous thromboembolism and its effect on survival among patients with common cancers. Archives of Internal Medicine. 166: 458–464.

56 Tapson VF (2008) Acute pulmonary embolism. The New England Journal of Medicine. 358: 1037–1052.

57 Stein PD and Firth J (2004) Ch. 15:54. Venous thromboembolism. In: DA Warrell et al. (eds) Oxford Textbook of Medicine (5e). Oxford University Press, Oxford.

58 Keeling DM et al. (2004) The diagnosis of deep vein thrombosis in symptomatic outpatients and the potential for clinical assessment and D-dimer assays to reduce the need for diagnostic imaging. British Journal of Haematology. 124: 15–25.

59 Wells PS et al. (2003) Evaluation of D-dimer in the diagnosis of suspected deep-vein thrombosis. The New England Journal of Medicine. 349: 1227–1235.

60 Kadlecek S and Rizi RR (2005) New diagnostic tests for pulmonary emboli. Academic Radiology. 12: 133–135.

61 BTS (2003) British Thoracic Society guidelines for the management of suspected acute pulmonary embolism. Thorax. 58: 470–483.

62 Reid JH (2004) Multislice CT pulmonary angiography and CT venography. British Journal of Radiology. 77 Spec No 1: S39–45.

63 Qaseem A et al. (2007) Current diagnosis of venous thromboembolism in primary care: a clinical practice guideline from the American Academy of Family Physicians and the American College of Physicians. Annals of Family Medicine. 5: 57–62.

64 Stein PD et al. (2006) Diagnostic pathways in acute pulmonary embolism: recommendations of the PIOPED II investigators. The American Journal of Medicine. 119: 1048–1055.

65 Seddighzadeh A et al. (2007) Venous thromboembolism in patients with active cancer. Thrombosis and Haemostasis. 98: 656–661.

66 Noble SI et al. (2008) Management of venous thromboembolism in patients with advanced cancer: a systematic review and meta-analysis. The Lancet Oncology. 9: 577–584.

67 Trujillo-Santos J et al. (2008) Predicting recurrences or major bleeding in cancer patients with venous thromboembolism. Findings from the RIETE Registry. Thrombosis and Haemostasis. 100: 435–439.

68 Mandala M et al. (2008) Management of venous thromboembolism in cancer patients: ESMO clinical recommendations. Annals of Oncology. 19 Suppl 2: ii126–127.

69 Agency for Health Care Policy and Research (1992) Acute pain management, operative or medical procedures and trauma 92-0032. In: Clinical Practice Guidelines Quick Reference Guide for Clinicians. AHCPR Publications, Rockville, Maryland, USA, pp. 1–22.

70 Lee A et al. (2003) Low molecular weight heparin versus a coumarin for the prevention of recurrent venous thromboembolism in patients with cancer. New England Journal of Medicine. 349: 146–153.

71 Noble SI and Finlay IG (2005) Is long-term low-molecular-weight heparin acceptable to palliative care patients in the treatment of cancer related venous thromboembolism? A qualitative study. Palliative Medicine. 19: 197–201.

72 Baglin T et al. (2006) Guidelines on the use and monitoring of heparin. British Journal of Haematology. 133: 19–34.

73 Dong B et al. (2006) Thrombolytic therapy for pulmonary embolism. Cochrane Database of Systematic Reviews. CD004437.

74 Kuderer NM et al. (2007) A meta-analysis and systematic review of the efficacy and safety of anticoagulants as cancer treatment: impact on survival and bleeding complications. Cancer. 110: 1149–1161.

75 Ihnat D et al. (1998) Treatment of patients with venous thromboembolism and malignant disease: should vena cava filter placement be routine? Journal of Vascular Surgery. 28: 800–807.

76 Stam J et al. (2002) Anticoagulation for cerebral sinus thrombosis. Cochrane Database of Systematic Reviews. CD002005.

77 Colman R and Rubin R (1990) Disseminated intravascular coagulation due to malignancy. Seminars in Oncology. 17: 172–186.

78 Spero J et al. (1980) Disseminated intravascular coagulation: findings in 346 patients. Journal of Thrombosis and Haemostasis. 43: 28–33.

79 O'Shaughnessy DF et al. (2004) Guidelines for the use of fresh-frozen plasma, cryoprecipitate and cryosupernatant. British Journal of Haematology. 126: 11–28.

80 Naschitz J et al. (1993) Thromboembolism in cancer. Cancer. 71: 1384–1390.

81 Bona R et al. (1995) The efficacy and safety of oral anticoagulation in patients with cancer. Journal of Thrombosis and Haemostasis. 74: 1055–1058.

82 Pineo G (1997) Decreased mortality in cancer patients treated for deep vein thrombosis with low molecular weight heparin as compared with unfractionated heparin (Abstract). Journal of Thrombosis and Haemostasis. Supp: 384.

83 Anonymous (1998) Low molecular weight heparins for venous thromboembolism. Drug and Therapeutics Bulletin. 36: 25–29.

84 Boneu B (1994) Low molecular weight heparin therapy: is monitoring needed? Journal of Thrombosis and Haemostasis. 72: 330–334.

8: NEUROLOGICAL SYMPTOMS

WEAKNESS

Localized
Localized weakness may be caused by:
- brain tumour, e.g. monoparesis, hemiparesis
- spinal cord compression, generally bilateral (see p.264)
- peripheral nerve lesions, e.g.:
  ▷ brachial plexus lesion
  ▷ Pancoast's tumour
  ▷ axillary recurrence
  ▷ lumbosacral plexus lesion
  ▷ lateral popliteal nerve palsy
- proximal limb muscle weakness, e.g.
  ▷ corticosteroid myopathy (see p.258)
  ▷ paraneoplastic myopathy and/or neuropathy
  ▷ paraneoplastic dermatomyositis
  ▷ LEMS (see p.262).

Peripheral neuropathy secondary to diabetes mellitus or vitamin B_{12} deficiency is occasionally seen in advanced cancer. Correction of hyperglycaemia or vitamin deficiency prevents further deterioration but improvement takes time. Corrective measures are unnecessary in patients close to death.

Generalized
Generalized progressive weakness may mean that the patient is close to death. Other possibilities should be considered (Table 8.1).

Management
When weakness relates to an easily correctable cause, specific measures should be considered (Table 8.1). If it relates mainly to disease progression and is troubling the patient, consider a 1 week trial of corticosteroids, e.g. dexamethasone 4mg once daily or

Table 8.1 Causes of generalized weakness in advanced cancer

Causes	Treatment possibilities
Cancer	
Progression of disease	Modify pattern of life; physiotherapy and occupational therapy
Anaemia	Haematinics, blood transfusion, epoetin
Hypercalcaemia	Bisphosphonate
Hypo-adrenalism ⎫	
Neuropathy ⎬	Corticosteroid (but can also cause myopathy; see below)
Myopathy ⎭	
Treatment	
Surgery ⎫	
Chemotherapy ⎬	Supervised rehabilitation
Radiotherapy ⎭	
Hypokalaemia	Potassium supplements
Debility	
Insomnia	Identify underlying psychological and/or physical causes and take corrective measures; possibly prescribe a night sedative (see p.203)
Prolonged bed rest	Physiotherapy
Pain ⎫	
Breathlessness ⎭	Relieve symptom
Dehydration	Hydration
Malnutrition	Dietary advice
Concurrent disorders	
Depression	Psychotherapy; antidepressant
Infection	Antibacterial
Hypothyroidism	Thyroid replacement therapy

prednisolone 20–30mg once daily. There is about a 50% chance of benefit lasting several weeks, sometimes longer.[1] However, often the best course is to help the patient adjust their goals, i.e. living within the constraints debility imposes and not hankering after the increasingly impossible. IV hyperalimentation is not indicated for weakness in advanced cancer; it only occasionally leads to weight gain but weakness persists.[2]

CORTICOSTEROID MYOPATHY

The onset of corticosteroid myopathy generally occurs in the third month of treatment with dexamethasone >4mg once daily or prednisolone >40mg once daily.[3,4] It can occur earlier and with lower doses.[5] An appropriate level of suspicion is the main prerequisite for diagnosis (Box 8.A). For example, a patient may walk into the consulting room with no difficulty but subsequently have difficulty getting up from the sitting position. If the chronological sequence fits with corticosteroid myopathy, a presumptive diagnosis should be made and the following steps taken:

- explanation to patient and family
- discuss the need to compromise between maximizing therapeutic benefit and minimizing undesirable effects
- halve the corticosteroid dose (generally possible as a single step)
- consider changing from dexamethasone to prednisolone (non-fluorinated corticosteroids are said to cause less myopathy)
- attempt further reductions in dose at intervals of 1–2 weeks
- arrange for physiotherapy (disuse exacerbates myopathy)
- emphasize that weakness should improve after 3–4 weeks
- review after 2–3 weeks to ensure that there is no further deterioration.

Box 8.A   Corticosteroid myopathy[6]

Symptoms
Generally insidious onset
Diffuse myalgia may occur
Breathlessness from respiratory
   muscle myopathy
Difficulty with
   climbing stairs } early
   standing up
   arm elevation
   holding head up } late
   distal extremities

Signs
Weakness   } generally
Wasting   } symmetrical
Hypercortisolism
   moonface
   ankle oedema
   abdominal striae

Normal
Sensation
Reflexes
Enzymes (AST, CPK, aldolase)

Differential diagnosis
Hypokalaemia
Hypophosphataemia
Paraneoplastic neuropathy/myopathy
Lumbosacral plexopathy
Spinal cord compression

PARANEOPLASTIC NEUROLOGICAL DISORDERS

In paraneoplastic neurological disorders a particular form of cancer is associated with a non-metastatic effect on the nervous system more frequently than expected by chance (Box 8.B).[7]

Only a limited number of cancers cause these disorders. The commonest is SCLC, in which the incidence is about 3%.[7] In the UK, there are about 250 new cases per year, but in practice the diagnosis is not always made. Other cancers commonly implicated in paraneoplastic neurological disorders are:

- breast
- ovarian

- neuroblastoma
- thymoma
- lymphoma.

The relationship between a neurological disorder and the associated cancer is complex. A particular disorder can occur with several different cancers, and a particular cancer may well be associated with several different disorders, e.g. SCLC (Table 8.2). The onset of the neurological disorder may precede the diagnosis of cancer by up to 5 years.

Box 8.B   Paraneoplastic neurological disorders

Cerebellar degeneration
Trunk and limb ataxia
Vertigo
Nausea
Diplopia (sometimes)

Encephalomyelitis
Sensory neuropathy[8]
Ataxia
Paresis
Autonomic dysfunction
Memory loss ⎤
Personality change ⎟
Depression ⎬ limbic form
Hallucinations ⎟
Seizures ⎦
Deafness ⎤
Diplopia ⎟
Vertigo ⎬ brain stem
Dysarthria ⎟ form
Central respiratory ⎟
   failure ⎦

LEMS (see below)

Myasthenia gravis
Fatigue
Muscle weakness which
worsens with exercise
   ocular
   limb
   bulbar
   respiratory

Neuromyotonia
Myoclonus (see p.279)
Myokymia
Muscle hypertrophy
Cramps
Sweating
Mood change, occasional
Hallucinations, occasional

Opsoclonus-myoclonus
Oscillopsia (jiggling eye
   movements, nystagmus)
Vertigo
Ataxia
Limb myoclonus

**Inflammatory dorsal
root ganglionopathy**
Painful
Symmetric or asymmetric

Retinopathy[9]
Generally bilateral
Early night blindness
Blurred vision

Stiff person syndrome[9]
Paraspinal and abdominal muscle
   rigidity
Muscle spasms triggered by
   movement or emotional upset

Pathogenesis
The presence of auto-antibodies and the partial response to immunotherapies suggest that most paraneoplastic neurological disorders are auto-immune. Similarities between

Table 8.2 Paraneoplastic neurological disorders and the more common associations[7,10]

Disorder	Associated cancer
Cerebellar degeneration	Breast Ovary SCLC NSCLC Hodgkin's lymphoma Thymoma Neuroblastoma
Encephalomyelitis	Breast SCLC Prostate Thymoma Neuroblastoma
Brain stem encephalomyelitis	NSCLC
Limbic encephalomyelitis	SCLC NSCLC Testicular cancer Thymoma Ovarian/thoracic teratoma
LEMS	SCLC
Myasthenia gravis	Thymoma
Neuromyotonia	SCLC Thymoma
Opsoclonus-myoclonus	Breast SCLC Neuroblastoma
Sensory neuropathy/neuronopathy	SCLC
Retinopathy	SCLC Melanoma
Stiff person syndrome	SCLC Breast
Autonomic neuropathy	SCLC Prostate Neuroblastoma

tumour antigens and antigens expressed on normal neural tissue may play a role ('molecular mimicry'). Antibodies raised against tumour antigens leads to aberrant recognition of the normal antigens, and damage to normal neural tissue.[10]

So far about 16 antibodies have been well or partially characterized, e.g. Anti-Hu (ANNA-1, antineural nuclear antibody), Anti-Yo (PCA-1, Pürkinje cytoplasmic antibody), Anti-VGCC (anti-voltage-gated calcium channels).[7] Specific antibodies do not always correlate with specific disorders, and are not always detectable. Thus, their absence does *not* exclude the diagnosis.

Clinical features
Symptoms are determined by the underlying pathological condition (Table 8.2). They are typically subacute in onset. More than one disorder may be present in the same patient.[10]

Management
The humoral-mediated disorders may respond to:
- plasma exchange
- IV immunoglobulin
- immunosuppressive treatment with prednisolone or cyclophosphamide[11]
- treatment of the cancer associated with:
  ▷ LEMS (most commonly SCLC)
  ▷ paraneoplastic cerebellar degeneration if Hodgkin's disease
  ▷ limbic encephalitis if teratoma.

Immunosuppression and cancer treatment are less effective in cell-mediated immune attack. Tacrolimus is sometimes beneficial. A combined approach may be required as in some disorders both humoral and cell-mediated immunity are involved.

Symptomatic therapy may also be used, particularly if the patient is too ill to receive immunosuppressive or cytotoxic treatment:
- opsoclonus, e.g. clonazepam, propranolol
- myoclonus (see below)
- stiff person syndrome, e.g. diazepam, clonazepam, baclofen.

Prognosis
Disorders such as LEMS and myasthenia gravis generally respond well to treatment of the underlying cancer and immunosuppression. This is because the neuromuscular junction can recover function if the underlying cause is removed. Disorders involving the CNS may at best stabilize when the underlying cancer is treated. Some disorders, e.g. opsoclonus-myoclonus, may resolve spontaneously.[10]

LAMBERT-EATON MYASTHENIC SYNDROME (LEMS)

LEMS is a disorder of neuromuscular transmission which occurs in 3% of patients with SCLC and occasionally with other cancers, e.g. NSCLC, breast, and lymphoma.[12] It also occurs spontaneously without any underlying cancer. LEMS is distinct from the myopathy of cachexia (see p.79).

Pathogenesis
In LEMS there is a pre-synaptic deficit in neuromuscular transmission caused by a reduction in the amount of acetylcholine released on arrival of nerve impulses at the motor nerve terminal. Neurological paraneoplastic disorders in SCLC often occur concurrently.[12] Thus, LEMS may present with one or more of the following:
- sensory neuropathy/neuronopathy
- cerebellar degeneration

- limbic encephalopathy
- myelopathy
- visual failure.

LEMS is associated with auto-immunity. Antibodies against SCLC are sometimes cross-reactive against the voltage-gated calcium channel, which regulates release of acetylcholine from the pre-synaptic terminal of the neuromuscular junction. SCLC is thought to be derived from neural crest tissue, and this is thought to explain the cross-reactivity with other neural tissues and the association with other paraneoplastic neurological disorders.

Clinical features
The common symptoms are:
- proximal muscle weakness:
    ▹ always present in the legs (and the presenting symptom in over 50%)
    ▹ seen in the arms in about 25% of cases
    ▹ onset generally insidious but can be abrupt
    ▹ often worse after exercise
- diplopia (generally transient)
- dry mouth (75%)
- erectile impotence
- constipation.

Signs include:
- a rolling or waddling gait associated with truncal and proximal weakness
- transient augmentation of strength after a few seconds of muscle contraction (post-tetanic potentiation)
- diminished or absent tendon reflexes at rest but which re-appear or increase after sustained (10sec) muscle contraction; this is pathognomonic of a pre-synaptic neuromuscular transmission deficit
- cranial nerve involvement with dysarthria, dysphagia, ptosis, diplopia, strabismus (uncommon, in contrast to myasthenia gravis)
- absence of sensory symptoms or signs.

Evaluation
Because at least 50% of cases of LEMS are paraneoplastic, a search for an underlying cancer must be undertaken in affected patients even in the absence of respiratory symptoms, particularly in smokers.

The diagnosis of LEMS is confirmed by electrophysiological tests.[13] In 90% of patients there is a positive assay for antibodies against the voltage-gated calcium channel.[14]

Patients with LEMS generally feel stronger if given edrophonium 10mg IM/IV. Edrophonium is an anticholinesterase with a duration of action of about 5min. A negative result does not exclude the diagnosis, and a positive result is also seen in myasthenia gravis.

Management
Successful anticancer treatment is often accompanied by improvement of the neurological symptoms. Unlike other paraneoplastic neurological disorders, LEMS generally responds to:
- immunosuppression
- symptomatic treatment to enhance neuromuscular transmission.[15]

Immunosupression
- prednisolone 1.5mg/kg once daily on alternate days, up to a maximum of 100mg
- IV immunoglobulin 400mg/kg for 5 days; improvement is seen within 2 weeks and lasts for up to 6 weeks[16]
- plasma exchange.

It is possible that some cachectic patients who benefit from corticosteroids may have an immune-mediated paraneoplastic disorder.

Enhanced neuromuscular transmission
- 3,4-diaminopyridine (DAP) inhibits potassium flux out of neurones and thereby prolongs acetylcholine release which enhances neuromuscular transmission. DAP 10mg q.d.s. is prescribed in the UK on a named patient basis, increasing up to 20mg q.d.s.[12] Most patients experience dose-related paraesthesias in association with periods of increased strength. The effects of an anticholinesterase and DAP are additive
- possibly add an anticholinesterase, e.g. pyridostigmine ≤60mg q4h.

SPINAL CORD COMPRESSION

Spinal cord compression (SCC) is a medical emergency which requires:
- a 'prevent-the-preventable' approach, i.e. make the diagnosis and provide treatment *before* the compression is sufficient to impair nerve function; this requires a high index of clinical suspicion, particularly in high-risk patients such as:
  ▷ those with breast cancer and increasing thoracic spine pain
  ▷ those with previously treated spinal epidural metastases
- urgent treatment to prevent further deterioration (the outcome in those with paraparesis is better than the outcome in those with complete paraplegia).

Malignant SCC is defined as compression of the dural sac and its contents (spinal cord and/or cauda equina) by an extradural tumour mass.[17] The minimum radiological evidence of SCC is indentation of the theca at a level consistent with the clinical features.[18] If radiological features are present but there are no accompanying clinical features, the SCC is classed subclinical.

Up to 40% of all cancer patients develop spinal metastases,[19] and 10–20% of these progress to symptomatic SCC.[20,21] However, in a large cancer population-based study, SCC was diagnosed in only 3% of patients with advanced cancer.[22] It is more likely in cancers which produce bone metastases. Thus cancers of the breast, bronchus and prostate account for more than 1/2 of all cases of SCC.[22] Myeloma, non-Hodgkin's lymphoma and renal cancer account for about 1/4.[22]

SCC is sometimes the presenting manifestation of cancer, e.g.:
- primary of unknown origin
- non-Hodgkin's lymphoma
- myeloma
- lung cancer.[23]

Survival
Survival after SCC is generally short, and this should be taken into account when decisions are being made about management. For patients who do not recover

mobility after treatment, the median survival is 1–3 months; for those able to walk, 5–8 months.[24,25] Decompressive surgery extends survival by less than 1 month.[26]

On the other hand, some patients survive 1–2 years, notably those with lymphoma or myeloma.[27] Prognosis is worse:
- in patients with multiple bone and/or visceral metastases
- a short interval between diagnosis and SCC (≤15 months)
- a rapid onset of functional deficit (≤2 weeks).[28]

Pathogenesis
The cancer itself is the most likely cause of SCC:
- a vertebral metastasis ± vertebral collapse (85%)
- an extravertebral tumour extending through the intervertebral foramina into the epidural space, e.g. lymphoma (10%)
- an intramedullary tumour (originates from within the spinal cord), e.g. ependymoma
- an intradural tumour, i.e. arising from the meninges or nerve roots
- an epidural blood-borne metastasis (Figure 8.1).

Rarely, a non-cancer cause may need to be considered:
- cervical disc prolapse
- spinal abscess, e.g. from epidural catheter.

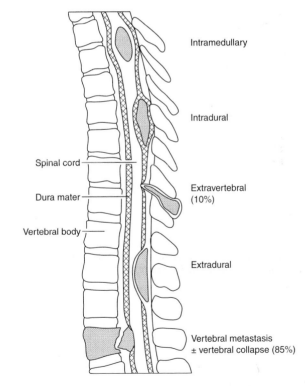

Figure 8.1 Mechanisms of spinal cord compression in cancer.

Compression leads sequentially to:
- venous stasis → venous hypertension
- white matter (axonal) vasogenic oedema
- decreased spinal cord blood flow → ischaemia → infarction.[23]

In vasogenic oedema, the number of macrophages increases as does the production of VEGF (vascular endothelial growth factor). This occurs in response to tissue hypoxia and is one possible mechanism of neural damage. The beneficial anti-inflammatory effects of dexamethasone may lead to a reduction in oedema and in the production of VEGF.

In the later stages of SCC, ischaemic-hypoxic neuronal damage and cytotoxic oedema predominates, which leads to the release of pre-synaptic glutamate and influx of Ca^{2+} through NMDA-receptor channels, with consequential neuronal injury and disintegration (excitotoxicity).[23]

Clinical features
The aim should be, if possible, to make the diagnosis and treat before the compression is sufficient to impair nerve function.

SCC is more common in the thoracic (60–80%) than the lumbosacral (15–30%) and cervical (<10%) spine. There is compression at more than one level in 30–50%.[23,29,30] If SCC is incomplete, there may only be unilateral neural signs.

Typically, there is a slow evolution of the clinical picture over weeks–months (caused by progressive compression by a slowly enlarging tumour), but occasionally the clinical features develop in just a few hours (caused by cord infarction as a result of spinal artery compression and thrombosis).

Increasing pain typically predates other symptoms and signs of SCC by several weeks or months. Pain may be caused by:
- vertebral metastasis
- root compression
- compression of the long tracts of the spinal cord (funicular pain).

Pain may be localized or referred, radicular or funicular, and related to position or movement. It may be worse after a period of lying down. Radicular and funicular pains are often exacerbated by neck flexion or straight leg raising, and by coughing, sneezing or straining. Funicular pain is generally less sharp than radicular pain, has a more diffuse distribution (like a cuff or garter around thighs, knees or calves) and is sometimes described as a cold unpleasant sensation.

Typical features include:
- pain >90%
- weakness >75% (2/3 of these are unable to walk)
- sensory level >50%
- bladder dysfunction >40%.

The spinal sensory level is generally 1–5 segments below the anatomical level of compression; radicular sensory loss or loss of a reflex are more reliable localizing signs.[23]

Examination
The neural signs of SCC are:
- in acute onset, flaccid paralysis/paraparesis
- progressing over time to spasticity (increased tone and hyperreflexia)

- plantar reflexes upgoing (but not if the cauda equina is involved)
- sensory loss with well-defined dermatomal level.

With compression of the cauda equina, there may only be asymmetrical 'saddle anaesthesia' around the anus and perineum, and reduced anal tone. When sensory loss is confined in this way to the sacrum or perineum, the patient may be unaware of it until examined.

Investigation

Unless the patient is too ill and close to death, urgent radiological investigations should be arranged to confirm the clinical diagnosis and identify the level(s) of compression:

- MRI of the whole spine to exclude multiple levels of SCC (found in about 1/3 of patients) is the investigation of choice
- CT if MRI is contra-indicated or not available.

If neither CT nor MRI is feasible, plain radiographs of the spine will show vertebral metastatic involvement and/or collapse at the anticipated level.

Management

SCC must be treated as an emergency; patients with paraparesis do better than those who are totally paraplegic.[17,30–32] Loss of bladder control is a bad prognostic sign.

Rapid onset of complete paraplegia (<48h) has a poor prognosis; it is almost always caused by infarction of the spinal cord secondary to tumour compression and thrombosis of a spinal artery.

The main therapeutic options are:

- corticosteroids (all)
- radiotherapy (most)
- surgery (carefully selected minority).

Corticosteroids

Corticosteroids inhibit inflammation, stabilize vascular membranes, and reduce spinal cord oedema. Thus, there is often a dramatic reduction in pain,[33] and an early improvement in the patient's physical status. Traditionally, dexamethasone has been used, with many centres giving the initial dose IV. However, given the high PO bio-availability of dexamethasone, this seems unnecessary. A typical PO regimen would be:

- a stat dose of 16mg PO
- continue with 16mg PO each morning for a further 3–4 days
- maintain on 8mg PO each morning until the completion of radiotherapy
- taper (and discontinue) over 2 weeks after the completion of radiotherapy.[20]

If there is neurological deterioration during the dose reduction, the dose should be increased again to the previous satisfactory dose, and maintained at that level for a further 2 weeks before attempting to taper the dose again. About 1/4 require maintenance dexamethasone in order to preserve neural function.

Very high initial doses of dexamethasone (96–100mg stat and once daily for 3 days, then tapering to zero over 2 weeks) are not justified. They provide little or no more benefit than 16mg,[34] but are associated with a definite risk of a major adverse event (>10%), particularly acute GI perforation (3%, at any level from the stomach to the sigmoid colon), GI haemorrhage, and sepsis, and possibly even death.[35–37]

Radiotherapy

Radiotherapy (together with corticosteroids) is widely used to treat SCC. Bony compression and spinal instability impact negatively on the outcome. Combined results from prospective non-randomized studies of radiotherapy for SCC revealed that ambulatory rates after radiotherapy in people without bony compression were >90% in those who were ambulatory before treatment, but only 63% in those who needed assistance before treatment. In those who were paraparetic and paraplegic before treatment, recovery of ambulation was <40% and 13% respectively.[17,38]

Reviews of non-randomized studies of a range of treatment schedules indicate that none is clearly superior.[17,39] Combined results from retrospective studies which suggested that longer courses of radiotherapy were associated with better local tumour control[28] have not been confirmed in a prospective, non-randomized evaluation of different radiation schedules. Thus, 40Gy in 20 fractions was not superior to 30Gy in 10 fractions.[40] Further, in patients with an estimated poor prognosis, an RCT which compared 'short course radiotherapy' (16Gy in 2 fractions 1 week apart) and 'split course radiotherapy' (30Gy in 8 fractions spread over 2 weeks) did not detect any significant differences between the two arms.[25] About 90% of patients maintained ambulation but <30% of paraparetic patients regained ambulation.

However, because of the risk of delayed onset post-radiation myelopathy, longer courses of radiotherapy should be considered for the small subset of patients with a better prognosis, e.g. patients with a haematological tumour, or with breast or prostate cancer without visceral metastases.

Surgery
Surgery can provide immediate relief of compression and mechanical stabilization of an unstable spine.[26] People who have recently lost the ability to walk are more than twice as likely to regain mobility with surgery compared with radiotherapy.[41]

However, it is important to remember that about 90% of those who are able to walk before radiotherapy (and corticosteroids) are still able to walk after irradiation.[17,41] Further, the longer survival reported after surgery amounts to <1 month.[26] The real extra benefit of surgical decompression would seem to be for the *non-ambulant* patient with a single site of cord compression and a prognosis of >3 months.

The following are other possible indications for surgery:
• unstable spine, this is a radiological diagnosis based on dividing the spine into three columns; involvement of only one column = stable, but involvement of ≥2 columns = unstable by definition, regardless of the extent of the neural impairment:
  ▷ *anterior column*: anterior longitudinal ligament, anterior half of the vertebral body and anterior portion of the annulus fibrosus
  ▷ *middle column*: posterior longitudinal ligament, posterior half of the vertebral body and posterior aspect of the annulus fibrosus
  ▷ *posterior column*: neural arch, ligamentum flavum, facet capsules and interspinous ligaments
• compression from intraspinal bony fragments or a collapsed vertebra (will not be corrected by radiotherapy)
• maximum radiotherapy already received
• neural symptoms and signs progress despite radiotherapy and dexamethasone
• the diagnosis is in doubt.[23]

Most cases of SCC require an anterior surgical approach, and the insertion of mechanical supports. A laminectomy (posterior decompression) should be avoided in these patients; it may simply create an unstable spine, and exacerbate the cord injury.[42]

Bladder management

Bladder dysfunction depends on the site and extent of damage to the sensory and motor tracts of the spinal cord, and may manifest as urinary retention, incontinence, and/or large post-voiding residual volumes (Box 8.C). Generally, patients presenting with paraplegia should be catheterized if unable to void by tapping or pressing on the lower abdomen or if the residual urine after voiding is ≥100mL.

Box 8.C Bladder function in paraplegia

Lesion above T12–L1

The cauda equina is intact, and the patient will have an upper motor neurone bladder (*suprasacral/reflex bladder*). The bladder reflexes are still intact, and when the bladder is full it may empty automatically. Since the nerves above the sacral section of the spinal cord are no longer connected to the brain, the patient will not have any awareness of the full bladder and will not have voluntary control.

The reflex can be triggered by tapping the lower abdomen, but may also be triggered by involuntary spasms or movement.

Lesion below T12–L1

The cauda equina (i.e. sacral nerves rather than spinal cord) is damaged; all reflexes are destroyed and the bladder has reduced muscle tone (*flaccid/floppy/areflexic bladder*). When the bladder is full, dribbling incontinence will occur.

In patients with a poor prognosis, continue to use an indwelling catheter. Silastic catheters generally need to be changed only every 3 months. In contrast, latex (Foley®) catheters need to be changed every 2–3 weeks. In men, the catheter tubing should be strapped onto the lower abdominal wall; in women, onto the inner thigh.

Normal bladder function may return in patients who respond well to dexamethasone and radiotherapy (or surgery). In patients with a suprasacral/reflex bladder and a good prognosis (≥6 months), consideration can be given to intermittent urinary catheterization q6h–q4h. Prerequisites include the ability to sit up, manual dexterity, cognitive awareness and sufficient bladder capacity. If dribbling occurs between catheterizations, in patients with a suprasacral lesion an antimuscarinic may be helpful, e.g. propantheline, oxybutynin, tolterodine.

Autonomic dysreflexia

Autonomic dysreflexia is a life-threatening complication of paraplegia above spinal cord level T7 (Box 8.D). It is most commonly caused by a distended bladder (but sometimes by another nociceptive stimulus *below* the level of the lesion) causing sympathetic autonomic overactivity resulting in vasoconstriction and hypertension. This stimulates parasympathetic overactivity *above* the lesion via the carotid and aortic baroceptors resulting in vasodilation and bradycardia. Thus, the patient may appear flushed above the level of the lesion and pale below, although this is not always obvious.

As a general rule, headache in someone with paraplegia/tetraplegia should lead to action: check the urinary catheter and, if draining satisfactorily, examine the anus (anal fissure?) and rectum (faecal impaction?).

Box 8.D Autonomic dysreflexia[43]

Typical features

Sudden uncontrolled rise in blood pressure:

- systolic pressures reaching up to 250–300mmHg, but 180–200mmHg is more typical
- diastolic pressures reaching up to 200–220mmHg, but 100–150mmHg is more typical.

Other features of autonomic imbalance vary, but may include:

- pounding headache
- sweating or shivering
- feelings of anxiety
- chest tightness
- blurred vision
- nasal congestion
- blotchy skin rash or flushed above the level of the spinal injury (due to parasympathetic activity)
- cold with goose pimples below the level of injury (due to the sympathetic activity).

Management

Confirm diagnosis (blood pressure >200/100 or 20–40mmHg higher than normal). Provided the spine is stable (see p.268), sit the patient up; avoid lying down.

For patients with catheter:

- check that the tubing is not blocked or kinked
- if blocked, remove the catheter, and re-catheterize using a lidocaine lubricant.

For patients without catheter:

- if bladder distended and patient unable to pass urine, insert catheter using a lidocaine lubricant.

If bladder distension excluded, gently examine the anus and rectum using a gloved finger lubricated with lidocaine jelly; remove any faeces.
If symptoms persist, give sublingual:

- nifedipine 5–10mg (empty out the contents of 1–2 capsules) *or*
- glyceryl trinitrate 300–600microgram (tablets) *or* 400microgram (spray).

If symptoms persist, repeat after 20min.
If blood pressure remains high, consider an IV hypotensive drug:

- hydralazine 20mg *or*
- diazoxide 20mg.

Continue to search for cause and monitor blood pressure.
Contact a Spinal Cord Injury Centre for further advice.
May require management on a high-dependency unit if the problem persists.

Bowel management

Guidelines: Bowel management in paraplegia and tetraplegia, p.272.

Management is governed to a certain extent by the level of the spinal cord lesion:[44]

- *above T12–L1*: cauda equina intact → spastic bowel with preserved sacral reflex; generally responds to digital stimulation of the rectum; the presence of an anal reflex suggests an intact sacral reflex

---

- *below T12–L1*: cauda equina involved → flaccid bowel; generally requires digital evacuation of the rectum
- a lesion at the level of the conus medullaris (the cone shaped distal end of the spinal cord, surrounded by the sacral nerves) may manifest a mixture of clinical features.

Determine the anal tone by:
- visual inspection
- stimulation of the anus with a pin.

Puckering around the anus and reflex contraction in response to pin prick indicate the presence of anal tone. However, some patients with a flaccid bowel will respond to the spastic bowel measures; and, similarly, some patients with a spastic bowel will need regular supplementary digital evacuation.

Rehabilitation

The functional outcome 1 month after treatment relates to:
- functional status at time of diagnosis; those still able to walk do best
- primary diagnosis:
  ▷ most radiosensitive do better, e.g. lymphoma, myeloma, breast, prostate, SCLC
  ▷ least radiosensitive do worse, e.g. lung cancer, melanoma
- speed of onset; there is little or no chance of improvement when paraplegia develops in ≤48h.[23,27,28]

Rehabilitation is an essential component of the care of patients with SCC. Patients will need help in adjusting to any degree of disability. There should be early referral to physiotherapy and occupational therapy. It is generally appropriate to involve specialist palliative care services. Advice for patients and families can be downloaded from the website of the Spinal Injuries Association.[45]

Patients see SCC as an indication of advancing cancer. Their concerns regarding disability are often secondary to those relating to the emotional and practical consequences of a life-threatening illness. During radiotherapy, there is generally hope that mobility will improve, and thus at this stage some will find it difficult to plan for permament paraplegia.[46]

As far as possible, problems should be pre-empted. This requires a multiprofessional team skilled in dealing with SCC. It is important to liaise with the appropriate community services before discharge because the full implications of the disability may be recognized by the patient only when they go home.[46]

After 1 month, 2/3 of those patients who were walking unaided at diagnosis are at home, compared with 1/3 of those who were unable to walk. Back ± nerve root pain remains an ongoing problem in 1/2 of patients.[27]

Recurrence

The risk of developing SCC at a new site or of a recurrence at the same site increases with survival:
- after 6 months, 10–20%
- after 2 years, 50%
- after 3 years, almost 100%.[23]

As already pointed out, few patients with SCC survive >1 year. However, in those who do, radiotherapy can often be repeated, with functional improvement in 40%.[28]

Guidelines: Bowel management in paraplegia and tetraplegia

Theoretically, management is determined by the level of the spinal cord lesion:
- above T12–L1 = cauda equina intact → spastic bowel with preserved sacral reflex; generally responds to digital stimulation of the rectum; the presence of an anal reflex suggests an intact sacral reflex
- below T12–L1 = cauda equina involved → flaccid bowel; generally requires digital evacuation of the rectum
- a lesion at the level of the conus medullaris (the cone shaped distal end of the spinal cord, surrounded by the sacral nerves) may manifest a mixture of clinical features.

However, in practice, management tends to follow a common pathway.

Aims

1 Primary: to achieve the controlled regular evacuation of normal formed faeces:
- every day in long-term paraplegia/tetraplegia, e.g. post-traumatic
- every 1–3 days in advanced cancer.

2 Secondary: to prevent both incontinence (faeces too soft, over-treatment with laxatives) and an anal fissure (faeces too hard, under-treatment with laxatives).

Oral laxatives

3 In debilitated patients with a poor appetite, a bulking agent is unlikely to be helpful, and may result in a soft impaction.

4 Particularly if taking morphine or another constipating drug, an oral contact (stimulant) laxative should be prescribed, e.g. senna 15mg b.d., bisacodyl tablets 5–10mg b.d. The dose should be carefully titrated to a level which results in normal faeces *in the rectum* but without causing an uncontrolled evacuation.

5 In relatively well patients with a good appetite (probably the minority):
- maintain a high fluid intake
- encourage a high roughage diet, e.g. wholegrain cereals, wholemeal foods, greens, bran or a bulk-forming laxative, e.g. ispaghula (psyllium) husk.

6 Beware:
- the prescription of docusate sodium, a faecal softener, may result in a soft faecal impaction of the rectum, and faecal leakage through a patulous anus
- oral bisacodyl in someone not on opioids may cause multiple uncontrolled evacuations, at the wrong time and in the wrong place.

Rectal measures

7 Initially, if impacted with faeces, empty the rectum digitally. Then, develop a daily routine:
- as soon as convenient after waking up in the morning, insert 2 glycerol suppositories, or 1–2 bisacodyl suppositories (10–20mg), or a micro-enema deep into the rectum, and wait for 1.5–2 hours
- because the bisacodyl acts only after absorption and biotransformation, bisacodyl suppositories must be placed against the rectal wall, and not into faeces

continued

- the patient should be encouraged to have a hot drink after about 1 hour in the hope that it will stimulate a gastrocolonic reflex
- if there is a strong sacral reflex, some faeces will be expelled as a result of the above two measures
- to ensure complete evacuation of the rectum and sigmoid colon, digitally stimulate the rectum:
  ▷ insert gloved and lubricated finger (either soap or gel)
  ▷ rotate finger 3–4 times
  ▷ withdraw and wait 5 minutes
  ▷ if necessary, repeat 3–4 times
  ▷ check digitally that rectum is fully empty.

8 Patients who are unable to transfer to the toilet or a commode will need nursing assistance. Sometimes it is easiest for a patient to defaecate onto a pad while in bed in a lateral position.

9 If the above measures do not achieve complete evacuation of the rectum and sigmoid colon, proceed to digital evacuation (more likely with a flaccid bowel). A pattern will emerge for each patient, allowing the rectal measures to be adjusted to the individual patient's needs and response.

CRAMP

Cramp is a painful involuntary muscle spasm lasting from a few seconds to many hours or days. However, some authorities refer to pain lasting >10min as painful muscle stiffness.[47]

Cramp is a universal experience. It occurs most commonly in a single muscle in the calf or foot. Cramp originates from spontaneous discharges of the motor nerves rather than from within the muscle itself.[48] Clinical features include:

- rapid onset of acute pain with a variable rate of improvement
- visible, palpable contraction generally in one muscle or part of a muscle
- triggered by trivial movements or forceful contractions
- eased by stretching the muscle
- residual soreness and swelling which may last several days
- an elevated serum creatinine kinase.[48]

Careful evaluation will help to:

- distinguish true cramp from local or generalized muscle pain, and non-painful muscle spasm
- identify sensory loss (suggests a polyneuropathy)
- identify the presence or absence of weakness, muscle wasting, fasciculation (suggests a lower motor neurone disorder), hyperreflexia and spasticity (suggests an upper motor neurone disorder).

Investigations will depend on the cause(s) considered likely.

Causes

There are many causes of cramp (Box 8.E). In patients with cancer, cramp may occur in muscles close to a painful bone metastasis, particularly when movement precipitates or exacerbates the pain.

Box 8.E   Causes of cramp[48]

Idiopathic
Exercise
Old age (nocturnal leg cramps)

Acute extracellular volume depletion
Diuretics
Excessive sweating ('heat cramps')
  generally with exertion
Haemodialysis
GI fluid loss (diarrhoea, vomiting)

Drugs (see Box 8F)

Endocrine
Hypo-adrenalism
Hypothyroidism
Pregnancy

Lower motor neurone disorders
MND/ALS
Neuropathy
Post-poliomyelitis
Radiculopathy

Metabolic
Cirrhosis
Hypomagnesaemia
Renal impairment

Miscellaneous
Auto-immune disease
  (antibodies to voltage-gated
  potassium channels)
Hereditary disorders

In 41/50 cancer patients with severe cramp referred to a neurology clinic it was possible to identify an underlying pathological condition.[49] Causes included:
- meningeal metastases
- nerve compression
- peripheral neuropathy
- polymyositis
- spinal degeneration.

In some patients, the peripheral neuropathy was secondary to diabetes mellitus. Cramp occurred in:
- legs only (40%)
- arms and legs (40%)
- arms only (about 10%)
- arms, legs and trunk (10%).

Most patients suffered frequent attacks, generally of brief duration (seconds → minutes). In patients with advanced cancer, cramp in the arm(s) in particular should alert the doctor to the possibility of an underlying neurological cause.

Cramp may be caused by drugs (Box 8.F). In the case of diuretics, cramp is triggered by volume depletion ± electrolyte imbalance, i.e. loss of Na^+ and Mg^{2+}. Cramp associated with cisplatin possibly relates to the combined impact of hypomagnesaemia and peripheral neuropathy. In many cases, the mechanism is not clear.

Management
Correct the correctable
When possible, treatment should be directed to the underlying cause, e.g. replacement of lost fluid and electrolytes such as Na^+ and Mg^{2+}. If feasible, causal drugs should be reduced in dose or stopped at least temporarily.

Box 8.F   Drug-induced cramps[48–51]

ACE inhibitors	Chemotherapy
enalapril	vincristine
ramipril	cisplatin
Amitriptyline	Cimetidine
Amphotericin B	Clofibrate
β_2-Agonists	Diuretics
salbutamol	Lithium
terbutaline	Statins
Bisphosphonates	Steroids
disodium pamidronate	beclometasone (by inhaler)
zoledronic acid	medroxyprogesterone acetate
Celecoxib	prednisolone

Non-drug treatment

Cramp cannot be induced or sustained in a stretched muscle.[52] Stretching movements (both active and passive) are an important non-drug measure. Exercise and/or stretching exercises three times a day, particularly before going to bed, often reduce the frequency and severity of nocturnal calf and foot cramps.[48] In debilitated patients, this is best done by a physiotherapist, nurse or relative.

Forced dorsiflexion of the foot for 5–10sec repeated for up to 5min stretches both calf and foot muscles. It is an uncomfortable procedure but the nocturnal benefit may outweigh the short-term discomfort in some but not all patients.[53,54]

Some patients may be fit enough to stretch their own muscles by leaning with both hands against a wall and with one leg bent to provide stability and the other stretched back with the dorsiflexed foot firmly on the floor. Stretching is aided by 'rocking' on the dorsiflexed foot. After stretching the muscles of one leg, the positions of the two legs are reversed and the procedure repeated.

Massage and relaxation therapy are particularly important for cramp associated with myofascial trigger points (see Figure 2.4, p.19).

Drug treatment

For more information, see PCF3.

Local

Trigger points are often made less sensitive by injection with a local anaesthetic, e.g. lidocaine 1% or bupivacaine 0.5%. If the trigger point is secondary to muscle trauma, injection of a depot preparation of a corticosteroid (methylprednisolone or triamcinolone) may help to disrupt the trigger.

IM injections of botulinum toxin have been reported of benefit in the inherited benign cramp-fasciculation syndrome.[55]

Systemic

In patients with advanced disease and recurrent or persistent cramp, diazepam 5mg at bedtime is probably the drug of choice. Alternatively, baclofen (see Table 8.4, p.278) can be tried. Both drugs work via a central inhibitory GABA mechanism, reducing muscle tone. In anxious patients, diazepam is of double benefit; it relaxes both muscles and mind.

Other drug options are summarized in Table 8.3, including certain drugs which have been used in specific circumstances. For example, in MND/ALS for mild fasciculations and cramp, magnesium and vitamin E are used; if severe, quinine or an anti-epileptic should be considered.[56]

Table 8.3 Alternative drugs for treating cramp

Class	Drug	Dose	Comment
Muscle relaxant	Quinine	200–300mg at bedtime	FDA advises against use for cramps because of risk of cardiac arrhythmias; MND/ALS if severe[56]
	Dantrolene	Start with 25mg once daily See Table 8.4, p.278	Of limited value because of need for slow dose titration
Anti-epileptic	Gabapentin	300mg at bedtime[57]	
	Carbamazepine	100–200mg at bedtime[48]	MND/ALS if severe[56]
	Phenytoin	100–200mg once daily[48]	
Miscellaneous	Magnesium	5mmol t.d.s.	Third trimester of pregnancy,[58] MND/ALS[56]
	Verapamil	120mg at bedtime	Nocturnal cramps in the elderly[59]
	Vitamin E	200mg t.d.s–400mg b.d.	Cirrhosis, haemodialysis,[60,61] MND/ALS[56]

SPASTICITY

Spasticity is a condition in which there is increased resistance to stretch of the passive skeletal muscles with exaggerated tendon reflexes.[62] This causes stiffness or tightness of the muscles and can interfere with gait, movement and speech.

Causes

Spasticity is generally caused by damage to the spinal cord or to the area of the brain which controls voluntary movement. Causes include:
- spinal cord injury
- multiple sclerosis
- MND/ALS
- brain injury, e.g. ischaemic stroke, anoxic brain damage, cerebral palsy.

Clinical features

Clinical features include:
- hypertonicity (increased muscle tone)
- clonus (a series of rapid contractions provoked by forcibly stretching the affected muscle)
- exaggerated deep tendon reflexes
- muscle spasms
- scissoring (involuntary crossing of the legs)
- fixed joints.

The degree of spasticity varies from mild muscle stiffness to severe painful uncontrollable muscle spasms which greatly interfere with daily activities.

Management

Non-drug treatment

As with cramp, physiotherapy is important in the management of spasticity. Exacerbating conditions such as infection or pain should be treated. In patients with chronic disease, surgery is sometimes of benefit, e.g. muscle and tendon lengthening, release of contractures, tendon transfers.[63,64]

Drug treatment

For more information, see PCF3.

The drug treatment of spasticity is similar to that for cramp.[65] However, quinine sulphate is of no value. Baclofen, diazepam, dantrolene and tizanidine are all currently approved for use in patients with spasticity (Table 8.4). There is no clear evidence that any one drug is superior to any other.[66,67] If there are no concurrent indications for a benzodiazepine, baclofen should generally be prescribed as the first-line drug, particularly if long-term treatment is likely. Gabapentin at doses of up to 900mg t.d.s. is also an effective treatment, although it has only been studied in the short-term.[68,69]

All skeletal muscle relaxants may reduce voluntary muscle power. Further, spastic muscle tone may enable some hemiplegics or paraplegics to walk or function more independently. Dose escalation to the maximum recommended dose should thus be carried out over 4–8 weeks to balance the benefits of reduced spasticity with possible loss of functional performance. These concerns do not apply to patients unable to use their limbs because of severe spasticity or paralysis. For these patients, sedation may limit the use of muscle relaxants.[70]

More invasive treatments include IT phenol. This is neurotoxic and can cause urinary and faecal incontinence. The use of indwelling devices to deliver IT baclofen has largely replaced the use of IT phenol.[65,69]

Botulinum toxin (BTX) injections are largely reserved for treatment of contractures. The BTX-type A light chain acts as a zinc endopeptidase and interferes with acetylcholine release.[71] The toxin is injected into each spastic muscle separately and reduces spasticity in a dose-dependent manner. Its use is rarely relevant in palliative care.

Table 8.4 Oral drugs used to treat spasticity

Agent	Starting dose	Maximum dose	Undesirable effects	Monitoring	Precautions
Baclofen	5mg once daily—t.d.s.	20mg q.d s.	Weakness, sedation, fatigue, dizziness, nausea, hepatotoxicity	Periodic LFTs	Abrupt cessation may result in rebound anxiety and psychosis; seizures may also occur
Dantrolene	25mg once daily	100mg q.d.s.	Weakness, sedation, diarrhoea, hepatotoxicity	Periodic LFTs	
Diazepam	5mg at bedtime	60mg/24h	Weakness, sedation, cognitive impairment, depression	Accumulation, prolongation of plasma halflife with cimetidine	Abrupt cessation may result in rebound anxiety and insomnia
Tizanidine[a]	2–4mg at bedtime	12mg t.d.s.	Drowsiness, dry mouth, dizziness, hepatotoxicity	Periodic LFTs	Do not use with antihypertensives or clonidine

a. tizanidine is relatively expensive, and generally regarded as a second- or third-line drug.

MYOCLONUS

Myoclonus is sudden, brief, irregularly repetitive shock-like involuntary muscular movements. Myoclonus is caused by either primary muscle activity or secondary to CNS stimulation. Myoclonus may be:
- focal (a single muscle or group of muscles), regional or multifocal (generalized)
- unilateral or bilateral (either asymmetrical or symmetrical)
- mild (twitching) or severe (jerking).

Secondary multifocal myoclonus is a central pre-epileptiform phenomenon and should not be ignored. It occurs mainly in moribund patients.

Causes
Myoclonus may be:
- physiological, e.g. associated with sleep or a startle reaction
- primary (essential)
- secondary to:
  ▷ neurological disorders, e.g. encephalopathies, epilepsy, intoxication
  ▷ biochemical disorders, e.g. hypoglycaemia, renal impairment
  ▷ drug toxicity, e.g. antimuscarinics, gabapentin, opioids (see Table 2.5, p.40).[72,73]

Management
If of recent onset, review medication and, if possible, reduce or stop causal drugs. If caused by an opioid, switching to an alternative opioid may be indicated (see p.39); likewise when treating neuropathic pain, switching from gabapentin to valproate. Symptomatic drug treatment comprises:
- clonazepam 0.5mg once daily increasing every 3 days to 1–2mg once daily as tolerated
- valproate 300mg once daily increasing by 300mg every 3 days as tolerated to a maximum of 600mg–3g.[74]

In moribund patients, consider:
- diazepam 5mg PR stat and 5–10mg PR at bedtime *or*
- midazolam 5mg buccal/SC p.r.n, and 10mg/24h by CSCI. Adjust the dose upwards if several p.r.n. doses are needed.

GENERALIZED CONVULSIVE SEIZURES

Epilepsy is defined as two or more seizures which are not provoked by other illnesses or circumstances.[75] Epileptic seizures may be classified as primary generalized seizures, or partial seizures which evolve to secondary generalized seizures.[76]

Seizures are relatively common in advanced cancer, and possibly in up to 25% of patients with brain metastases.[77] Seizures caused by structural brain lesions are initially partial, although these are often unrecognized.

Causes

Seizures in advanced cancer can either be provoked (Box 8.G) or relate to long-standing epilepsy. Common provoked causes include:
- previous stroke
- brain tumour, primary or secondary
- biochemial disturbance, e.g. renal impairment, severe hyponatraemia, alcohol intoxication.

Box 8.G Causes of provoked seizures

Cancer
Primary brain tumour
Brain metastases

Drugs
TCAs
Thiazide diuretics
Antipsychotics
Theophylline
Levodopa
Withdrawal of
  anti-epileptics
  benzodiazepines

Infective
Septicaemia
Meningitis
Encephalitis
Brain abscess
Tuberculosis
HIV
Malaria
Creutzfeld-Jacob disease

Cardiac
Arrhythmias   } cause
Severe aortic stenosis } hypoxia

Substance abuse
Alcohol withdrawal
Amphetamines
Cocaine

Metabolic
Hypoglycaemia
Hypo/hypernatraemia
Hypo/hypercalcaemia
Uraemia

Neurological
Stroke
Neurodegenerative diseases
  Alzheimer's
  multi-infarct dementia
Multiple sclerosis
Head trauma

Herbal remedies
Ginkgo bilboa

Other
Porphyria
Systemic lupus erythematosus
Sarcoid

Evaluation

Diagnosis is based largely on history from the patient, family and/or friends, and any eye-witnesses. There are two questions to answer:
- did the patient have a seizure?
- was the seizure provoked or does the patient have epilepsy?

Epilepsy is more likely if:
- there are precipitating factors (e.g. television, sleep deprivation), prodrome/aura, unilateral symptoms (more likely in partial seizures)

- *during the seizure*:
  - ▷ tongue biting, particularly at edge of tongue
  - ▷ faecal incontinence (urinary incontinence is less specific)
  - ▷ paroxysmal stereotypic movements, e.g. the body becomes rigid (tonic phase) possibly followed by regular muscle jerking (clonic phase)
  - ▷ apnoeic episodes with cyanosis
- *after the seizure*:
  - ▷ sleepiness
  - ▷ confusion
  - ▷ amnesia
  - ▷ muscle aches.

The main differential diagnoses of generalized seizures are syncope and psychogenic seizures. Syncope may be preceded by 'wooziness' but no aura or unilateral symptoms. Loss of consciousness is much briefer (<20sec), and the patient rapidly returns to normal. Muscle jerks may occur secondary to hypoxia.[75]

In psychogenic seizures, the patient may have a psychiatric history. The patient may be motionless and have fluttering eye movements with forceful eye closure. Unusual or erratic movements may be seen, e.g. pelvic thrusting, out-of-phase limb thrashing. Breathing is more likely to be continuous and cyanosis is not seen. Incontinence and tongue biting are uncommon. It is often refractory to treatment.[75]

In relatively fit patients, the cause of the seizure(s) should generally be investigated:
- FBC
- urea, creatinine, electrolytes, LFTs, calcium, magnesium, glucose
- ECG and chest radiograph
- CT/MRI
- consider lumbar puncture
- EEG.

Management
Epilepsy
If epilepsy is diagnosed, seek the advice of a neurologist about the most appropriate oral anti-epileptic. Combination treatment should be avoided until at least two trials with a single drug have been ineffective.[76,78] With combination treatment:
- there is an increased likelihood of drug interactions
- toxicity may be enhanced.

Monitoring of the plasma drug concentration should be carried out in accordance with standard guidelines.

Provoked seizures
An anti-epileptic may be required to suppress provoked seizures. In palliative care, an anti-epileptic is often commenced after a first seizure (rather than waiting until after a second seizure) because the underlying cause (e.g. brain tumour) makes further seizures probable. The choice of anti-epileptic depends on the seizure type.

However, if the underlying cause of the seizure can be treated, e.g. meningitis or alcohol withdrawal, it should be possible subsequently to stop the anti-epileptic.

If a patient has a generalized seizure lasting ⩾5min, or ⩾3 seizures in 1h, give a benzodiazepine, e.g.:
- diazepam 10–20mg solution PR; if not settled, repeat after 15min *or*
- midazolam 10mg SC/IV, buccal, intranasal; if not settled, repeat after 15min.

If these measures fail, see below.

Status epilepticus

Status epilepticus is defined as a continuous seizure lasting more than 30min, or $\geqslant 2$ discrete seizures between which the patient does not recover consciousness.[76] Figure 8.2 summarizes current UK recommendations for the management of status epilepticus.[78,79] It is also important to:

- check the blood glucose
- administer glucose solution 50% 50mL IV and thiamine 250mg IV (e.g. Pabrinex® 2 vials), if the patient is malnourished or if any suggestion of alcohol abuse.

Many palliative care services do not stock fosphenytoin but do have an emergency supply of phenobarbital.

Fosphenytoin is a pro-drug of phenytoin (1.5mg of the former is equivalent to 1mg of the latter). The dose is expressed as phenytoin sodium equivalent (PE). It can be given more rapidly than phenytoin. Ideally, heart rate, blood pressure and respiratory function should be monitored during and for 30min after administration of

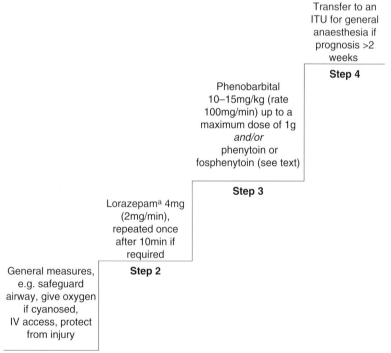

Figure 8.2 Management of status epilepticus.

a. if unavailable, clonazepam 1mg over 2min or midazolam 10mg are alternatives. If venous access cannot be obtained give midazolam 10mg buccally or SC, clonazepam 1mg SC or diazepam 10–20mg PR (for more information, see *PCF3*).

fosphenytoin 20mg(PE)/kg (100–150mg(PE)/min). IV phenytoin sodium 18mg/kg (50mg/min) can be used instead, preferably with ECG monitoring.

If resuscitation facilities are poor, PR paraldehyde is a useful option because it causes little respiratory depression. Paraldehyde 20mL is administered from a glass syringe (*it dissolves plastic*) as an enema, 1 part paraldehyde to 9 parts 0.9% saline.

After the seizures have been controlled, treatment should be continued with an appropriate maintenance regimen.

Moribund patients

When patients are no longer able to swallow, convert to PR diazepam or midazolam by CSCI. Although, higher doses may be necessary, maintenance treatment in moribund patients typically comprises:

* diazepam 10–30mg PR at bedtime or b.d. *or*
* midazolam 30–60mg/24h by CSCI *or*
* phenobarbital 200–600mg/24h by CSCI.

If some hours have elapsed since the last PO dose, it may be wise to give a stat dose of diazepam 10mg PR or midazolam 10mg SC. Remember:

* phenytoin and sodium valproate have long plasma halflives and will be present in the patient for some time after stopping oral treatment. The continuing but diminishing effects of phenytoin and sodium valproate supplement the benzodiazepine
* phenobarbital sodium for injection is made up in 90% propylene (200mg/1mL). If given by CSCI:
  ▷ dilute with water for injection
  ▷ give separately on its own
  ▷ *never mixed with another drug.*

NON-CONVULSIVE STATUS EPILEPTICUS

Non-convulsive status epilepticus (NCSE) is characterized by seizure activity on an EEG but without associated physical seizures. NCSE occurs in about 6% of cancer patients with no evidence of brain metastases.[80] Its incidence is likely to be higher in patients with primary brain tumours or brain metastases. Sometimes NCSE occurs in a patient with known epilepsy. It can be caused by any of the conditions that lead to generalized convulsive seizures (see above).

Because its clinical features (Box 8.H) may mimic those of dementia, delirium, other psychiatric disorders or coma, NCSE should be considered in the differential diagnosis

---

Box 8.H Possible clinical features of non-convulsive status epilepticus

Cognitive symptoms	Motor signs
Confusion	Automatisms
Dysphasia	Fluctuating pupil size (hippus)
Personality change	Nystagmus
Fear	Mild clonus of an extremity
Paranoid ideation	
Psychosis	

---

of all these conditions. Presenting features may have a fluctuating course and persist over hours, days, or weeks.[81,82] A high index of suspicion is needed to diagnose NCSE. Diagnosis can be confirmed only by EEG.

Treatment for NCSE is less urgent than that for convulsive status epilepticus:
- if patient conscious and able to swallow safely, continue or, if recently stopped, re-instate anti-epileptic
- if patient unconscious, apply general measures and give IV benzodiazepines (see above) preferably under EEG control
- if appropriate, transfer the patient to hospital for monitoring and further treatment[76] or
- seek advice from a neurologist.

PATULOUS EUSTACHIAN TUBE

The Eustachian tube is normally closed and opens only temporarily during swallowing. When the tube is patulous (i.e. remains open), free passage of air and sound occurs between the nasopharynx and the middle ear. The air causes flapping of the tympanic membrane and this is responsible for the annoying auditory discomfort linked to breathing.

The Eustachian tube becomes patulous particularly in pregnant women and in association with a rapid marked loss of weight. The incidence in advanced cancer is not known; possibly 2–3% of patients. It is often misdiagnosed as otitis media.

Clinical features
Symptoms are either continuous or intermittent, and vary from a minor annoyance to a major cause of distress:
- a feeling of aural fullness/pressure, generally interpreted as a blocked ear which is not relieved by swallowing
- blowing sound in ear(s) synchronous with breathing
- crackling sound when chewing
- voice sounds excessively loud and hollow, resembling an echo (autophony)
- postural variation: symptoms often diminish or disappear when patient is supine.

Auroscopy generally shows movement of the tympanic membrane synchronous with nasal inspiration and expiration.

Management
Symptoms are not often severe and explanation alone is generally adequate. Patients benefit by discovering that in certain positions the symptoms remit, e.g. when supine. A sharp forceful sniff may also bring temporary relief. Other options include:
- nasal drops containing hydrochloric acid, chlorbutanol, benzyl alcohol and propylene glycol[83]
- intratubal injection of:
  ▷ atropine
  ▷ liquid paraffin
  ▷ gelatine sponge
  ▷ Teflon®
- insertion of a grommet (ventilating tube) in the tympanic membrane under local anaesthetic by an ENT specialist.

STOPPING DEXAMETHASONE IN PATIENTS WITH INTRACRANIAL MALIGNANCY

Most patients stop taking dexamethasone when they become moribund and can no longer swallow. However, some centres administer parenteral dexamethasone instead.[84] If dexamethasone is withdrawn abruptly, the patient may need diamorphine/ morphine by CSCI to prevent distressing headaches and PR diazepam/SC midazolam to prevent seizures.

Occasionally, a patient with a brain tumour or multiple brain metastases requests that dexamethasone is stopped because, despite its continued use, there is progressive physical deterioration and/or cognitive impairment. In this circumstance, it is often best to reduce the dexamethasone step by step on a daily basis. This gives the patient time to reconsider. Extra analgesics should be prescribed in case headache develops as the intracranial pressure increases:

- if already taking paracetamol, prescribe a weak opioid or a weak opioid-paracetamol combination p.r.n.
- if already taking a weak opioid, prescribe morphine 10–20mg PO or morphine 5–10mg SC p.r.n.
- if >2 p.r.n. doses have been given in the last 24h, increase the regular analgesic dose
- if the patient becomes drowsy or swallowing becomes difficult, consider changing PO anti-epileptics to SC midazolam, and possibly give both morphine and midazolam by CSCI.

If the patient becomes semicomatose and cannot communicate clearly, the presence of headache may manifest as grimacing or general restlessness. However, as in all moribund patients, it is important to exclude other common reasons for agitation, e.g. a full bladder or rectum, and discomfort and stiffness secondary to immobility.

1 Bruera E et al. (1985) Action of oral methylprednisolone in terminal cancer patients: a prospective randomized double-blind study. Cancer Treatment Reports. 69: 751–754.
2 Bozzetti F (1996) Guidelines on artificial nutrition versus hydration in terminal cancer patients. Nutrition. 12: 163–167.
3 Dropcho EJ and Soong S-J (1991) Steroid induced weakness in patients with primary brain tumours. Neurology. 41: 1235–1239.
4 Eidelberg D (1991) Steroid myopathy. In: DA Rottenberg (ed) Neurological Complications of Cancer Treatment. Butterworth-Heineman, Boston, pp. 185–191.
5 Vecht C et al. (1994) Dose-effect relationship of dexamethasone on Karnofsky performance in metastatic brain tumors. A randomized study of doses of 4, 8 and 16mg per day. Neurology. 44: 675–680.
6 van Balkom RH et al. (1994) Corticosteroid-induced myopathy of the respiratory muscles. The Netherlands Journal of Medicine. 45: 114–122.
7 de Beukelaar JW and Sillevis Smitt PA (2006) Managing paraneoplastic neurological disorders. The Oncologist. 11: 292–305.
8 Graus F et al. (2001) Anti-Hu-associated paraneoplastic encephalomyelitis: analysis of 200 patients. Brain. 124: 1138–1148.
9 Lorusso L et al. (2004) Immunological features of neurological paraneoplastic syndromes. International Journal of Immunopathology and Pharmacology. 17: 135–144.
10 Darnell RB and Posner JB (2003) Paraneoplastic syndromes involving the nervous system. The New England Journal of Medicine. 349: 1543–1554.
11 Vernino S et al. (2004) Immunomodulatory treatment trial for paraneoplastic neurological disorders. Neuro-oncology. 6: 55–62.
12 Elrington G (1992) The Lambert-Eaton myasthenic syndrome. Palliative Medicine. 6: 9–17.
13 Newsom-Davis J and Murray N (1984) Plasma exchange and immunosuppressant drug treatment in the Lambert-Eaton Myasthenic Syndrome. Neurology. 34: 480–485.
14 Motomura M et al. (1995) An improved diagnostic assay for Lambert-Eaton Myasthenic syndrome. Journal of Neurology, Neurosurgery and Psychiatry. 58: 85–87.

15 Newsom-Davis J (1998) A treatment algorithm for Lambert-Eaton Myasthenic Syndrome. *Annals of the New York Academy of Sciences.* **841**: 817–822.
16 Bain P *et al.* (1996) Effects of intravenous immunoglobulin on muscle weakness and calcium-channel autoantibodies in the Lambert-Eaton myasthenic syndrome. *Neurology.* **47**: 678–683.
17 Loblaw DA *et al.* (2005) Systematic review of the diagnosis and management of malignant extradural spinal cord compression: the Cancer Care Ontario Practice Guidelines Initiative's Neuro-Oncology Disease Site Group. *Journal of Clinical Oncology.* **23**: 2028–2037.
18 Laperriere NJ (1996) *The Management of Spinal Cord Compression.* Princess Margaret Hospital, Toronto, Ontario.
19 Wong DA *et al.* (1990) Spinal metastases: the obvious, the occult, and the impostors. *Spine.* **15**: 1–4.
20 Klimo P, Jr. and Schmidt MH (2004) Surgical management of spinal metastases. *Oncologist.* **9**: 188–196.
21 Schaberg J and Gainor BJ (1985) A profile of metastatic carcinoma of the spine. *Spine.* **10**: 19–20.
22 Loblaw DA *et al.* (2003) A population-based study of malignant spinal cord compression in Ontario. *Clinical Oncology (Royal College of Radiologists).* **15**: 211–217.
23 Prasad D and Schiff D (2005) Malignant spinal-cord compression. *The Lancet Oncology.* **6**: 15–24.
24 Helweg-Larsen S *et al.* (2000) Prognostic factors in metastatic spinal cord compression: a prospective study using multivariate analysis of variables influencing survival and gait function in 153 patients. *International Journal of Radiation Oncology, Biology, Physics.* **46**: 1163–1169.
25 Maranzano E *et al.* (2005) Short-course versus split-course radiotherapy in metastatic spinal cord compression: results of a phase III, randomized, multicenter trial. *Journal of Clinical Oncology.* **23**: 3358–3365.
26 Patchell RA *et al.* (2005) Direct decompressive surgical resection in the treatment of spinal cord compression caused by metastatic cancer: a randomised trial. *Lancet.* **366**: 643–648.
27 Conway R *et al.* (2007) What happens to people after malignant cord compression? Survival, function, quality of life, emotional well-being and place of care 1 month after diagnosis. *Clinical Oncology (Royal College of Radiologists).* **19**: 56–62.
28 Rades D *et al.* (2006) Prognostic factors for local control and survival after radiotherapy of metastatic spinal cord compression. *Journal of Clinical Oncology.* **24**: 3388–3393.
29 Chamberlain MC and Kormanik PA (1999) Epidural spinal cord compression: a single institution's retrospective experience. *Neuro-oncology.* **1**: 120–123.
30 Cowap J *et al.* (2000) Outcome of malignant spinal cord compression at a cancer center: implications for palliative care services. *Journal of Pain and Symptom Management.* **19**: 257–264.
31 White BD *et al.* (2008) Diagnosis and management of patients at risk of or with metastatic spinal cord compression: summary of NICE guidance. *British Medical Journal.* **337**: a2538.
32 NICE (2008) Metastatic spinal cord compression: diagnosis and management of patients at risk of or with metastatic spinal cord compression. (Clinical guideline 75.). National Institute for Health and Clinical Excellence, London. Available from: www.nice.org.uk/CG75
33 Greenberg HS *et al.* (1980) Epidural spinal cord compression from metastatic tumor: results with a new treatment protocol. *Annals of Neurology.* **8**: 361–366.
34 Vecht C *et al.* (1989) Initial bolus of conventional versus high-dose dexamethasone in metastatic spinal cord compression. *Neurology.* **39**: 1255–1257.
35 Graham PH *et al.* (2006) A pilot randomised comparison of dexamethasone 96mg vs 16mg per day for malignant spinal-cord compression treated by radiotherapy: TROG 01.05 Superdex study. *Clinical Oncology (Royal College of Radiologists).* **18**: 70–76.
36 Heimdal K *et al.* (1992) High incidence of serious side effects of high-dose dexamethasone treatment in patients with epidural spinal cord compression. *Journal of Neuro-Oncology.* **12**: 141–144.
37 Sorensen S *et al.* (1994) Effect of high-dose dexamethasone in carcinomatous metastatic spinal cord compression treated with radiotherapy: a randomised trial. *European Journal of Cancer.* **30A**: 22–27.
38 George R *et al.* (2007) Interventions for the treatment of metastatic extradural spinal cord compression in adults. *Cochrane Database of Systematic Reviews.* CD006716.
39 Falkmer U *et al.* (2003) A systematic overview of radiation therapy effects in skeletal metastases. *Acta Oncologica.* **42**: 620–633.
40 Rades D *et al.* (2004) A prospective evaluation of two radiotherapy schedules with 10 versus 20 fractions for the treatment of metastatic spinal cord compression: final results of a multicenter study. *Cancer.* **101**: 2687–2692.
41 Klimo P, Jr. *et al.* (2005) A meta-analysis of surgery versus conventional radiotherapy for the treatment of metastatic spinal epidural disease. *Neuro-oncology.* **7**: 64–76.
42 Siegal T and Siegal T (1985) Surgical decompression of anterior and posterior malignant epidural tumours compressing the spinal cord: a prospective study. *Neurosurgery.* **17**: 424–432.
43 Gall A and Turner-Stokes L (2008) Chronic spinal cord injury: management of patients in acute hospital settings. *Clinical Medicine.* **8**: 70–74.
44 Bhattacharjee S and Poonnoose P (2003) Management of paraplegia in palliative care. *Indian Journal of Palliative Care.* **9**: 14–18.

45 Spinal Injuries Association (2008) Factsheets. Available from: www.spinal.co.uk
46 Eva G et al. (2009) Patients' constructions of disability in metastatic spinal cord compression. Palliative Medicine. **23**: 133–140.
47 Jansen P et al. (1991) Clinical diagnosis of muscle cramp and muscle cramp syndromes. European Archives of Psychiatry and Clinical Neuroscience. **241**: 98–101.
48 Miller TM and Layzer RB (2005) Muscle cramps. Muscle Nerve. **32**: 431–442.
49 Steiner I and Siegal T (1989) Muscle cramps in cancer patients. Cancer. **63**: 574–577.
50 Siegal T (1991) Muscle cramps in the cancer patient: causes and treatment. Journal of Pain and Symptom Management. **6**: 84–91.
51 Lear J and Daniels R (1993) Muscle cramps related to corticosteroids. British Medical Journal. **306**: 1169.
52 Layzer R (1994) The origin of muscle fasciculations and cramps. Muscle and Nerve. **17**: 1243–1249.
53 Daniell HW (1979) Simple cure for nocturnal leg cramps. The New England Journal of Medicine. **301**: 216.
54 Coppin RJ et al. (2005) Managing nocturnal leg cramps–calf-stretching exercises and cessation of quinine treatment: a factorial randomised controlled trial. The British Journal of General Practice. **55**: 186–191.
55 Bertolasi L et al. (1997) Botulinum toxin treatment of muscle cramps: a clinical and neurophysiological study. Annals of Neurology. **41**: 181–186.
56 Oliver D and Borasio GD (2004) Diseases of motor nerves. In: R Voltz et al. (eds) Palliative Care in Neurology. Oxford University Press, Oxford, p.84.
57 Serrao M et al. (2000) Gabapentin treatment for muscle cramps: an open-label trial. Clinical Neuropharmacology. **23**: 45–49.
58 Dahle LO et al. (1995) The effect of oral magnesium substitution on pregnancy-induced leg cramps. American Journal of Obstetrics and Gynecology. **173**: 175–180.
59 Boltodano et al. (1988) Verapamil vs quinine in recumbent nocturnal leg cramps in the elderly. Archives of Internal Medicine. **148**: 1969–70.
60 Konikoff F et al. (1991) Vitamin E and cirrhotic muscle cramps. Israel Journal of Medical Sciences. **27**: 221–223.
61 Roca AO et al. (1992) Dialysis leg cramps. Efficacy of quinine versus vitamin E. American Society for Artificial Internal Organs Journal. **38**: M481–485.
62 Noth J and Fink GR (2004) Spasticity. In: R Voltz et al. (eds) Palliative Care in Neurology. Oxford University Press, Oxford.
63 Kasdon D (1986) Controversies in the surgical management of spasticity. Clinical Neurosurgery. **35**: 523–529.
64 Doraisamy P (1992) The management of spasticity – a review of options available in rehabilitation. Annals of the Academy of Medicine of Singapore. **21**: 807–812.
65 Kita M and Goodkin D (2000) Drugs used to treat spasticity. Drugs. **59**: 487–495.
66 Chou R et al. (2004) Comparative efficacy and safety of skeletal muscle relaxants for spasticity and musculoskeletal conditions: a systematic review. Journal of Pain and Symptom Management. **28**: 140–175.
67 Shakespeare DT et al. (2003) Anti-spasticity agents for multiple sclerosis. Cochrane Database of Systematic Reviews. CD001332.
68 Paisley S et al. (2002) Clinical effectiveness of oral treatments for spasticity in multiple sclerosis: a systematic review. Multiple Sclerosis. **8**: 319–329.
69 Royal College of Physicians (2004) Multiple Sclerosis: National clinical guidelines foe diagnosis and management in primary and secondary care. Available from: www.rcplondon.ac.uk/pubs/books/MS/MSfulldocument.pdf
70 Noth J and Fink GR (2004) Spasticity. In: R Voltz et al. (eds) Palliative Care in Neurology. Oxford University Press, Oxford, p. 154.
71 Brin M (1997) Dosing, administration and a treatment algorithm for use of botulinum toxin A for adult-onset of spasticity. Muscle and Nerve. **Supplement 6**.
72 Lauterbach E (1999) Hiccup and apparent myoclonus after hydrocodone: Review of the opiate-related hiccup and myoclonus literature. Clinical Neuropharmacology. **22**: 87–92.
73 Zhang C et al. (2005) Gabapentin-induced myoclonus in end-stage renal disease. Epilepsia. **46**: 156–158.
74 Weil S and Noachtar S (2004) Epileptic seizures and myoclonus. In: R Voltz et al. (eds) Palliative Care in Neurology (No. 69). Oxford University Press, Oxford, p. 154.
75 French JA and Pedley TA (2008) Clinical practice. Initial management of epilepsy. The New England Journal of Medicine. **359**: 166–176.
76 Stokes T et al. (2004) Modified from: Commission on Classification and Terminology of the International League Against Epilepsy. Proposal for revised clinical and electroencephalographic classification of epileptic seizures in: Clinical Guidelines and Evidence Review for the Epilepsies: diagnosis and management in adults and children in primary and secondary care. Royal College of General Practitioners, London. Available from: http://guidance.nice.org.uk/CG20/guidance/pdf/English/download.dspx
77 Posner JB (1992) Management of brain metastases. Revue Neurologique (Paris). **148**: 477–487.
78 NICE (2004) The clinical effectiveness and cost effectiveness of newer drugs for epilepsy in adults. In: Technology appraisal. National Institute for Clinical Excellence. Available from: www.nice.org.uk/page.aspx?o=ta076guidance

79 BNF (2008) Section 4.8.1 Control of epilepsy. In: *British National Formulary* (No. 55). British Medical Association and Royal Pharmaceutical Society of Great Britain, London. Current BNF available from: www.bnf.org/bnf/bnf/current/

80 Cocito L *et al.* (2001) Altered mental state and nonconvulsive status epilepticus in patients with cancer. *Archives of Neurology.* **58**: 1310.

81 Walker M (2005) Status epilepticus: an evidence based guide. *British Medical Journal.* **331**: 673–677.

82 Lorenzl S *et al.* (2008) Nonconvulsive status epilepticus in terminally ill patients-a diagnostic and therapeutic challenge. *Journal of Pain and Symptom Management.* **36**: 200–205.

83 DiBartolomeo J (1993) Correspondence. *American Journal of Otology.* **14**: 313.

84 Rousseau P (2004) Sudden withdrawal of corticosteroids: a commentary. *The American Journal of Hospice and Palliative Care.* **21**: 169–171.

9: URINARY SYMPTOMS

DEFINITIONS

Frequency
Voiding too often (>8 times in 24h).[1]

Nocturia
Waking at night to void.[1]

Urgency
A sudden compelling desire to void which is difficult to delay.[1]

Urge incontinence
The involuntary leakage of urine associated with urgency.

Overactive bladder syndrome
Urgency ± urge incontinence, frequency, and nocturia in the absence of urinary tract infection (UTI) or other obvious pathological cause, generally caused by detrusor overactivity.[1] Also known as *urge syndrome* or *urgency-frequency syndrome*. Prevalence increases with age, and is exacerbated by cognitive impairment. Detrusor overactivity is the second most common cause of urinary incontinence in women.

Stress incontinence
The involuntary loss of urine associated with coughing, sneezing, laughing or lifting.

Genuine stress incontinence (urethral sphincter incompetence)
The involuntary leakage of urine when the intravesical pressure exceeds maximum urethral pressure in the absence of detrusor activity. The fault always lies in the sphincter mechanisms of the bladder, and is associated with multiparity, after the menopause and after hysterectomy.

One or more of the following features will be present:
• descent of urethrovesical junction outside the intra-abdominal zone of pressure
• decrease in urethral pressure due to loss of urethral wall elasticity and contractility
• short functional length of the urethra.

Urethral sphincter incompetence is the most common cause of urinary incontinence in women.

Dysuria
Pain during and/or after voiding. Often urethral in origin (a burning sensation) but may be caused by bladder spasm (intense suprapubic and urethral pain), or both.

Hesitancy
A prolonged delay between attempting and achieving voiding.

BLADDER INNERVATION

'You pee with your parasympathetics. You stop with your sympathetics.'

The sphincter relaxes when the detrusor (bladder muscle) contracts, and vice versa (Table 9.1). Thus, antimuscarinics not only cause contraction of the bladder neck sphincter but also relax the detrusor. Detrusor sensitivity is also:
- increased by PGs
- decreased by NSAIDs.

The urethral sphincter, under voluntary control, is innervated by the pudendal nerve (S2–4).

Table 9.1   Autonomic innervation of the bladder and its effects

Innervation	Neurotransmitter	Sphincter	Detrusor
Sympathetic (T10–12, L1)	Noradrenaline (norepinephrine)	Contracts (α)	Relaxes (β)
Parasympathetic (S2–4)	Acetylcholine	Relaxes	Contracts

Morphine and other opioids have several effects on bladder function:
- bladder sensation *decreased*
- sphincter tone *increased*
- detrusor tone *increased*
- ureteric tone and amplitude of contractions *increased*.

These are generally asymptomatic. Occasionally hesitancy or retention occurs.

FREQUENCY AND URGENCY

The incidence in cancer patients is not known.

Causes
There is overlap between the causes of frequency, urgency, and urge incontinence (Box 9.A). The precipitating factor in urge incontinence is delayed voiding relative to need. Delay is associated with:
- weakness and difficulty in getting to a commode

- disinterest:
  - ▷ depression
  - ▷ dejection
- lack of awareness:
  - ▷ confusion
  - ▷ drowsiness.

The differential diagnosis includes:
- genuine stress incontinence
- retention with overflow
- urinary fistula
- flaccid sphincter (presacral plexopathy)
- detrusor hyperreflexia with external sphincter dyssynergia, after the resolution of spinal shock (generally 2–12 weeks) caused by complete thoracic or cervical cord compression.[2]

Box 9.A   Causes of urgency and urge incontinence

Cancer
Pain
Hypercalcaemia (polyuria)
Intravesical   }   mechanical
Extravesical   }   irritation
Bladder spasms
Sacral plexopathy

Treatment
Radiation cystitis
Drugs
    cyclophosphamide
    diuretics
    tiaprofenic acid

Debility
Infective cystitis

Concurrent
Idiopathic detrusor instability
Central neurological disease
    post-stroke
    multiple sclerosis
    dementia

Uraemia
Diabetes mellitus   }
Diabetes insipidus   }   cause polyuria

Management
Prevent the preventable

Tiaprofenic acid (an NSAID) can cause severe cystitis presenting months, or even years, after starting treatment.[3-5] Tiaprofenic acid should not be given to patients with urinary tract disorders.[6] Patients prescribed tiaprofenic acid should be advised to stop taking it and to report to their doctor promptly if they develop urinary tract symptoms, e.g. frequency, nocturia, urgency, dysuria, haematuria.

Correct the correctable
- stop tiaprofenic acid
- reduce or change diuretic
- treat infective cystitis with the appropriate antibacterial
- for prophylaxis against cystitis, recommend cranberry juice 150mL b.d. or 300mL once daily.[7-10]

- alternatively, prescribe a urinary antiseptic long-term:
  ▷ methenamine (hexamine) hippurate 1g b.d.–t.d.s.[11]
  ▷ nitrofurantoin 50–100mg at bedtime.[12]

Cranberry juice
For more information, see *PCF3*.

Cranberry juice contains fructose and pro-anthocyanidins which inhibit bacterial adherence to the uro-epithelium *in vitro*. It reduces the frequency of symptomatic UTIs in women at risk of this infection.[13]

The INR of patients taking warfarin should be monitored more frequently because cranberry juice may increase the INR.[10,14]

Urinary antiseptics
For more information, see *PCF3*.

In catheterized patients, methenamine hippurate reduces sediment and catheter blockage, and doubles the interval between catheter changes.[15]

Both methenamine hippurate and nitrofurantoin are ineffective against acute *upper* UTI, and both can cause dyspepsia, nausea and vomiting.

Non-drug treatment
Patients with mild symptoms may respond to regular time-contingent voiding, e.g. every 1–3h. They will also be helped by:
- proximity to the toilet
- ready availability of a bottle or commode
- a rapid response by nurses to requests for help
- abstaining from caffeine and alcohol (both are diuretics).[16]

Drug treatment
For more information, see *PCF3*.

Antimuscarinics are the drugs of choice[17] although treatment may be limited by other antimuscarinic effects. Various other drugs may also be helpful (Box 9.B).

Oxybutynin and tolterodine reduce urinary frequency by about 15–30%, and incontinence episodes by 50–80%.[21–23] Solifenacin, a new long-acting M_3-receptor selective antimuscarinic given once daily, is of comparable efficacy to m/r tolterodine, with a similar incidence of undesirable effects.[17,24]

Post-menopausal urge incontinence and frequency is sometimes helped by the prescription of an oestrogen (unlicensed use), preferably topically, or PO.[25] Oestrogens do not improve stress incontinence.[16]

Bumetanide 1mg 4–6h before bedtime (e.g. 1800h) may also decrease episodes of nocturia, unless nocturia is related to benign prostatic hyperplasia.[16,26]

Box 9.B   Drugs for urinary frequency and bladder spasms

Antimuscarinics
- oxybutynin 2.5–5mg b.d.–q.d.s.; also has a topical anaesthetic effect on the bladder mucosa[18]
- tolterodine 2mg b.d. is as effective as oxybutynin 5mg t.d.s. but has fewer antimuscarinic effects;[19] it is more expensive
- amitriptyline 25–50mg at bedtime
- imipramine 25–50mg at bedtime[20]
- propantheline 15–30mg b.d.–t.d.s.

Sympathomimetics, e.g. terbutaline 5mg t.d.s.

Musculotropic drugs, e.g. flavoxate 200–400mg t.d.s.

NSAIDs, e.g. naproxen 250–500mg b.d. (a possible co-antispasmodic, rather than a primary treatment)

Topical analgesics, e.g. phenazopyridine 100–200mg t.d.s. (not UK)

Vasopressin analogues, e.g. desmopressin, are of value in refractory nocturia, but hyponatraemia is a common complication (>10%).[16]

BLADDER SPASMS

Bladder (detrusor) spasms are transient, often excruciating, sensations felt in the suprapubic region and urethra/penis. They are generally secondary to irritation or hyperexcitability of the trigone.

Causes
Bladder spasms may relate to local cancer or other factors (Box 9.C).

Box 9.C   Causes of bladder spasms

Cancer		Debility
Intravesical	} irritation	Anxiety
Extravesical		Infective cystitis
		Indwelling catheter
Treatment		mechanical irritation by catheter balloon
Radiation fibrosis		catheter sludging with partial retention

Management
Correct the correctable
Treatment options for reversible causes are listed in Table 9.2.

Drug treatment
For more information, see *PCF3*.

Systemic analgesics should be used to control any constant background pain and, as with overactive bladder syndrome, an antimuscarinic given to reduce or prevent the spasms. Alternatives include:

- hyoscine (Quick Kwells®) 300microgram SL b.d.–q.d.s.
- hyoscyamine 150microgram b.d.–q.d.s. or m/r 375microgram b.d. (not UK); twice as potent as hyoscine
- belladonna and opium suppositories (B & O Supprettes®) up to hourly (not UK); each B & O Supprette® contains either 30mg (No. 15A) or 60mg (No. 16A) of powdered opium and approximately 200microgram of belladonna alkaloids.

If the above measures are ineffective, consider:

- hyoscine butylbromide 60–160mg/24h by CSCI
- intravesical morphine (10–20mg t.d.s. or diamorphine 10mg t.d.s. diluted in 0.9% saline to 20mL);[27] instil through an indwelling catheter and clamp for 30min
- bupivacaine t.d.s. (0.5% bupivacaine 10mL diluted in 0.9% saline to 20mL) used alone or with intravesical morphine[28]
- spinal analgesia, e.g. epidural morphine and 0.5% bupivacaine.

Table 9.2   Management of reversible causes of bladder spasms

Cause	Treatment option
Catheter irritation	Change catheter Reduce volume of balloon
Catheter sludging	Bladder washouts (100mL) Continuous bladder irrigation
Blood clots (haematuria)	see p.241
Infection (cystitis)	Bladder washouts (if catheterized) Change indwelling catheter Switch to intermittent catheterization q6h–q4h Encourage oral fluids Antibacterials, systemic or by instillation Urinary antiseptics, e.g. methenamine hippurate Cranberry juice

VOIDING DIFFICULTIES

Voiding difficulties is a term encompassing three closely associated symptoms, namely, hesitancy, slow stream and terminal dribble. Voiding difficulties may be associated with urinary storage symptoms, e.g. frequency, nocturia, urgency, retention.

Causes
Voiding difficulties have many possible causes (Box 9.D).[29]

Management
Correct the correctable
Treatment options for reversible causes of hesitancy are listed in Table 9.3.

> **Box 9.D**   Causes of voiding difficulties
>
> **Cancer**
> Malignant enlargement of prostate
> Infiltration of bladder neck
> Presacral plexopathy
> Spinal shock
> Cauda equina or sacral nerve
>   root compression
>
> **Treatment**
> Antimuscarinics
> Morphine (occasionally)
> Spinal analgesia (particularly with bupivacaine)
> Intrathecal nerve blocks
>
> **Debility**
> Loaded rectum
> Inability to stand to void
> Generalized weakness
>
> **Concurrent**
> Benign prostatic hyperplasia

Table 9.3   Management of reversible causes of hesitancy

Cause	Treatment
Antimuscarinics	Stop if possible, or replace with a less antimuscarinic alternative
Loaded rectum	Suppositories / Enema / Digital evacuation } → oral laxative regimen
Inability to void lying down	Nursing assistance → more upright posture
Benign prostatic hyperplasia	Transurethral resection

Non-drug treatment
Generally, drug treatment should take precedence over non-drug treatment, i.e. catheterization. However, in debilitated bedbound patients, a trial of catheterization may be preferable. In such patients, per urethral catheterization will be the norm. For patients who have several months to live, suprapubic catheterization should be considered.

Drug treatment
For more information, see *PCF3*.

Several options are available for the treatment of symptoms suggestive of benign prostatic hyperplasia. α_1-Adrenoceptor antagonists remain the treatment of choice, preferably m/r tamsulosin 400microgram once daily.[30–32] Other options include:
- a 5α-reductase inhibitor e.g. finasteride 5mg once daily (alone or with an α_1-adrenoceptor antagonist)[30]
- a parasympathomimetic, e.g. bethanechol 10–25mg b.d.–q.d.s; use with caution
- an anticholinesterase, e.g. distigmine 5mg once daily.

Added benefit can be obtained by combining either a parasympathomimetic or an anticholinesterase with an α_1-adrenoceptor antagonist.

---

1 International Continence Society (2005) Factsheet 2: Overactive Bladder. Available from: www.icsoffice.org
2 Shah DK and Badlani GH (2004) Ch. 25. Urological symptoms. In: R Voltz et al. (eds) Palliative Care in Neurology. Oxford University Press, Oxford, p. 264.
3 McCaffery M (1981) Nursing Management of the Patient with Pain (seconde). Lippncott, Philadelphia.
4 Bateman D (1994) Tiaprofenic acid and cystitis. British Medical Journal. 309: 552–553.
5 Mayall F et al. (1994) Cystitis and ureteric obstruction in patients taking tiaprofenic acid. British Medical Journal. 309: 599.
6 BNF (2008) Section 10.1.1 Tiaprofenic acid. In: British National Formulary (No. 55). British Medical Association and the Royal Pharmaceutical Society of Great Britain, London. Current BNF available from: www.bnf.org/bnf/current/
7 Avorn J et al. (1994) Reduction of bacteriuria and pyuria after ingestion of cranberry juice. Journal of the American Medical Association. 271: 751–754.
8 Harkins K (2000) What's the use of cranberry juice? Age and Ageing. 29: 9–12.
9 Jepson R et al. (2000) Cranberries for preventing urinary tract infections. Cochrane Database of Systematic Reviews. 2: CD001321.
10 DTB (2005) Cranberry and urinary tract infection. Drug and Therapeutics Bulletin. 43: 17–19.
11 Cronberg S et al. (1987) Prevention of recurrent acute cystitis by methenamine hippurate: double blind controlled crossover longterm study. British Medical Journal. 294: 1507–1508.
12 Brumfitt W et al. (1981) Prevention of recurrent urinary infections in women: a comparative trial between nitrofurantoin and methenamine hippurate. Journal of Urology. 126: 71–74.
13 Kontiokari T et al. (2001) Randomised trial of cranberry-lingonberry juice and Lactobacillus GG drink for the prevention of urinary tract infections in women. British Medical Journal. 322: 1571.
14 Welch JM and Forster K (2007) Probable elevation of INR from cranberry juice. Journal of Pharmacy Technology. 23: 104–107.
15 Norberg A et al. (1980) Randomized double-blind study of prophylactic methenamine hippurate treatment of patients with indwelling catheters. European Journal of Clinical Pharmacology. 18: 497–500.
16 NICE (2006) Urinary incontinence: the management of urinary incontinence in women. In: Clinical Guidelines. National Institute for Health and Clinical Excellence. Available from: http://guidance.nice.org.uk/CG40
17 DTB (2007) Update on drugs for overactive bladder syndrome. Drug and Therapeutics Bulletin. 45: 44–48.
18 Robinson T and Castleden C (1994) Drugs in focus: 11. Oxybutynin hydrochloride. Prescribers' Journal. 34: 27–30.
19 Hills C et al. (1998) Tolterodine. Drugs. 55: 813-820.
20 Castledon C (1988) Imipramine: possible alternative to current therapy for urinary incontinence in the elderly. Journal of Urology. 22: 525–533.
21 Anderson RU et al. (1999) Once daily controlled versus immediate release oxybutynin chloride for urge urinary incontinence. OROS Oxybutynin Study Group. The Journal of Urology. 161: 1809–1812.
22 Chancellor M et al. (2000) Tolterodine, an effective and well tolerated treatment for urge incontinence and other overactive bladder symptoms. Clinical Drug Investigation. 19: 83–91.
23 Sand PK et al. (2004) A comparison of extended-release oxybutynin and tolterodine for treatment of overactive bladder in women. International Urogynecology Journal and Pelvic Floor Dysfunction. 15: 243–248.
24 Chapple CR et al. (2005) A comparison of the efficacy and tolerability of solifenacin succinate and extended release tolterodine at treating overactive bladder syndrome: results of the STAR trial. European Urology. 48: 464–470.
25 Moehrer B et al. (2003) Oestrogens for urinary incontinence in women. Cochrane Database of Systematic Reviews. CD001405.
26 Pedersen PA and Johansen PB (1988) Prophylactic treatment of adult nocturia with bumetanide. British Journal of Urology. 62: 145–147.
27 McCoubrie R and Jeffrey D (2003) Intravesical diamorphine for bladder spasm. Journal of Pain and Symptom Management. 25: 1–3.
28 Chiang D et al. (2005) Management of post-operative bladder spasm. Journal of Paediatrics and Child Health. 41: 56–58.
29 Crawford ED (2005) Management of lower urinary tract symptoms suggestive of benign prostatic hyperplasia: the central role of the patient risk profile. BJU International. 95 Suppl 4: 1–5.
30 Schulman CC (2003) Lower urinary tract symptoms/benign prostatic hyperplasia: minimizing morbidity caused by treatment. Urology. 62: 24–33.
31 Milani S and Djavan B (2005) Lower urinary tract symptoms suggestive of benign prostatic hyperplasia: latest update on alpha-adrenoceptor antagonists. BJU International. 95 Suppl 4: 29–36.
32 Wilt TJ et al. (2003) Tamsulosin for benign prostatic hyperplasia. Cochrane Database of Systematic Reviews. CD002081.

10: OEDEMA IN ADVANCED CANCER

OEDEMA

Oedema is a common feature of advanced cancer. There are multiple causes which may co-exist (Box 10.A). Lymphatic failure is inevitable in immobile patients who sit for many hours day after day and have little or no exercise ('armchair legs'). This is because muscle activity is essential to maintain both venous and lymph return from dependent limbs.

Extra load placed on the lymphatics as a result of venous incompetence also leads to lymphatic failure. Thus, patients with chronic venous leg ulcers and swelling have a combination of venous oedema and lymphatic failure, often called lymphovenous stasis.

Box 10.A   Causes of oedema in advanced cancer

General

Drugs
  salt and water retention,
    e.g. NSAIDs, corticosteroids
  vasodilation, e.g. nifedipine
Hypo-albuminaemia
Malignant ascites, associated with
  secondary hyperaldosteronism
  (see p.127)
Anaemia
CHF
End-stage renal failure

Local

Venous obstruction
  extrinsic venous compression by
    cancer
  DVT (see p.244)
  IVC obstruction
  SVC obstruction (see p.361).
Lymphovenous stasis
  immobility and dependency
  paralysis, e.g. hemiplegia,
    paraplegia
Lymphatic obliteration/obstruction
  surgery
  radiotherapy
  repeated infections
  metastatic cancer in lymph nodes

Leg oedema can occur in ascites, particularly when associated with secondary hyperaldosteronism (see p.127). In this circumstance, drainage of the ascites or use of spironolactone (an aldosterone antagonist) can lead to a reduction of the leg oedema.

LYMPHOEDEMA

For more general accounts of lymphoedema management, see either a comprehensive textbook[1] or the international consensus document.[2] A booklet for patients is available from CancerBACUP.[3]

Lymphoedema is tissue swelling caused by a failure of lymph drainage. It results from an imbalance between the influx and efflux of the lymphatic system. It can occur in any part of the body but generally it affects one or more limbs $\pm$ the adjacent trunk. In the UK, cancer and cancer treatment account for 1/4 of the cases of chronic oedema/lymphoedema.[4] Risk factors include:
• axillary or groin surgery
• postoperative infection
• radiotherapy
• lymph node metastases, e.g. axillary, groin, intrapelvic or retroperitoneal.[5]

A combination of two or more of these factors greatly increases the likelihood of lymphoedema. After radical hysterectomy for cancer of the cervix (which includes excision of the pelvic lymph nodes) and postoperative radiotherapy, about 40% of women develop lymphoedema.[6]

Although described as 'protein-rich', the protein content of chronic lymphoedema is about 5g/L lower than that of interstitial fluid in the contralateral normal limb.[7] Further, the protein content is relatively low in early lymphoedema (10–20g/L) compared with long-established lymphoedema (>30g/L).[8] However, the protein content of lymphoedema is much higher than the protein content of cardiac and venous oedemas (<5g/L and 5–10g/L respectively).[8] The protein in lymphoedema stimulates low-grade chronic inflammation; this leads to interstitial fibrosis and fat deposition.[9]

CLINICAL FEATURES

Symptoms include:
• tightness
• heaviness
• a bursting feeling if there is an acute exacerbation
• pain caused by:
  ▷ shoulder strain (caused by the weight of the lymphoedematous arm)
  ▷ inflammation
  ▷ brachial or lumbosacral plexopathy (caused by the associated cancer)
• impaired function/mobility
• psychosocial distress:
  ▷ altered body image
  ▷ problems in obtaining well-fitting clothes or shoes.

The impact on the patient psychosocially is not always obvious. Specific enquiry is needed to elicit the extent of the patient's distress.

Unlike other types of oedema, chronic lymphoedema results in changes in the skin and subcutis. Clinical signs include:
- persistent swelling of part or all of the limb which over time becomes non-pitting as a result of the interstitial fibrosis and fat deposition, and which does not decrease with elevation overnight
- increased tissue turgor
- Stemmer's sign (the inability to pick up a fold of skin at the base of the second toe or middle finger); *the absence of this sign does not necessarily exclude more proximal lymphoedema*
- distorted limb shape
- lymphangiectasia (dilated skin lymphatics which look like blisters)
- deep skin creases associated with cutaneous fibrosis
- hyperkeratosis (a build-up of surface keratin resulting in a warty scaly skin)
- papillomatosis (a cobblestone effect caused by dilated skin lymphatics surrounded by fibrosis)
- cellulitis/AIEs (see p.312)
- lymphorrhoea (leakage of lymph).

Hyperkeratosis and papillomatosis are seen mainly in lower limb lymphoedema. Lymphorrhoea is more common in lymphovenous stasis, IVC obstruction and CHF. Ulceration is uncommon unless there is associated venous or arterial disease.

When the trunk is involved:
- the subcutis feels thickened on palpation
- when a fold of skin is pinched up simultaneously on both sides on the trunk, the skin is more difficult to grip on the affected side
- underwear leaves deeper markings on the affected side
- in unilateral lower limb lymphoedema, the ipsilateral buttock is bigger when examined with the patient standing
- in women, there may be genital wetness from leaking lymphangiectasia.

Radiotherapy also causes subcutaneous thickening but it is qualitatively different from that in lymphoedema, i.e. it is firmer and completely non-pitting.

EVALUATION

In advanced cancer, particularly with lower limb swelling, there may be more than one cause (see Box 10.A). If the clinical features do not suggest a likely cause, investigations should be considered:
- FBC
- plasma albumin concentration
- plasma electrolytes and creatinine concentrations
- chest radiograph.

Also, if the prognosis is more than 3–6 months, consider:
- ultrasound to determine venous function
- CT or MRI to determine disease status, and whether there is lymphadenopathy.

EXPLANATION

When caused by cancer, unless there is a likelihood of a complete remission with radiotherapy or chemotherapy, patients should be told that the lymphoedema cannot be cured.

The aim of treatment is to make the affected limb(s) more comfortable. This can be achieved in most cases by measures which reduce the tension in the swollen tissues, and prevent further deterioration as a result of cellulitis/AIEs and immobility. In advanced cancer, reduction in the size of a lymphoedematous limb may *not* be possible. Thus, patients need to be educated about:

- the importance of daily skin care to improve and maintain skin integrity (see below), and thus to minimize the likelihood of infection (AIEs, see p.312)
- the reasons why they are susceptible to AIEs, e.g. skin crevices harbour bacteria, stagnant fluid, reduced immunity[10]
- the consequences of AIEs, i.e. increased swelling, more fibrosis, decreased response to treatment for reducing limb size
- reducing risk by reducing the swelling,[11] protecting hands when gardening, cleaning cuts, treating fungal infections and ingrowing toenails
- the importance of seeking prompt medical attention and treatment if symptoms or signs suggest the onset of an AIE
- the importance of limb movement and exercise (see p.305)
- the need for a compression garment (see p.304).

MANAGEMENT

Emphasis should be placed on relieving discomfort and preventing deterioration (Box 10.B).

Box 10.B   Palliative lymphoedema management

Correct the correctable	Drug treatment
Skin care	Analgesics
	Corticosteroids
Non-drug treatment	Diuretics (only if associated with fluid retention)
Positioning	
Containment	**Management of complications**
Exercise	Prevention and treatment of infection
Massage	Ulceration
Pneumatic compression	Lymphorrhoea

Correct the correctable
Skin care
Guidelines: Dry skin in lymphoedema, p.302.

The aim of skin care is to prevent debilitating infections (AIEs) which exacerbate the oedema. In chronic lymphoedema the skin becomes dry, warty and discoloured. A break in the skin, often invisible, enables bacteria to gain access to stagnant protein-rich lymph, an ideal growth medium. Infection accelerates fibrosis and causes more damage to the lymphatics. Careful hygiene reduces the risk of infection by reducing the bacteria resident on the skin. After washing, preferably every day, the swollen limb should be dried carefully, paying particular attention to between the digits and any skin folds (Box 10.C).

Box 10.C Written information for patients about skin care[12]

General information

Keep the skin supple by applying oil or bland (unperfumed) cream, e.g. aqueous cream BP, Diprobase®.

Swollen arm: protect the hand and arm with a glove and long sleeve when cooking, washing up or gardening; wear a thimble when sewing.

Swollen leg: wear protective footwear at all times; do not walk in bare feet.

Avoid excessive heat (e.g. very hot showers/baths, saunas, sunbeds) and sunburn on the affected area because these can increase the swelling.

Dry well between digits after washing to protect from fungal infections.

If shaving within the affected area, use an electric razor to avoid cuts.

Take care when cutting toe or finger nails; use clippers rather than scissors; do not push back nail cuticles.

Treat cuts or grazes promptly by washing and applying an antiseptic; cover with a dressing.

See your GP immediately if the limb becomes hot or more swollen.

Other important points about the swollen limb:
• do not allow your blood pressure to be taken on it
• do not have needles stuck into it (blood tests, injections, acupuncture).

Summer advice

Avoid insect bites; use insect repellent cream/spray; treat bites with antiseptics and/or antihistamines.

Protect the swollen limb from the sun:
• sit in the shade when possible
• use a high-factor sun block, e.g. 30–50.

Equipment to take on holiday:
• emollient
• high-factor sun block
• insect repellent cream/spray
• antihistamine tablets
• antiseptic solutions, e.g. Savlon®, TCP®.

If you have had recurrent infections, take antibiotics with you when you go on holiday in case of need.

Guidelines: Dry skin in lymphoedema

In lymphoedema, a healthy skin reduces the risk of local infection (acute inflammatory episodes/AIEs); moisturizing the skin regularly is essential.

I Emollients (moisturizers) soothe, smooth and hydrate the skin. They are indicated for all causes of dry skin and scaling disorders. Because the effect is short-lived, emollients should initially be applied t.d.s.–q.d.s. Less frequent application, once daily–b.d., should continue indefinitely. When compression garments are worn, application once daily at bedtime minimizes seepage into the garment.

2 The choice of emollient depends mainly on the condition of the skin.

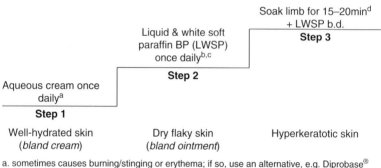

a. sometimes causes burning/stinging or erythema; if so, use an alternative, e.g. Diprobase®
b. ointments are generally not necessary for more than a few days
c. some people prefer coconut oil BP because it has a skin-cooling effect; use the plain variety because added fragrance occasionally causes allergic dermatitis
d. after soaking in a bucket of warm water (to which 15–20mL of LWSP has been added) and after drying the limb, apply LWSP using a circular motion; this helps lift off hyperkeratotic skin.

3 Other options for hyperkeratotic skin:
- use a jacuzzi or shower spray to penetrate into the crevices
- to reduce bacterial and fungal colonization in the crevices, add potassium permanganate tablets or granules to a bucket of warm water, sufficient to achieve a rose wine colour; in practice, it is easier initially to make a concentrated solution in a disposable cup and then add that to the bucket of water (note: potassium permanganate stains skin and material brown)
- if culture of a skin swab indicates superficial infection with *Pseudomonas*, add vinegar 10mL per litre of water; saturate some gauze and apply a double layer for 10 minutes to the affected area
- if there is fungal infection, apply terbinafine cream once daily for 2 weeks to the affected areas.

continued

4 For areas resistant to treatment, consider applying LWSP and covering with a hydrocolloid dressing (Comfeel®, Granuflex®) for 2 days and then soak, etc.

5 Ointments can cause folliculitis if massaged into the hair follicles; the likelihood of this is reduced by applying the ointment in the direction of hair growth.

6 Avoid the use of emollients which:
- are strongly scented (can cause allergic dermatitis)
- are expensive, e.g. E45®cream (costs several times more than aqueous cream BP).

7 Soap should not be used because it dries the skin; use aqueous cream as a soap substitute, but note that this tends to make the bath or shower surfaces slippery.

8 Use an emollient liquid bath additive, e.g. Balneum®(soya), or Oilatum®(light liquid paraffin).

Risk factors for infection include cracked or macerated interdigital skin, contact dermatitis, limb wounds (including leg ulcers), and weeping lymphangiectasia (leaking lymph blisters on the skin surface). Fungal infection between the toes is common, e.g. Tinea pedis (Athlete's foot), and should be treated with an appropriate antifungal agent (e.g. terbinafine cream once daily–b.d. for 2 weeks).

A bland emollient (moisturizer) should be applied daily to prevent drying and cracking, e.g. aqueous cream BP, Diprobase®. However, when used as a topical application (in contrast to its use as a soap substitute), aqueous cream may cause burning/stinging ± erythema.[13] If the skin is flaky or scaly, additional topical measures may be necessary.

Non-drug treatment
Positioning
Keeping the affected limb elevated as much as possible reduces venous hypertension and enhances drainage of the venous and lymphatic systems, thereby reducing swelling. Maximum benefit is achieved by elevation to the level of the heart. Arms should not be raised above 90% because further elevation reduces the space between the clavicle and the first rib, and may obstruct venous return.

In ambulant patients with arm oedema, avoid the use of a sling as much as possible because it tends to cause pooling of fluid at the elbow and stiffness of the elbow and shoulder joints.[14] However, in ambulant patients with gross arm oedema and weakness from brachial plexopathy, a broad arm sling (e.g. Lancaster® sling) to take the weight off the shoulder and neck and distribute it across the back provides comfort, and may also improve mobility by improving balance. Do not use a collar and cuff sling; it does not provide enough support and tends to act as a tourniquet.

When the patient is not ambulant, the sling should be removed and the full length of the arm supported, preferably with some elevation. Patients often benefit by placing the arm in specially made foam supports so that the limb, including the hand, is fully supported in a horizontal position.[15]

Similarly, elevation of the legs with support is comforting to patients with lymphoedema of the legs. The patient's back also needs to be well supported to prevent back pain, possibly by using a reclining chair. In very ill patients, swollen limbs should be supported with pillows to provide comfort.

Containment

Decongestive Lymphoedema Therapy (DLT)[11] and Manual Lymphatic Drainage (MLD)[16] have little place in the management of a swollen limb in advanced cancer. However, a wrapping or compression garment to help prevent (or 'contain') further swelling of limb is still important for many patients.

Unlike containment measures in patients with peripheral vascular disease and ulceration, in patients with lymphoedema there is little value in determining the ankle-brachial pressure index (ABPI). It may well be impossible to obtain a reading at the ankle, and the validity of measurements in the presence of gross oedema has not been confirmed.[17]

In practice, particularly in palliative care, an appropriate wrapping or compression garment should be applied on a trial basis:
• if the limb shape is still fairly normal and the patient is ambulant, apply a short-stretch bandage or an elastic low compression garment (Table 10.1)[2].
• if the limb is misshapen and the patient is ambulant, use a single layer of Shaped Tubigrip®
• if the limb is misshapen and the patient is immobile, apply a light support bandage daily (e.g. crepe) which is neither short-stretch nor elasticated.[18]

Table 10.1 Compression garments classification (mmHg)[19]

	Low	Medium	High	Very high
Upper limb	14–18	20–25	25–30	–
Lower limb	14–21	23–32	34–46	49–70

It is important to ensure that Shaped Tubigrip® does not form ridges or roll down the limb and act as a tourniquet, thereby exacerbating the swelling and increasing discomfort. Shaped Tubigrip® is often uncomfortable if the foot or hand is very swollen; *it should not be used if the digits are swollen*. If the wrapping causes pain, it should be removed and replaced by something which exerts less pressure (Table 10.1).

Compression garments should fit snugly around the limb to prevent:
• a tourniquet effect if too tight, particularly if there are deep skin folds or crevices
• the collection of fluid if too loose.

Garments are worn all day and removed at night. It is worth spending time finding a suitable garment because a patient will not wear it unless it is comfortable.

Modern garments are lightweight, extremely strong and machine washable. Most sleeves last 3 months, and stockings for 4–6 months. Garments can have their life extended if allowed to 'rest' for a week every month; in this way they regain some elasticity.

In patients with swelling of the fingers, a compression glove should be worn. Leotard or bodice-style garments are available for patients with lymphoedema affecting part of the torso, but these are generally not ideal for patients with advanced cancer. Some women benefit from custom-made bras. For men, a scrotal support can be used when indicated.[20] Compression garments do not fit comfortably on awkwardly shaped limbs; padding and bandaging may need to be used instead.[21]

In patients with fungating breast cancer affecting the axilla or chest wall, the application of pressure to the adjacent swollen arm may improve lymph drainage from the arm and increase the load on the neighbouring superficial lymphatics around the shoulder and chest wall. With damaged lymphatics exposed to the surface in fungating tumours, increased flow will result in increased leakage. In these circumstances, it may still be appropriate to use containment to relieve symptoms but the patient should be warned that the discharge from the chest wall or axilla may increase. In addition, the district nurse should be advised that the dressings may need to be changed more than once daily, at least in the short-term.

In advanced pelvic malignancy with bilateral leg swelling and genital and truncal oedema, compression of the legs may increase truncal and genital swelling. Compression garments can be used to provide support to the genitalia, e.g. support tights, maternity garments (panty girdles), cycling shorts.

Exercise
The skin is so designed that the health of the outer 0.3mm of its surface (mainly the epidermis) is maintained by low amplitude body movements.[22] These are the kind of movements which occur during normal activity, e.g. blinking, yawning, stretching, walking. Yawning, stretching and abdominal breathing all alter the intrathoracic pressure and help to empty the thoracic and abdominal lymphatics. Walking and other limb movements help to empty the peripheral lymphatics. Static activity, e.g. carrying a heavy object for more than a few metres, should be discouraged because it reduces both venous and lymphatic return.

Movement of the skin also helps the superficial non-contractile initial lymphatics to empty into the deeper muscular contractile collecting lymphatics. Normal use of the affected limb and gentle active movements should be encouraged. On the other hand, vigorous exercise damages the superficial fine vasculature with consequential overload of the lymphatics and should be avoided.

Specific exercises should be carefully tailored to the patient's abilities and general condition:
- joints are put through a full range of movements to maintain, and possibly improve, function
- limb muscles are used to improve lymph drainage
- fibrosis may be disrupted.

If active exercises are impossible, passive exercises should be carried out at least b.d. Passive movements of a swollen limb (including hand and fingers or feet and toes) in a severely ill, bedbound patient can reduce stiffness and discomfort. In more active patients, exercise may maintain rather than improve function. A complex exercise regimen is inappropriate in advanced cancer.[23]

To enable patients to continue to function as normally as possible with severely swollen limbs, various appliances may be helpful, e.g.:
- aids for walking and dressing for those with swollen legs
- special cutlery, tin openers, scissors, etc. for those with swollen hands and arms.

Massage
Massage of the skin with associated deep breathing is an important component of lymphoedema management. It is the only way of reducing truncal lymphoedema but is not possible in areas of cutaneous metastasis, e.g. en cuirass spread in breast cancer.

Specialized forms of massage are used in lymphoedema clinics.[24,25] These are generally inappropriate in patients with a short prognosis; instead a more straightforward form of self-massage should be encouraged. 'Self-massage' includes massage by a relative, close friend or carer.

When contained by a bandage or compression garment, limb movements automatically massage the limb. Self-massage is therefore confined to the trunk. It is appropriate even if there is no detectable truncal oedema because it clears the abdominal and thoracic lymphatics, and thus facilitates the movement of lymph from the limbs into the empty truncal lymphatics. Truncal massage takes about 20min. The following points should be noted:

- the patient should lie in a comfortable position with the head supported with a pillow or cushion but leaving the neck free
- hands should be clean and dry if they are to move the skin effectively (use non-scented talcum powder if sweaty); always keep the hands in contact with the skin
- movements should be light, slow and rhythmic; the hands, fingers and wrists are kept straight with the movement coming from the arms and body
- use only enough pressure to move the skin over the underlying tissue; massage should not cause any reddening of the skin or discomfort to the patient
- the neck should always be massaged first, i.e. empty the neck lymphatics into the venous system via the thoracic duct
- in unilateral limb oedema, the contralateral upper half of the trunk is massaged next, followed by the ipsilateral side before proceeding to the lower half
- the area adjacent to a lymphoedematous limb is massaged last
- as well as a practical demonstration, the patient should be given written instructions (Box 10.D and Figure 10.1; Box 10.E and Figure 10.2).

Deep abdominal breathing is an important part of the massage. To help the patient do this effectively, ask the patient to bend their knees and then:

- place your flat hand in the centre of their abdomen to offer a little resistance
- ask the patient to inhale so that their abdomen balloons out, and pushes against your hand
- ask them to exhale and let your hand sink
- ask them to inhale again and repeat several times.

Pneumatic compression

Guidelines: Pneumatic compression therapy, p.311.

In advanced cancer, pneumatic compression may soften a hard oedema and ease discomfort. There is a risk of increasing truncal or genital oedema if used alone. Care should also be taken if the patient has a history of CHF, or has impaired sensation. The following are absolute contra-indications:

- extensive cutaneous metastases around the upper arm and shoulder, or upper thigh and groin
- infection (it is too painful)
- recent venous thrombosis (may dislodge thrombus).

Trunk oedema is a relative contra-indication because fluid in the limb is pushed from the limb into an already congested area.

Pneumatic compression is particularly useful in non-obstructive leg oedema:

- lymphovenous stasis:
  ▷ immobility
  ▷ venous incompence
- hypo-albuminaemia.

Pneumatic compression therapy is less helpful in chronic lymphoedema.[26]

Box 10.D Self-massage for arm lymphoedema: advice to patients

Recline comfortably but, before starting the session, make sure that the hands and the area to be massaged are free of oils and creams so as to allow good contact between the hand and the skin.

The hand moves the skin over the underlying tissues:
- if you just glide over the surface of the skin, you are not being firm enough
- if the skin reddens, you are being too firm.

The massage is slow and gentle with the hand moving the skin in semicircles away from the affected arm, and then allowing the elasticity of the skin to return the hand to the starting position.

Both sides of the neck below the ears are massaged for 2 minutes using a slow circular motion (Figure 10.1a).

Massage the hollows above the collar bones for 1 minute.

Place the hand of your unaffected arm behind your head and massage the unaffected axilla for 1 minute (Figure 10.1b).

Starting close to the unaffected arm (Figure 10.1c), massage across the chest towards the swollen arm, changing hands when you cross the midline (Figure 10.1d); this takes 5–10 minutes. Finish by massaging over the affected shoulder.

If someone can help you, ask them to do the same across the upper back starting close to the unaffected arm, moving across towards the swollen arm; this takes 5–10 minutes.

Finish with abdominal breathing to clear the deep lymphatic channels. Place both hands in the gap between your ribs (Figure 10.1e). Without arching the back, breathe in slowly and deeply. You should feel your fingers rise as your abdomen expands. Count '1 and 2', then breathe out slowly. Repeat 4 times, then relax for a few minutes before getting up.

Pneumatic compression consists of an inflatable sleeve connected to a motor driven air pump. The limb is inserted into the sleeve which inflates and deflates cyclically. A multichamber sequential intermittent pneumatic compression pump is preferable. A compression pump used on low pressure, i.e. 20–30mmHg, can help by massaging the legs.

Various makes and models are available, e.g. Centromed®, Flowtron®, Lymphapress®, Jobst®, Talley®, ranging from small portable pumps with a single chamber sleeve to larger models with multichamber sleeves which inflate and deflate sequentially. The smaller models generally operate on a predetermined inflation/deflation cycle whereas the larger models offer a selection of cycle times. The machines have a pressure dial which may range from 20mmHg to as high as 300mmHg.

The ripple effect of a multichamber sequential pump is more effective at shifting fluid than the simple squeezing effect of single chamber pumps. Single chamber pneumatic compression has no direct effect on lymph flow; it simply forces fluid out of the limb via tissue planes and veins. The sequential action of multichamber pneumatic compression may also help to disrupt tissue fibrosis.

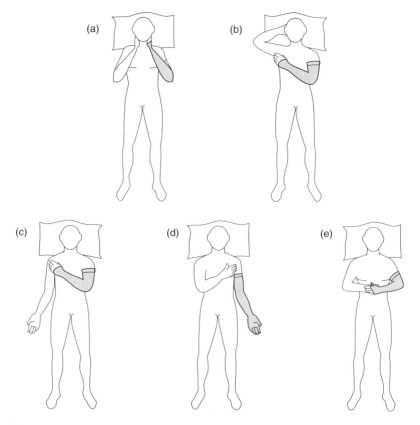

Figure 10.1 Self-massage for arm lymphoedema.

Compression pumps can be used for as many hours as is practical but most patients will not cope with more than about 4h/day.[26] In non-obstructive oedema, treatment overnight may be the best way of achieving a rapid result.[27]

Allow the patient to find the highest comfortable pressure; this may be only 20–30mmHg but could be 40–60mmHg. Pressures higher than this may result in the obstruction of blood flow, increased venous leakage and increased lymph production. Particularly with single chamber pumps, high pressure may lead to oxygen deprivation and, if prolonged, this may cause nerve damage.[28,29]

A containment garment should be used between treatments to prevent the over-stretched tissues rapidly refilling. Use a low pressure garment, e.g. Shaped Tubigrip®.

Remember:
- do not apply pneumatic compression for 6 weeks after a venous thrombosis
- generally do not use pressures higher than 30–40mmHg
- fit compression garments, Shaped Tubigrip® or support bandages to the limb between treatments
- monitor closely, particularly initially.

> **Box 10.E**   Self-massage for leg lymphoedema: advice to patients
>
> Recline comfortably but, before starting the session, make sure that the hands and the area to be massaged are free of oils and creams so as to allow good contact between the hand and the skin.
>
> The hand moves the skin over the underlying tissues:
> * if you just glide over the surface of the skin, you are not being firm enough
> * if the skin reddens, you are being too firm.
>
> The massage is slow and gentle with the hand moving the skin in semicircles away from the affected leg, and then allowing the elasticity of the skin to return the hand to the starting position.
>
> Both sides of the neck below the ears are massaged for 2 minutes using a slow circular motion (Figure 10.2a).
>
> Place the hand of one arm, behind your head and massage the lymph glands under the arm in the same way for 1 minute; repeat with the other arm (Figure 10.2b).
>
> Massage your chest on the side of the unaffected leg, starting from below the collar bone and progressing down to the groin (Figure 10.2c); this takes 5–10 minutes.
>
> The lymph glands in the groin of the unaffected leg are massaged for 1 minute. Repeat on the affected side.
>
> If someone can help you, ask them to do the same on the upper back, progressing downwards; this takes 10–15 minutes.
>
> Finish with abdominal breathing to clear the deep lymphatic channels. Place both hands in the gap between your ribs (Figure 10.2d). Without arching the back, breathe in slowly and deeply. You should feel your fingers rise as your abdomen expands. Count '1 and 2', then breathe out slowly. Repeat 4 times, then relax for a few minutes before getting up.

Drug treatment
Chemotherapy
Palliative chemotherapy should be considered for cancers which may be chemo-sensitive, e.g. breast, lymphoma.

Analgesics
For more information, see *PCF3*.

Analgesics should be prescribed for pain associated with lymphoedema in advanced cancer. Because of a reported association between skin infections, NSAIDs and necrotizing fasciitis, paracetamol and opioids are the preferred analgesics.[30] If analgesics are of little benefit, review and optimize non-drug measures; e.g. resting the arm in a well-supported position. This generally provides significant relief.

Corticosteroids
For more information, see *PCF3*.

If lymphoedema is associated with cancer infiltrating regional lymph nodes, a trial of dexamethasone 8–12mg once daily for 1 week should be considered. By reducing peritumour inflammation, lymphatic obstruction may be reduced. If the swelling

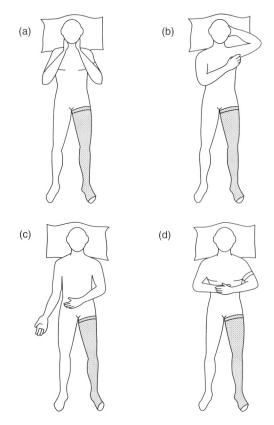

Figure 10.2 Self-massage for leg lymphoedema.

improves, dexamethasone 2–4mg once daily can be continued indefinitely. Occasionally, in breast and prostate cancer or lymphoma, corticosteroids have a more specific anticancer effect.

Diuretics

Diuretics are *not* of value in lymphoedema unless:

* the swelling has developed or increased since the prescription of an NSAID or a corticosteroid
* there is a cardiac or venous component.

In these circumstances, prescribe furosemide 20–40mg once daily for 1 week initially; the dose is then adjusted according to response.

Guidelines: Pneumatic compression therapy

Intermittent pneumatic compression is used mainly *for leg swelling other than lymphoedema*; it must be medically prescribed and monitored. For use in lymphoedema, seek the advice of your local Lymphoedema Clinic.

1 Centromed Macro pptt®(10 chambers) sequential compression pump can operate three compression garments simultaneously, e.g. two stockings and one abdominal girdle:
   - fixed options for treatment duration: 20, 30, 60 minutes or continuous
   - cycle time: 40, 60 or 120 seconds (*normally 60*)
   - pressure: variable.

2 Explain the procedure to the patient:
   - advise the patient to empty their bladder
   - ensure that the patient is in a comfortable lying position with the affected limb supported
   - during treatment the patient should wear Tubifast® (cylindrical cotton bandage) or pyjama trousers or light-weight trousers.

3 External compression should be maintained between treatments during the day, using Shaped Tubigrip® or compression garments; the foot of the bed should be elevated at night.

4 First session: pressure 20–30mmHg for 30 minutes on the swollen leg(s); use the session to familiarize the patient with the multichamber stockings and pump, and to make sure that the treatment is comfortable.

5 Subsequent sessions: pressure 40mmHg for 60 minutes b.d. on the swollen leg(s), but not all patients can tolerate this.

6 If the limb size does not reduce, consider increasing pressure to 60mmHg for 1–2 hours t.d.s.; overnight is also a possibility.

7 Hygiene: the inflatable garments should be cleaned with disinfectant wipes between use by different patients.

8 Stop the treatment and contact a doctor:
   - if the patient becomes breathless when using the pump
   - if the limb becomes red, hot or painful.

9 Reconsider if swelling develops around:
   - the shoulder or chest wall (with arm oedema)
   - the groin, genitalia or buttock (with leg oedema).

10 Monitor progress by making circumferential limb measurements before starting the treatment and then once or twice a week using three fixed points, e.g.:
   - 10cm proximal to the base of the nail of the big toe
   - 30cm above the base of the heel (inner aspect)
   - 60cm above the base of the heel (inner aspect).
   It is not necessary to measure limb volume.

MANAGEMENT OF COMPLICATIONS

Cellulitis/AIEs

Guidelines: Cellulitis/acute inflammatory episodes (AIEs) in lymphoedema, p.314.

AIEs are common in lymphoedema, and must be treated promptly with antibacterials to limit morbidity from increased swelling and accelerated fibrosis. Unlike cellulitis in a non-lymphoedematous limb (typically caused by *Staphylococcus aureus*), most AIEs are probably caused by Group A *Streptococcus*.[31–34] Some patients recall an accidental skin puncture, e.g. a gardening injury or an insect bite, which preceded the attack but most do not.

Because the presentation varies considerably, the diagnosis may be missed. In practice, AIEs are classified as either mild or severe:

- *mild*: pain, increased swelling and (often) blotchy erythema
- *severe*: increased swelling, extensive well-defined erythema, with blistering and weeping skin.

The skin redness varies from multifocal inflamed spots to confluent erythema. Pain may occur without obvious inflammation and constitutional upset may be minimal. Sometimes the condition 'grumbles' in a chronic manner for weeks and a firm diagnosis is made only with recovery after prolonged antibacterial treatment.

A severe AIE is often accompanied by pain, malaise, fever, rigors, headache, nausea and vomiting, and sometimes delirium. When the leg is affected, there may also be difficulty in walking.[33] Prompt treatment with antibacterials is required. If there is a significant constitutional upset, bed rest and limb elevation are crucial in addition to IV antibacterials.

AIEs tend to recur. The interval between episodes may be several months or just a few weeks. With each attack, a stepwise deterioration in the lymphoedema occurs as a result of fibrosis and further damage to lymphatics.

Treatment of AIEs

Antibacterial treatment should be based on the supposition that the AIE is caused by Group A *Streptococcus*, even though in practice it is often impossible to isolate the responsible pathogen. The advice of the British Lymphology Society/Lymphoedema Support Network (www.thebls.com) is summarized in Table 10.2. Because of variation in local antibacterial policies, alternative antibacterials may have to be used. Where this is the case, it is crucial that the policy makers are aware that the likely infective agent is *Streptococcus* and not *Staphylococcus*.[35]

The advice of a microbiologist should be obtained in unusual circumstances, e.g. an AIE developing shortly after an animal lick or bite, and when the inflammation fails to respond to the recommended antibacterials. Because lymphoedema is stagnant, treatment should be for a minimum of 2 weeks.

With patients who have repeated episodes of infection, long-term prophylaxis is the best way of preventing recurrent attacks and minimizing fibrosis secondary to infection.

AIEs are painful: analgesics should be prescribed regularly and p.r.n. Because of a possible association between skin infections (particularly *Streptococcal*), NSAIDs and necrotizing fasciitis, the preferred analgesics are paracetamol and opioids.[36–38]

Table 10.2 Antibacterials for AIEs[a]

Situation	First-line antibacterial	If allergic to penicillin	Second-line antibacterial	Comment
Acute AIE + septicaemia (inpatient admission)	Amoxicillin 2g IV q8h[b] or benzylpenicillin 1.2–2.4g IV q6h[c]	Clindamycin 600mg IV q6h[39]	Clindamycin 600mg IV q6h (if poor or no response by 48h)	Switch to amoxicillin 500mg q8h or clindamycin 300mg q6h when: • temperature down for 48h • inflammation much resolved • falling CRP Then continue as below
Acute AIE (home care)	Amoxicillin 500mg q8h[d]	Clindamycin 300mg q6h	Clindamycin 300mg q6h; if fails to resolve, convert to IV regimen in row 1 above	Give for a minimum of 2 weeks. Continue antibacterials until the acute inflammation has completely resolved; this may take 1–2 months
Prophylaxis if 2+ AIEs per year	Phenoxymethylpenicillin 500mg once daily (1g if weight >75kg)	Erythromycin or clarithromycin 250mg once daily	Clindamycin 150mg or clarithromycin 250mg once daily	After 1 year, halve the dose of phenoxymethylpenicillin; if an AIE develops after discontinuation, treat the acute episode and then commence life-long prophylaxis
Emergency supply of antibacterials 'in case of need' (when away from home)	Amoxicillin 500mg q8h	Clindamycin 300mg q6h	If fails to resolve, or constitutional symptoms develop, convert to IV regimen as in row 1 above	

a. PO unless stated otherwise
b. amoxicillin is associated with Clostridium difficile enteritis, and its use is discouraged in some centres
c. if the anogenital region is involved, add gentamicin 5mg/kg IV once daily for 1 week, dose adjusted according to renal function
d. if Staphylococcus aureus infection suspected (folliculitis, pus formation, crusted dermatitis), add flucloxacillin 500mg q6h.

Guidelines: Cellulitis/acute inflammatory episodes (AIEs) in lymphoedema

Cellulitis/AIEs are common in lymphoedema. If severe, they are associated with septicaemia (e.g. fever, flu-like symptoms, hypotension, tachycardia, delirium, nausea and vomiting). It is often difficult to identify the infective agent, but *Streptococcus* is the mostly likely pathogen.

Evaluation

1 Clinical features
  • mild: pain, increased swelling, erythema (well-defined or blotchy)
  • severe: extensive erythema with well-defined margins, increased swelling, blistering and weeping skin; often accompanied by fever, nausea and vomiting, pain and, when the leg is affected, difficulty in walking.

2 Diagnosis is based on pattern recognition and clinical judgement. The following information should be solicited:
  • present history: date of onset, precipitating factor (e.g. insect bite or trauma), treatment received to date
  • past history: details of previous AIEs, precipitating factors, antibacterials taken
  • examination: include sites of lymphatic drainage to and from inflamed area.

3 Establish a baseline
  • extent and severity of rash: if well demarcated, outline with pen and date
  • level of systemic upset: temperature, pulse, BP, CRP, WBC
  • swab cuts or breaks in skin for microbiology before starting antibacterials.

4 Arrange admission to hospital for patients with septicaemia or who deteriorate or fail to improve despite antibacterials.

Antibacterials

5 To prevent increased swelling and accelerated fibrosis, AIEs should be treated promptly with antibacterials for at least 2 weeks on the supposition that the AIE is caused by Group A *Streptococcus* and not *Staphylococcus*. Continue antibacterials until the acute inflammation has completely resolved; this may take 1–2 months.

6 The advice of a microbiologist should be obtained in unusual circumstances, e.g. an AIE developing shortly after an animal bite, and when the inflammation fails to respond to the recommended antibacterials.

7 Standard treatment at home (PO):

		Admit to hospital
		Step 3
	Clindamycin 300mg q6h PO for 2+ weeks	
	Step 2	
Amoxicillin[a] 500mg q8h ± flucloxacillin[b] 500mg q6h PO for 2+ weeks		
Step 1 *Initial treatment*	*Infection not resolving after 48h*	*Infection not resolving after 48h*

a. if a history of penicillin allergy, start on Step 2
b. add if features suggest *Staphylococcus aureus* infection, e.g. folliculitis, pus, crusted dermatitis.

continued

8 Standard treatment in hospital (IV): Choice of antibacterials may vary with local policy. The following are the recommendations of the British Lymphology Society and Lymphoedema Support Network. Switch to PO amoxicillin or clindamycin when no fever for 2 days, inflammation settling and CRP falling (see 7 above).

Consult microbiologist

		Step 3
	IV Clindamycin 600mg q6h	
	Step 2	
IV Amoxicillin[a,b] 2g q8h		
Step 1		
Initial treatment	*Infection not resolving after 48h*	*Infection not resolving after 48h*

a. IV benzylpenicillin 1.2–2.4g q6h is an alternative to IV amoxicillin
b. if a history of penicillin allergy, start on Step 2.

9 If ≥2 AIEs/year, review skin condition and skin care regimen, and consider further steps to reduce limb swelling. Start antibacterial prophylaxis with:
- phenoxymethylpenicillin 500mg (1g in patients >75kg) once daily for 2 years; halve the dose after 1 year if no recurrence
- if allergic to penicillin, erythromycin or clarithromycin 250mg once daily
- if an AIE develops despite antibacterials, switch to clindamycin 150mg or clarithromycin 250mg once daily
- if an AIE develops after discontinuation of antibacterials after 2 years, treat the acute episode, and then commence life-long prophylaxis.

General

10 Remember:
- if severe, bed rest and elevation of the affected limb on pillows is essential
- AIEs are painful; analgesics should be prescribed regularly and p.r.n.
- because of a possible association between skin infections, NSAIDs and necrotizing fasciitis, paracetamol and opioids are the preferred analgesics
- compression garments should not be worn until limb is comfortable
- daily skin hygiene should be continued; washing and gentle drying
- emollients should not be used in the affected area if the skin is broken.

11 Patients should be educated about:
- why they are susceptible to AIEs, i.e. skin crevices harbour bacteria, stagnant fluid, reduced immunity
- the consequence of AIEs, i.e. increased swelling, more fibrosis, decreased response to treatment
- the importance of daily skin care to maintain skin integrity
- reducing risk, e.g. by reducing the swelling, protecting hands when gardening, cleaning cuts, treating fungal infections (terbinafine cream once daily for 2 weeks) and ingrowing toenails
- obtaining prompt medical attention if an AIE occurs
- if a history of AIEs, taking a 2-week supply of amoxicillin 500mg q8h (or clindamycin 300mg q6h) for emergency use when away from home.

Cellulitis/AIEs continued
Note:
- compression garments should not be worn until the limb is comfortable
- daily skin hygiene should be continued; washing and gentle drying
- emollients should not be used in the affected area if the skin is broken
- if severe, bed rest is essential with the affected limb elevated in a comfortable position and supported on pillows.

Ulceration
Ulceration is more a feature of venous and arterial disease.[40] When it occurs in lymphoedema in advanced cancer, it is generally associated with:
- fragile skin and/or skin damage as a result of a poorly fitting compression garment or poorly applied support bandaging
- severe infection with blistering and desquamation
- fungating cutaneous secondaries.

If the skin is thin and fragile, the shearing forces created when putting on an elastic compression garment and taking it off can tear the skin and make matters worse. In this situation, light support is more appropriate, e.g. Shaped Tubigrip®.

With fragile skin, any dressings should be non-adherent, and will need to be soaked off with sterile saline to avoid further skin damage. Haemostatic dressings may be needed to control bleeding (e.g. calcium alginate) or topical adrenaline (epinephrine) solution 1mg/1mL (1 in 1,000) applied when dressings are changed (see Box 7.E, p.236).

Lymphorrhoea
Lymphorrhoea refers to leakage of lymph through the skin surface. If severe, lymphorrhoea can soak through dressings and pool in shoes. It occurs mainly when the skin is thin and fragile. It may also occur in an acute exacerbation when the skin is rapidly stretched. Apart from the discomfort and inconvenience, lymphorrhoea increases the risk of infection. Treatment comprises:
- normal skin care, including emollients
- elevation of the limb to reduce venous hypertension and to increase venous return
- the application of absorbent pads to soak up leakage
- bandaging to apply pressure and thus to minimize further leakage while the skin heals.

Lymphorrhoea generally responds to these measures in a few days. The bandages should be applied round the clock but replaced when they become soaked.

FLUID DRAINAGE

Severe discomfort from a swollen limb can sometimes be eased by draining fluid from the limb. This can be done by inserting needles into the limb and allowing free drainage for several days.[41,42] Such an approach is not new; its use was recorded 2,000 years ago, and again in the late 19th century.[43-45] It has always been a 'last resort' intervention.

Note: inserting needles into a lymphoedematous limb is generally *bad practice*. Fluid drainage should be reserved for patients with advanced cancer who remain distressed despite the appropriate use of the full range of standard approaches.

Fluid drainage is likely to be of greater benefit when the main cause of the swelling is *not* lymphoedema (see Box 10.A, p.297). In one patient with lower limb oedema secondary to hypo-albuminaemia, >30L was drained off in 6 days.[46] With chronic lymphoedema alone, the amount drained off is likely to be much less, e.g. 3–4L over 2–3 days. The main risk is infection (cellulitis/AIE) but this was not a problem in a group of patients who survived for a median of 2 weeks after drainage.[41]

Techniques vary. Some centres use winged needle infusion sets, whereas others prefer plastic cannulas because larger diameter ones are generally more readily available, and they seem to interfere less with mobility. However, in patients already restricted by the gross debility of end-stage disease, mobility is not significantly affected if only 1–2 winged needles are used. The general approach is as follows (Figure 10.3):

- consider the use of local anaesthetic cream (e.g. EMLA®) topically or a local dermal injection of lidocaine 1–2% before the insertion of the needles

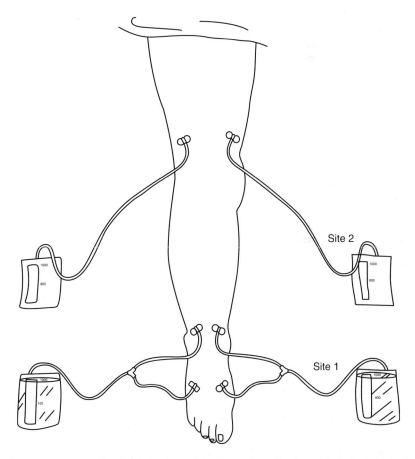

Figure 10.3 Needle placement for SC drainage of swollen lower limb. Reproduced from American Journal of Hospice and Palliative Medicine with permission.[41]

- prepare insertion sites with alcohol wipes
- with the point directed rostrally, place the needles/cannulas in the distal part of the limb, e.g. the foot and/or ankle
- ideally, in chronic obstructive lymphoedema, use a 16G needle, although an 18G may be satisfactory
- unlike SC needle placement for CSCI, the tubing must *not* be looped (a standard precaution against dislodgement); looping creates significant resistance to drainage
- 'reverse wrap' the limb with bandages to encourage efflux, i.e. bandage proximal to distal rather than distal to proximal, but do not bandage over the needles/cannulas.

Also note that:

- drainage is better from dependent legs
- loose wadding placed under the leg(s) may sometimes be preferable to a drainage bag
- SC needles/cannulas have been used to relieve distressing swelling limited to the scrotum and vulva[47,48]
- when the needles/cannulas are removed, fluid will often continue to leak out, and it may help to attach stoma bags over the drainage sites[46]
- to limit leakage, apply pressure with absorbent pads and bandaging (see Lymphorrhoea, p.316)
- in a patient with a prognosis of only a few weeks, subsequent compression with Shaped Tubigrip®, low compression garments or bandaging (see p.304) may prevent gross fluid re-accumulation.

1 Twycross RG et al. (2000) Lymphoedema. Radcliffe Medical Press, Oxford.
2 Lymphoedema Framework (2006) Best Practice for the Management of Lymphoedema. International consensus. MEP Ltd, London.
3 CancerBACUP (2004) Understanding Lymphoedema. British Association of Cancer United Patients, London.
4 Moffatt CJ et al. (2003) Lymphoedema: an underestimated health problem. QJM: Monthly Journal of the Association of Physicians. 96: 731–738.
5 Kissin M et al. (1986) The risk of lymphoedema following treatment of breast cancer. British Journal of Surgery. 73: 580–584.
6 Werngren-Elgstrom M and Lidman D (1994) Lymphoedema of the lower extremities after surgery and radiotherapy for cancer of the cervix. Scandinavian Journal of Plastic Reconstruction and Hand Surgery. 28: 289–293.
7 Bates D et al. (1993) Change in macromolecular composition of interstitial fluid from swollen arms after breast cancer treatment, and its implications. Clinical Science. 86: 737–746.
8 Crockett D (1956) The protein levels of oedema fluids. Lancet. ii: 1179–1182.
9 Brorson H et al. (1999) High content of adipose tissue in chronic arm lymphoedema – an important factor limiting treatment outcome. Lymphology. 32 (suppl): 52–54.
10 Mallon E et al. (1997) Evidence for altered cell-mediated immunity in postmastectomy lymphoedema. The British Journal of Dermatology. 137: 928–933.
11 Ko DS et al. (1998) Effective treatment of lymphedema of the extremities. Archives of Surgery. 133: 452–458.
12 Linnitt N (2000) Skin management in lymphoedema. In: RG Twycross et al. (eds) Lymphoedema. Radcliffe Medical Press, Oxford, pp. 118–129.
13 Cork MJ et al. (2003) An audit of adverse drug reactions to aqueous cream in children with atopic eczema. The Pharmaceutical Journal. 271: 747–748.
14 Badger CMA (1987) Lymphoedema management of patients with advanced cancer. Professional Nurse. 2: 100–102.
15 O'Brien A and Hickey J (1995) Poster. British Lymphogy Interest Group Annual Conference, Oxford.
16 Badger C et al. (2004) Physical therapies for reducing and controlling lymphoedema of the limbs. Cochrane Database of Systematic Reviews. CD003141.
17 Lymphoedema Framework (ed) (2006) Best Practice for the Management of Lymphoedema. International consensus. MEP Ltd, London, p. 12.
18 Crooks S et al. (2007) Palliative bandaging in breast cancer-related arm oedema. Journal of Lymphoedema. 2: 20–54.
19 Lymphoedema Framework (ed) (2006) Best Practice for the Management of Lymphoedema. International consensus. MEP Ltd, London, pp. 44, 46.

20 Lymphoedema Framework (ed) (2006) *Best Practice for the Management of Lymphoedema. International consensus.* MEP Ltd, London, p. 46.

21 Todd J (2000) Containment in the management of lymphoedema. In: RG Twycross *et al.* (eds) *Lymphoedema.* Radcliffe Medical Press, Oxford, pp. 165–202.

22 Ryan T (1998) The skin and its response to movement. *Lymphology.* **31**: 128–129.

23 Hughes K (2000) Exercise and lymphoedema. In: RG Twycross *et al.* (eds) *Lymphoedema.* Radcliffe Medical Press, Oxford, pp. 140–164.

24 Bellhouse S (2000) Self-massage appendix. In: RG Twycross *et al.* (eds) *Lymphoedema.* Radcliffe Medical Press, Oxford, pp. 223–235.

25 Leduc A and Leduc O (2000) Manual lymphatic drainage. In: RG Twycross *et al.* (eds) *Lymphoedema.* Radcliffe Medical Press, Oxford, pp. 203–216.

26 Gray B (1987) Management of limb oedema in advanced cancer. *Nursing Times.* **83**: 39–41.

27 Holt P and Bennett R (1972) Pneumatic stockings to treat 'rheumatic oedema'. *Lancet.* **ii**: 688–689.

28 Rydevik B *et al.* (1981) Effects of graded compression on intraneural blood flow. *The Journal of Hand Surgery.* **6**: 3–12.

29 Ogata K and Naito M (1986) Blood flow of peripheral nerve effects of dissection, stretching and compression. *The Journal of Hand Surgery.* **11**: 10–14.

30 Anonymous (2007) Necrotising fasciitis, dermal infections and NSAIDs: caution. *Prescrire International.* **16**: 17.

31 Sabouraud R (1892) Sur la parasitologie de l'elephantiasis nostras. *Annales de dermatologie et de syphiligraphie.* **3**: 592.

32 Stevens FA (1954) The behavior of local foci causing recurrent streptococcal infections of the skin, subcutaneous tissues, and lymphatics. *Surgery, Gynecology & Obstetrics.* **99**: 268–272.

33 Mortimer P (2000) Acute inflammatory episodes. In: RG Twycross *et al.* (eds) *Lymphoedema.* Radcliffe Medical Press, Oxford, pp. 130–139.

34 Chambers J and McGovern K (2004) Dental work as a cause of acute inflammation of a lymphoedematous limb. *Palliative Medicine.* **18**: 667–668.

35 Badger C *et al.* (2004) Antibiotics/anti-inflammatories for reducing acute inflammatory episodes in lymphoedema of the limbs. *Cochrane Database of Systematic Reviews.* CD003143.

36 Hasham S *et al.* (2005) Necrotising fasciitis. *British Medical Journal.* **330**: 830–833.

37 Malani AK *et al.* (2006) Family history in necrotising fasciitis. *Lancet.* **368**: 1573; author reply 1573.

38 Tillett RL *et al.* (2006) Group A streptococcal necrotising fasciitis masquerading as mastitis. *Lancet.* **368**: 174.

39 Bisno AL and Stevens DL (1996) Streptococcal infections of skin and soft tissues. *The New England Journal of Medicine.* **334**: 240–245.

40 Chant A (1992) Hypothesis: Why venous oedema causes ulcers and lymphoedema does not. *European Journal of Plastic Surgery.* **6**: 427–429.

41 Clein LJ and Pugachev E (2004) Reduction of edema of lower extremities by subcutaneous, controlled drainage: eight cases. *The American Journal of Hospice & Palliative Care.* **21**: 228–232.

42 Faily J *et al.* (2007) The use of subcutaneous drainage for the management of lower extremity edema in cancer patients. *Journal of Palliative Care.* **23**: 185–187.

43 Celsus AC *et al.* (1528) *De re medica, libri octo eruditissimi* Vol 3. J. Secerium, Haganoae.

44 Southey R (1877) Traitment de l'anasarque generale par une drainage capillaire. *Transactions of the Clinical Society of London.* **10**: 152.

45 Fiese MJ and Thayer JM (1950) Value of Southey-Leech tubes in rapid relief of massive edema. *Archivio Di Medicina Interna.* **85**: 132–143.

46 Palliativedrugs.com Bulletin Board. Available from: www.palliativedrugs.com

47 White PD and Monks JP (1933) *Journal of the American Medical Association.* **101**: 1632.

48 Rainford DJ (1970) Southey's tubes and vulval oedema. *British Medical Journal.* **4**: 538.

11: SKIN CARE

PRURITUS

Pruritus is an unpleasant sensation which provokes the desire to scratch (synonym: itch).[1,2] Although limited to skin, conjunctivae or a mucous membrane (including the upper respiratory tract), the cause is not always local. Pruritus is characteristic of dry skin and various skin diseases (e.g. atopic dermatitis, psoriasis), but also occurs in the presence of normal skin.[3]

Histamine is a causal factor (pruritogen) only in pruritus of cutaneous or mucosal origin. A neuro-anatomical classification of pruritus serves to emphasize this (Box 11.A). Antihistamines (H_1-receptor antagonists) have no place in the management of central itch.

Box 11.A A neuro-anatomical classification of pruritus

Peripheral causes
Cutaneous ('pruritoceptive'), e.g.
  skin diseases
  urticaria (most)
  stinging nettle rash
  insect bite reactions
  drug rash
  cutaneous mastocytosis (rare)
Neuropathic, e.g.
  post-herpetic neuralgia

Mixed peripheral and central causes
Uraemia

Central causes
Neuropathic, e.g.
  brain injury[4]
  brain abscess
  brain tumour[5]
  multiple sclerosis
Neurogenic, e.g.
  opioid
  cholestasis
  paraneoplastic
Psychogenic

Neurophysiology

Pruritus is a distinct sensation, even though the neuro-anatomy of pruritus is similar to that of pain.[6] The afferent nerve fibres mediating pruritus are a subset of C-fibres.[7,8] Their terminals are more superficial than the nociceptive C-fibres, close to the junction between the epidermis and the dermis, and they are stimulated by histamine and other pruritogens (Box 11.B). They project to a distinct subset of secondary neurones in the dorsal horn of the spinal cord. The nerve endings mediating pruritus tend to be clustered around discrete 'itch points'.

Box 11.B Chemical mediators of pruritus (pruritogens)

Amines, e.g.
  histamine
  serotonin
Opioids
Eicosanoids[a]
Cytokines
Proteases
Growth factors

Neuropeptides, e.g.
  substance P
  calcitonin-gene-related peptide (CGRP)
  bradykinin
  somatostatin
  vaso-active intestinal polypeptide (VIP)
  cholecystokinin

a. collective term for metabolites of arachidonic acid, including prostanoids and leukotrienes.

Heat-induced vasodilation exacerbates pruritus, whereas cold-induced vasoconstriction reduces it. It is also increased by attention, anxiety and boredom, and decreased by distraction and relaxation.

Histamine

Histamine is the most important chemical mediator of pruritus of *cutaneous* origin. It reproducibly causes itching when applied to damaged skin or injected intradermally. Endogenous histamine released in the skin is mostly from mast cells. In addition to the direct stimulation of neuronal H_1-receptors, histamine probably stimulates the formation of other mediators.[9] However, the response to histamine decreases when it is injected repeatedly at the same site, casting doubt over the role of histamine in chronic pruritus of peripheral origin.[10]

Serotonin

Serotonin/5HT can also cause pruritus,[11] but is a weaker pruritogen than histamine. Pruritus associated with spinal opioids is relieved by $5HT_3$-receptor antagonists.[12,13] Paradoxically, SSRIs (which have a serotonin/5HT *agonistic* effect) relieve pruritus associated with primary biliary cirrhosis[14,15] and paraneoplastic pruritus.[16]

Opioids

Endogenous opioids have a regulatory effect on pruritus and, depending on the circumstances, naloxone can either increase or decrease pruritus.[17] Morphine and other opioids can cause pruritus particularly if given spinally.[18,19] Naltrexone, an oral opioid antagonist, relieves cholestatic pruritus.[20] There is also RCT evidence that methylnaltrexone (a quaternary opioid which does not cross the blood-brain barrier) in a dose of *20mg/kg PO* may be helpful.[21] However, although parenteral methylnaltrexone is now available, PO doses of this magnitude are impractical and would be prohibitively expensive (around £2,000/dose, using multiple 12mg ampoules).

Pruritus associated with spinal opioids may be limited to just the face, affect the lower half of the body, or be even more generalized. It is definitely *not* histamine-mediated; it is a central phenomenon and does not respond to H_1-antihistamines.[22,23] In opioid-naïve patients, pruritus is more common with epidural morphine (about 40%) than epidural hydromorphone (about 10%).[24] Switching from morphine to another opioid generally leads to resolution of morphine-related pruritus.[25] Clinical experience suggests that the incidence of pruritus with opioids by non-spinal routes is uncommon. However, in an RCT in 19 patients, the incidence with IV morphine was 15%.[26]

Pathogenesis

About 10% of the population have dermographia, i.e. an exaggerated 'weal and flare' response to a firm linear stroke across the skin. Such people are more likely to develop a vicious circle of pruritus → scratching → more pruritus → more scratching.

Dry skin is a common cause of pruritus in palliative care patients, and may be associated with the increased expression of cytokines which occurs when the skin's integrity is damaged by cutaneous dehydration.[27,28] Wet macerated skin is also pruritogenic.

Primary skin disease

Pruritus is a common feature of skin disease, e.g.:
- atopic dermatitis
- contact dermatitis (Table 11.1)
- urticaria
- psoriasis
- scabies
- lice (pediculosis).

Table 11.1 Some potential skin allergens to which patients may be exposed

Allergen	Comment
Preservatives (particularly parabens and chlorocresol)[a]	In many creams
Emulsifying agents and ointment bases[a]	In many creams and ointments
Wool fat derivatives (including lanolin)[a]	In many creams and ointments
Topical local anaesthetics	
Neomycin	
Ethyl alcohol	In some preparations and skin wipes
Rubber additives (plasticizers, preservatives)	Undersheets, elastic stockings, etc.
Latex	In latex bladder catheters
Paraphenylenediamine, chromates	In leather
Tea tree oil[29]	

a. section 13.1.3 of the BNF lists potential sensitizers which mainly fall into these categories.

Systemic disease

Pruritus may occur in many systemic conditions (Box 11.C).

Drugs

Most drugs can cause a pruritic rash (Box 11.D).

Box 11.C Systemic disease associated with pruritus[30]

Renal
Chronic renal failure

Hepatic
Primary biliary cirrhosis
Cholestasis
Hepatitis

Haematological
Lymphomas
Leukaemias
Multiple myeloma
Polycythaemia rubra vera
Mastocytosis

Endocrine
Hyperthyroidism
Hypothyroidism
Carcinoid syndrome
Diabetes mellitus (associated
    with genital candidosis)

Other
Cancer
AIDS
Multiple sclerosis

Psychiatric
Psychosis

Box 11.D Common cutaneous drug reactions

Morbilliform drug rashes
Cephalosporins
Penicillins
Phenytoin
Sulphonamides

Urticaria
Cephalosporins
Penicillins
Radio-opaque dyes
Sulphonamides

Toxic epidermal necrolysis
Allopurinol
Carbamazepine
Penicillins
Phenylbutazone
Sulphonamides

Pseudolymphoma
Phenytoin

Multiple causes

Pruritus is sometimes multifactorial (Box 11.E). In patients with renal failure complicated by secondary hyperparathyroidism, correction of hypercalcaemia leads to the rapid relief of pruritus. In other circumstances, hypercalcaemia is not associated with pruritus.

Evaluation

Visual appearance, pattern recognition and probability generally indicate the cause. Contact dermatitis can be caused by many different topical applications. Preservatives and perfumes in an emollient may be the cause, and sometimes lanolin (wool fat).

Scabies can be difficult to diagnose. Both over-diagnosis and under-diagnosis is a problem. In addition to the typical clinical features of interdigital burrows, papules, and excoriation, a positive scraping (yielding microscopic confirmation of the presence of the causal mite) should be regarded as essential for diagnosis.

> **Box 11.E** Causal factors in pruritus
>
> **Old age**
> Dry skin
> Increased mast cell degranulation[31]
> Increased skin sensitivity to histamine[31]
>
> **Paraneoplastic**[a]
> Histamine release from basophils
> Increased release of serotonin
> Immune reaction
>
> **Cholestasis**[a]
> Increased endogenous opioids
> Increased release of serotonin
>
> **Renal failure**[a]
> Cytokines
> Mast cell proliferation
> Increased skin vitamin A
> Altered balance between μ- and
>   κ-opioid receptors
> Increased release of substance P
> Increased skin divalent ions
>   (Ca^{2+}, Mg^{2+}, PO_4^{2-})

a. dry skin is often an important concurrent factor.

Management
Correct the correctable
Most patients with advanced cancer and pruritus have a dry skin. Even when there is a definite endogenous cause, rehydration of the skin may obviate the need for specific measures (see p.329).

Review the patient's medication:
- is the pruritus caused by a drug-induced rash? With oral penicillins, this may not develop until several days after the end of the course of the antibacterial (Box 11.D)
- has an opioid been recently prescribed?

If a drug is the likely cause, it should be stopped if possible.

Scabies is treated with topical permethrin or malathion. Both are toxic, and to treat the whole immediate family (as is good practice) with one of these substances is not entirely risk-free, and should be undertaken only when the diagnosis is 'beyond reasonable doubt'.

Cholestatic pruritus secondary to obstruction of the common bile duct resolves if the jaundice is relieved by inserting an intraductal stent via endoscopic retrograde cholangiopancreatography (ERCP), or other drainage procedure.

Non-drug treatment
Non-drug treatment includes the following measures:
- discourage scratching but allow gentle rubbing
- keep finger nails filed short
- avoid prolonged hot baths
- add 500mg of soda to a late evening bath; the soda reacts with the skin and forms a smooth protective layer which maintains skin hydration for several hours, and in some patients improves sleep by reducing nocturnal pruritus associated with dry skin[32]
- dry the skin gently by 'patting' with a soft towel and/or by using a hair dryer on a cool setting

---

- avoid overheating and sweating; this can be a particular problem at night if a winter duvet is used in the summer or with nocturnal central heating
- increase air humidity in the bedroom to avoid skin drying.

Drug treatment

For more information, see *PCF3*.

Topical

Whenever possible, the treatment of pruritus should be cause-specific.[2] For example:
- scabies → treat patient and the whole family with permethrin or malathion
- atopic dermatitis → topical corticosteroid (+ emollient)
- contact dermatitis → topical corticosteroid, identify causal substance and avoid further contact.

A topical antipruritic can be considered when more specific options have been exhausted, e.g. in the treatment of pruritus of unknown cause. Although it is generally not practical to apply topical products to the whole body, many patients with generalized pruritus have patches of more intense discomfort, and may benefit from more selective application.

Because pruritus is often associated with dry skin, an emollient (moisturizer) should be tried first. Aqueous cream BP often suffices with mild–moderate degrees of dryness. If this is not acceptable to the patient, a proprietary product can be tried instead, e.g. Diprobase® cream. Products containing colloidal oatmeal (e.g. Aveeno®) are popular because of their silky feel.

Traditional topical antipruritics include phenol, menthol and camphor. Phenol acts by anaesthetizing cutaneous nerve endings, whereas menthol and camphor act as counter-irritants. Several topical products which contain these substances are available OTC.[33] The benefit of calamine lotion probably relates to its phenol content.

Generally, emollients and topical antipruritics should be applied after washing in the morning and again in the evening. In areas of skin damage/maceration, a barrier cream may be indicated. If inflamed, 1% hydrocortisone cream may help.

The topical use of antihistamine and local anaesthetic creams should be discouraged because prolonged use may lead to contact dermatitis. If being used and the skin becomes inflamed, discontinue, and apply 1% hydrocortisone cream until the inflammation has settled.

Crotamiton 10% (Eurax®) cream has mild antiscabetic properties but, as an antipruritic, it is no better than placebo.[34]

Systemic

Pruritus is generally worse at bedtime and through the night. A night sedative may well be necessary. A benzodiazepine is generally as effective as a sedative antihistamine.[35] However, anecdotal reports suggest that diazepam given to an alcoholic with pruritus may exacerbate pruritus.

If the skin is inflamed as a result of scratching (but not infected), consider a corticosteroid, e.g. dexamethasone 2–4mg each morning or prednisolone 10–20mg each morning, for 1 week.

Table 11.2 Management of pruritus in non-skin diseases with weight of evidence[a,b]

Condition	Step 1	Step 2	Step 3
Uraemia[c]	UVB phototherapy **A**[41] or capsaicin cream 0.025–0.075% once daily–b.d. (if localized) **A**[42]	Naltrexone 50mg once daily **A**[d,43,44]	Thalidomide 100mg at bedtime **A**[e,45]
Cholestasis[f]	Naltrexone 12.5–250mg once daily **A**[46]	Rifampicin 75–300mg once daily **A**[47] or sertraline 50–100mg once daily **A**[15]	Methyltestosterone 25mg SL once daily (not UK) **C**[48,49] or danazol 200mg once daily–t.d.s. **U**[g]
Lymphoma[h]	Prednisolone 10–20mg t.d.s.	Cimetidine 800mg/24h **A**[50]	Mirtazapine 15–30mg at bedtime **U** or carbamazepine 200mg b.d. **U**
Polycythaemia vera[h]	Aspirin 100–300mg once daily **A**[51]	Paroxetine 5–20mg once daily **A**[52]	Sedative, e.g. benzodiazepine
Spinal opioid-induced pruritus[i]	Give spinal bupivacaine concurrently **A**[53]	Ondansetron 8mg IV stat **A**[13,54]	Switch opioid, e.g. morphine → hydromorphone **B**[24]
Systemic opioid-induced pruritus[j]	Stat dose of H_1-antihistamine, e.g. chlorphenamine 4–12mg; if after 2–3h there is definite benefit, prescribe 4mg t.d.s.; if not, proceed to Step 2 **U**	Switch opioid[k], e.g. morphine → oxycodone **U**[55]	Ondansetron 8mg b.d.

continued

Table 11.2 Continued

Condition	Step 1	Step 2	Step 3
Paraneoplastic pruritus[h]	Paroxetine 5–20mg once daily **A**[16]	Mirtazapine 15–30mg at bedtime **U**	Thalidomide 100mg at bedtime **U**[e] or carbamazepine 200mg b.d. **U**
Other causes or origin unknown	Paroxetine 5–20mg once daily **U**	Mirtazapine 15–30mg at bedtime **U**	Thalidomide 100mg at bedtime **U**[e]

a. weight of evidence based on the system used by the Agency for Healthcare Policy and Research, USA: **A** ≥1 RCT, **B** non-randomized studies, **C** based on expert opinion and consensus reports, **U** unclassified, based on single case reports or small series
b. given PO unless stated otherwise
c. after the haemodialysis regimen has been optimized
d. controlled trials give contradictory results (much benefit vs. no benefit)
e. thalidomide is unlicensed and may cause severe neuropathy if used long-term
f. in total bile duct obstruction, where bile duct stenting is impossible or unwanted
g. androgens may be hepatotoxic and may increase cholestasis while reducing pruritus
h. assuming that anticancer treatment is impossible or unwanted
i. other postoperative options include diclofenac 100mg PR **A**[56] or tenoxicam 20mg IV (not UK) **A**[57], but any benefit may relate to the lower dose of opioid needed when these NSAIDs are given concurrently
j. pruritus after systemic opioids is uncommon, and poorly documented. Although some cases may be caused by cutaneous histamine release[25] and may be self-limiting (see main text), the most distressing cases are long-lasting and antihistamine-resistant[55]
k. methylnaltrexone has been used but the large doses required make it impractical and inordinately expensive.[21]

In *en cuirass* breast cancer complicated by inflammation, local pruritus and pain, an NSAID (a cyclo-oxygenase inhibitor) may reduce both pruritus and pain (tumour-related PGs sensitize nerve endings to pruritogenic substances).[36]

Drugs for pruritus associated with non-skin internal disease include the SSRIs and mirtazapine. However, more specific measures are indicated in specific circumstances (Table 11.2). The inclusion of carbamazepine (or oxcarbazepine) as an option for the treatment of pruritus associated with lymphoma or with cancer is based on its successful use in four patients (three with B-cell lymphoma and one with myeloma).[37] It has also been used with good effect in patients with multiple sclerosis.[38]

With histamine-mediated pruritus, prescribe a sedative antihistamine either just at bedtime or round the clock, depending on need. Either an H_1-receptor antagonist or a phenothiazine with antihistaminic properties can be used:

- chlorphenamine 4mg t.d.s.–12mg q.d.s.; useful for rapid dose escalation to determine if an antihistamine is of benefit
- cetirizine 5mg b.d. or 10mg once daily; a non-sedative antihistamine useful for maintenance treatment
- promethazine 25–50mg b.d.
- hydroxyzine 10–25mg b.d.–t.d.s.; 25–100mg at bedtime
- alimemazine (trimeprazine) 5–10mg b.d.–t.d.s.; 10–30mg at bedtime
- levomepromazine 12.5mg SC; if beneficial convert to 6–25mg PO at bedtime.[39]

Doxepin, a TCA and potent H_1- and H_2-receptor antagonist, is a further alternative. TCAs generally have antihistaminic properties, but none is as potent as doxepin.[40]

DRY SKIN

Rough scaly skin, either fine or coarse (synonym: xerosis).

Pathogenesis
The most superficial layer of the skin (stratum corneum or keratin layer) needs to be hydrated in order to function as a protective layer. Water is held in the layer of oil secreted by sebaceous glands. Dried out keratin contracts and splits, exposing the dermis and forming fine scales which flake off. The exposed dermis becomes inflamed and itchy, possibly as a result of increased cytokine expression.[27,28] Scratching increases inflammation and a vicious circle is created. This is broken by adding moisture and retaining it in a lubricant (emollient), enabling the keratin layer to reconstitute.

Management
Apply an emollient to the skin. The greater the concentration of oil the more wetting power a product has.[58] Aqueous cream once daily or b.d. is generally adequate and generally much cheaper than a proprietary product. However, aqueous cream when applied as an emollient, rather than used as a soap substitute, sometimes causes burning/stinging ± erythema.[59] When this is the case, an alternative such as Diprobase® can be used.

For mobile patients, if the emollient is applied at bedtime, it is fully absorbed before the next morning. An ointment may be needed indefinitely. Other measures include:
- stop using soap
- use a non-detergent soap substitute, e.g. aqueous cream BP
- add an emollient to bath water, e.g. Balneum® bath oil
- wet wrapping of localized pruritic area:
  ▹ apply emollient cream
  ▹ cover with a wet dressing
  ▹ cover wet dressing with a dry dressing.

WET SKIN

Wet skin means maceration, often compounded by blisters, exudate or pus from secondary infection.

Pathogenesis

Because the skin is wet, the epidermal keratin absorbs water, swells and becomes macerated. Once the protective barrier is broken, infection follows, commonly with yeasts and less commonly with *Staphylococcus* and/or *Streptococcus*. The result is inflammation and pruritus.

Maceration occurs particularly where two layers of skin are apposed. For example:
- perineum
- between buttocks } particularly in incontinent bedbound patients
- groins
- under pendulous breasts
- between fingers, particularly if arthritic.

Maceration may also occur around stomas and ulcers if effluent or transudate leaks onto healthy skin for prolonged periods.

Management

The first step is to dry excess moisture:
- pat with a soft towel
- use a hair dryer on a cool setting
- dust carmellose (Orahesive®) powder over the affected area
- apply an aqueous solution topically t.d.s., either alone or as a compress, and allow it to dry out completely:
  ▹ if infected, use an antifungal solution, e.g. clotrimazole 1%
  ▹ if very inflamed, use 1% hydrocortisone solution for 3–4 days.

Be careful with adsorbent powders, e.g. starch, talc, zinc oxide; in excess they can form a hard abrasive coating on the skin. However, the use of a proprietary product such as Ster-Zac® dusting powder is often satisfactory.

Particularly where two areas of skin are apposed, protect with an appropriate barrier:
- a wipe-on protective skin barrier, e.g. CliniShield®, Peri-Prep®; these contain an alcohol and sting if the skin is excoriated
- Cavilon No Sting Barrier Film®; this is sprayed on and does not sting on broken skin

- a barrier cream, e.g. 3M Durable®, Comfeel®, Drapolene®, or ointment, e.g. Morhulin®(zinc oxide 38%)
- a dry piece of linen, cotton, or folded lint to separate the skin surfaces.

Although a barrier cream or ointment is of little value if the excess moisture is caused by sweating, a wipe-on protective skin barrier may help. Barrier creams and ointments should not be used under the breasts or in the groin unless it is to protect the skin from exudate from a local ulcer or from urine.

Monitor for allergic contact dermatitis secondary to topical agents; this may look like the initial problem. Morhulin®, Comfeel® and Drapolene® all contain lanolin.

SKIN CARE DURING RADIOTHERAPY

Guidelines: Advice for radiotherapy patients about skin care, p.332.

In the past, excessively strict advice about skin care was given to patients receiving radiotherapy. Particularly with symptomatic palliative radiotherapy, it is important not to burden patients with unnecessary restrictions but, at the same time, providing them with clear instructions. More detailed advice should be obtained from your local/regional radiotherapy department for patients undergoing more intensive radiotherapy, or who develop a major skin reaction.

SWEATING

Sweat is skin moisture which has been secreted by sweat glands. Sweating (synonyms: diaphoresis, hydrosis) is a normal part of thermoregulation and aids cooling by evaporation from the skin surface.

Sweating also occurs in response to noxious stimuli, fear and embarrassment. In cancer patients, sweating ranges from mild–severe. Severe sweating (hyperhydrosis) necessitates a change of clothing or bedlinen, or both.[60] It can also lead to dehydration.

Physiology
Two types of gland secrete moisture onto the surface of the body:
- apocrine
- eccrine.

Apocrine glands develop at puberty and their ducts empty into hair follicles. They occur in the scalp, axillae, around the nipples and in the anogenital area. Secretions contain proteins and complex carbohydrates, and are under adrenergic control.[61]

Eccrine glands secrete sweat, a watery fluid containing chloride, lactic acid, fatty acids, glycoproteins, mucopolysaccharides and urea, directly onto the skin surface. There are two functionally separate sets of eccrine glands. One set populates the entire skin except the palms and soles and is responsible for thermal regulation; secretion is controlled by muscarinic post-ganglionic sympathetic fibres. The other set is confined to the palms, soles and axillae and is controlled by adrenergic fibres. Those on the palms and soles respond mostly to emotion whereas those in the axillae respond to both heat and emotion.

Guidelines: Advice for radiotherapy patients about skin care

Your treatment may result in some soreness of the skin overlying the part of the body being treated. The risk of this happening should be discussed with your radiotherapy doctor and radiographer, but in most cases skin reactions are mild. They develop some days after starting treatment and may well worsen until the end of treatment. In most cases the reaction heals within 4 weeks.

1 Bath or shower using warm (*not* hot) water for no more than 5 minutes.

2 Do not use soap in the area being irradiated.

3 Pat your skin dry with a soft towel, do not rub it. You may blow-dry your skin with a hairdryer on a cool setting.

4 Dust lightly with baby talc if you like to use powder.

5 Do not put anything else on the skin unless recommended by the radiotherapy staff. Certain products may irritate your skin, so please ask the staff before using anything on the treatment area.

6 Use an electric shaver, not a razor for shaving in the treatment area.

7 Wear loose clothing next to the skin in the treatment area. Underwear made from natural fibres are best, e.g. cotton.

8 Protect your skin from wind, sun and direct heat. You risk making the skin in the treatment area very sore if you expose it to direct sunshine, hot water bottles, electric blankets, etc.

Remember
- always ask for advice if you develop a problem
- it may be necessary to change this general advice in certain situations
- if you have any questions, please ask.

These guidelines may be relaxed when the reaction is diminishing, generally about 2 weeks after finishing treatment. Continue to avoid exposure of treated skin to intense sunlight either by keeping it covered or by using a sun-barrier cream.

Evaporation of secretions occurs constantly from the skin and the mucous membranes of the mouth and respiratory tract. The basal level of 'insensible' water loss is about 50mL/h, i.e. about 1,200mL/24h.[62] The maximum possible secretion from the 3–4 million eccrine glands in the skin is 2–3L/h.[63]

Causes
A high ambient temperature, exercise, emotion and fever are the common causes of sweating. In some patients, sweating is a paraneoplastic phenomenon. It ranges in severity from a mild nuisance to a major symptom with repeated drenching sweats, particularly during the night. Paraneoplastic sweating may or may not be associated with a remittent temperature. Several hypotheses have been adopted to explain the phenomenon:
- the release of pyrogens as a result of leucocyte infiltration or tumour necrosis
- a substance released by the tumour which acts either directly on the hypothalamus or indirectly via endogenous pyrogens.

The pyrogens then induce a PG cascade which results in sweating ± fever.[63–65]

Drugs are sometimes responsible for sweating, either *ab initio* or by exacerbating a concurrent cause:
- alcohol (vasodilation)
- TCAs (paradoxical effect)
- morphine.

Metastatic hepatomegaly and morphine may be a combined risk factor for sweating.

Sweating also occurs at the menopause as a hormone deficiency phenomenon distinct from hot flushes.[66] Sweating occurs in men after chemical or surgical castration.

Management
Correct the correctable
- lower the ambient temperature:
  - ▷ reduce heating
  - ▷ increase ventilation
  - ▷ use fan
  - ▷ use cotton clothing and cotton bed linen (linen aids surface evaporation; duvets can cause patients to become hot and sweaty)
- treat infection with the appropriate antibacterial
- hormone deficiency after castration, prescribe one of the following:
  - ▷ medroxyprogesterone 5–20mg b.d.–q.d.s ⎫
  - ▷ megestrol acetate 20–40mg each morning[67] ⎬ effect manifests
  - ▷ diethylstilbestrol 1mg each morning ⎬ after 2–4 weeks
  - ▷ cyproterone (has weak progestogen activity)[68] ⎬
  - ▷ clonidine 100microgram at bedtime[69] ⎭
- if a TCA or an SSRI is the cause, switch to mirtazapine or venlafaxine
- if morphine is the cause, consider switching to an alternative strong opioid (see p.39).

Non-drug treatment
Bed linen, sleep wear and undergarments manufactured specifically with a high 'wicking' property are available, e.g. from www.dermatherapyfabrics.com, and hiking shops. These do not prevent sweating, but draw the sweat away from the skin to keep patients warm and dry.

Although local treatment with aluminium chloride hexahydrate (axillae) and formalin or gluteraldehyde (feet) are of value in emotional sweating,[70] they are generally irrelevant in advanced cancer. Such treatments work by blocking or destroying sweat glands. Iontophoresis,[71] botulinum toxin and surgical approaches such as undercutting the axillary skin, excision and sympathectomy, are also irrelevant.[72,73]

Drug treatment
For more information, see *PCF3*.

Drug treatment is summarized in Box 11.F.

Box 11.F   Symptomatic drug treatment of paraneoplastic pyrexia and sweating

Begin by prescribing an antipyretic:
- paracetamol 500mg–1g q.d.s. or p.r.n. (generally less toxic than an NSAID)
- NSAID, e.g. ibuprofen 200–400mg t.d.s. or p.r.n. (or the locally preferred alternative).

If the sweating does not respond to an NSAID, prescribe an antimuscarinic:
- amitriptyline 25–50mg at bedtime (may cause sedation, dry mouth and other antimuscarinic effects)
- hyoscine hydrobromide 1mg/3 days TD[74]
- glycopyrronium up to 2mg PO t.d.s.

If an antimuscarinic fails, other options include:
- propranolol 10–20mg b.d.–t.d.s.
- cimetidine 400–800mg b.d.[75]
- olanzapine 5mg b.d.[76]
- thalidomide 100mg at bedtime.[77,78]

Thalidomide is generally seen as the last resort even though the response rate appears to be high.[78] This is because it can cause an irreversible painful peripheral neuropathy, and may also cause drowsiness.

STOMAS

A stoma is an artificial opening in the GI tract, created surgically to divert the flow of faeces and/or urine.[79] About 5% of patients with advanced cancer have one:
- permanent colostomy after resection of the rectum or to palliate incontinence associated with a rectovaginal or rectovesical fistula
- permanent ileostomy after total colectomy or panproctocolectomy
- temporary loop colostomy or ileostomy to divert faeces away from anastomosis or outlet when an obstruction is present
- gastrostomy for venting or feeding
- urostomy (ileal conduit) after cystectomy.

An ileostomy in particular can cause problems. The distal part of an ileostomy may get infected, resulting in an offensive loose watery effluent, and increased flatus. Absorption of some drugs, zinc, and vitamin B_{12} can be disturbed. Vitamin B_{12} absorption will cease completely if an ileostomy excludes the distal 90–120cm of

---

ileum. However, body stores are generally adequate for several years. Long-term metabolic complications of an ileostomy, such as urolithiasis and cholelithiasis, are not seen in advanced cancer because of the short prognosis.

Management
In the UK, a patient with a stoma will receive advice and support from a trained stoma care nurse.[80–82] In some oncology departments and palliative care units other nurses may develop a special interest in stoma care. In the community, district nurses provide much ongoing support.

Stoma care includes:
- psychological support
- choosing the right appliance
- skin care
- dietary advice
- flatus control
- managing stomal complications
- rehabilitation/adaptation.

Psychological support
Psychological preparation *before* the stoma operation is important and is the key to postoperative rehabilitation. Explanation about the use of stomas in various conditions helps the patient to feel less strange and less isolated from 'normal' people. Contact with other stoma patients before and after the stoma operation helps. Several support organizations have been established in the UK, generally run by patients (or former patients) for patients, including:
- Colostomy Association (www.colostomyassociation.org.uk)
- The Ileostomy and Internal Pouch Support Group (www.iasupport.org)
- National Association of Laryngectomee Clubs (www.laryngectomy.org.uk)
- Urostomy Association (www.uagbi.org).

In addition to these national organizations there are self-financing local groups or fellowships for ostomy patients in most counties and the large metropolitan areas.

Choosing the right appliance
Different appliances suit different people. A key decision is whether to use a 1-piece appliance or a 2-piece one. A 2-piece appliance means that, every time the bag is emptied, the skin is not affected because the base of the appliance may well remain unchanged for 2–3 days, or even longer. Some patients find the 2-piece too rigid and prefer the flexibility of a 1-piece.

Skin care
Care of the peristomal skin includes the careful replacement of a new appliance. Mild solvents, e.g. Clear Peel®, Lift Plus®, can be used to reduce discomfort in patients with sensitive skin. Warm water is used to clean the surrounding skin. The skin is dried by placing paper tissues or kitchen roll over the stoma and pressing lightly with an open hand over the stoma and surrounding area. Any residual mucus from the stoma should be dabbed away; if it gets under the flange it reduces the bonding of the adhesive to the skin.

A skin barrier, e.g. Comfeel® barrier cream, may be applied sparingly if the effluent is liquid or if the appliance/flange is being changed more than once daily. It is gently rubbed in and any excess wiped off. A barrier product is also useful around the anus in patients with an anal discharge despite having a defunctioning colostomy.

A template/cutting guide should be used to help prepare the opening for the stoma in the flange of the appliance. This reduces the chance of a poorly fitting appliance and is particularly helpful when several different people are involved in the care of the stoma. All modern appliances have hydrocolloid in the flange which helps to protect the skin. In the UK, patients can receive their own personalized supply precut by the manufacturers.

Serious skin problems are uncommon with modern standards of care and are mainly the result of liquid faeces coming into contact with the skin (Box 11.G). Poorly fitting appliances can lead to 'pancaking', i.e. liquid faeces ooze into a gap between the flange of the appliance and the skin and become trapped there. (But note: because diet affects faecal consistency, dietary modification is likely to be part of the solution; see p.337.)

Box 11.G   Risk factors for peristomal skin problems

Skin-related problems
Poor skin hygiene
Skin reactions
Sweating

Other
Abdominal radiotherapy
Diarrhoea
Poorly fitting appliance

Stoma problems
Herniation
Prolapse
Retraction
Stenosis

If the skin becomes red and sore, there is a reason for it. Steps must be taken immediately to stop fluid leaking onto the skin. The use of a wipe-on skin barrier, e.g. CliniShield®, Peri-Prep®, is often sufficient to allow resolution of early skin changes. Skin wipes may also be used prophylactically. The wipes dry quickly and do not leave a greasy surface.

Because they contain alcohol, wipes should not be applied to excoriated skin; Cavilon No Sting Barrier Film® should be used instead. This is a polymeric solution containing two siloxanes and acrylate copolymer which dries about 30sec after application. The film is colourless, transparent and is permeable to oxygen and moisture vapour, and acts as a barrier against irritation from body fluids, protecting intact or damaged skin from urine and/or faecal incontinence, digestive juices and wound drainage. It also reduces skin damage by adhesives, friction and shear. Cavilon No Sting Barrier Film® can be applied to apposing skin surfaces provided the surfaces are held apart and the coating allowed to dry before the surfaces are in contact again.

When used as a protection against body fluids or incontinence, Cavilon No Sting Barrier Film® should be applied at the time of each stoma-related nursing intervention. If necessary, a 2-piece appliance can be used until the skin has healed; the flange is left in place for 4–5 days before removal, facilitating healing.

To help appliances adhere to moist areas, Orahesive® powder (carmellose, gelatin and pectin) can be dusted onto raw skin. The powder adheres to the raw surface; excess powder is removed by blowing.

If the peristomal skin remains red and sore despite the above measures, this suggests infection. If confirmed, an appropriate local and/or systemic antibacterial should be prescribed.

Dietary advice

After stoma surgery, many patients think they will have to totally change their diet and restrict their food intake. This is not the case, but patients need to be advised about the expected faecal consistency from the stoma, and adapt their diet accordingly.

Most patients with a distal colostomy achieve normal faecal consistency spontaneously or with the help of a hydrophilic bulking agent. Consistency and quantity also depend on diet. With an ileostomy normal faeces are never possible; the aim is an effluent with the consistency of soft porridge.

The average effluent from an ileostomy is about 700mL/24h. Sodium and water loss is only about three times greater than from the faeces of normal subjects. Normal dietary intake can compensate for such losses. However, a high output (>1L/24h) from an ileostomy leads to sodium and water depletion. These can be corrected by prescribing oral rehydration salts, e.g. Diorylate®, Rehidrat® (contain potassium as well as sodium salts).

Other options are Boot's Isotonic® powder (contains no potassium) and Lucozade®. For patients paying their own prescription charges, a home-made rehydration solution is cheaper (Box 11.H).

Box 11.H Home-made rehydration solution: instructions for patients

Make a fresh solution every day:

glucose	6 × flat 5mL spoonfuls	
sodium chloride	1 × flat 5mL spoonful	in 1L of tap water.
sodium bicarbonate	1 × heaped 2.5mL spoonful	

You can buy these from any community pharmacy and some supermarkets.
Sodium chloride is table salt which you have already.
Sodium bicarbonate is also known as bicarbonate of soda.

Output can be reduced with an opioid antidiarrhoeal such as loperamide. Although PO hydrophilic bulking substances do not reduce ileostomy output, adding a sachet of a bulking agent, e.g. Fybogel®, Regulan®, to the ostomy bag makes the effluent firmer and more manageable. Vernagel® sachets, marketed to solidify urine standing in a urine bottle, are even more effective.

If an ostomy patient complains of troublesome diarrhoea:
- review the patient's medication (see Box 3.X, p.122)
- identify foods which increase stoma output and remove them from the diet (Table 11.3 and Table 11.4)
- encourage foods which decrease output (Table 11.3 and Table 11.4)
- recommend marshmallows 5–6 b.d.; these make faeces more solid
- if the diarrhoea persists, culture the faeces for possible infection (likely to be anaerobic which should respond to metronidazole).

Table 11.3   Foods which definitely affect stoma function

Increase output/watery flow	Increase flatus	Increase malodour	Undigested: may block stoma and/or cause pain[a]
Beans	Beans	Beans	Cabbage (raw)
Beer and alcohol	Beer/lager	Brassicas	Carrot (raw)
Fruit juices	Brassicas	Eggs	Celery
Greens	Carbonated drinks	Fish	Coconut
Spicy foods	Chick peas	Garlic	Fibrous fruit and vegetables, e.g. pineapple
	Cucumber	Onion	Fruit skins (raw)
	Dahl		Mushroom
	Garlic		Nuts
	Greens		Potato skins
	Lentils		Raisins
	Onion		Sweetcorn
			Tomato skins and pips

a. these foods in particular must be chewed well.

Table 11.4   Foods which *may* affect stoma function

Increase output/watery flow	Decrease output	Peristomal skin irritation	Increase flatus
Caffeinated beverages	Apple sauce	Citrus fruits and juices	Apricots
Chocolate	Bananas	Coconut	Aubergines
Fruits (raw)	Boiled rice	Nuts	Carrots
Wholegrain cereals	Cheese	Oriental vegetables	Ghee
Wholemeal food	Marshmallows	Some raw fruits and vegetables, e.g. apples, celery, coleslaw, oranges, sweetcorn	Instant coffee
	Noodles		Milk and milk products
	Pasta		Molasses
	Peanut butter		Peppers
	Potatoes		Prunes
	Suet pudding		Red wine
	Tapioca		
	Weetabix® (dry)		
	White bread		

Constipation with a colostomy generally relates to:
• the use of analgesics and other constipating drugs
• an inadequate fluid intake
• a failure to eat a moderately high fibre diet
• immobility

- depression
- obstruction caused by cancer.

If receiving an opioid or other constipating drug, in the first instance recommend oral laxatives. However, digital examination of the colostomy is necessary before proceeding to suppositories or an enema. If indicated, a phosphate enema is almost always effective. With faecal impaction, an oil enema may be necessary first.

Flatus is normal but is influenced by various factors, including diet. If problematic, discussion about foods, fluids and eating habits which increase the volume of flatus may help to reduce the unwanted embarrassment.[83] Habits which contribute to flatulence include:

- rushed eating
- chewing gum
- smoking
- breathlessness
- missing meals
- eating and drinking at the same time
- certain types of foods (Table 11.3 and Table 11.4)
- carbonated drinks.

All 1-piece and 2-piece systems have an integrated charcoal filter which adsorbs flatus and odour. Some appliances contain deodorant pellets. If malodour remains a problem, adding a de-odourizer to the appliance bag is preferable to oral medication, e.g. Atmocol®, Citrus Fresh®, Limone® (Table 11.5). If two puffs of a de-odourizer into the bag are not sufficient, they can also be used as room sprays. However, with such agents there should be no malodour except when the bag is changed.

Table 11.5   Selected agents for odour control in colostomy patients

Formulation	Name
Tablets	Amplex-C®
	Chlorophyll
	Charcoal
	Lactobacillus acidophilus[a]
Capsules	Peppermint oil (Colpermin®, Mintec®)
Spray[b]	Atmocol®
	Citrus Fresh®
	Limone®
	NaturCare®
Liquid[b]	Chironair liquid®
	Forest Breeze oil drops®
	Nilodor®
	Noroma®
Powder[b]	Ostobon®

a. alters the intestinal flora and reduces the number of colonic bacteria
b. put in the appliance bag or, if liquid, it can be put onto a tissue inserted into the bag.

Most so-called de-odourizers are in fact counter-odours. In contrast, NaturCare® is an odourless deodorant. It works in a confined space by chemically denaturing malodourous organic molecules. Because it does not harm normal or damaged skin, NaturCare® can be sprayed around an ostomy appliance or a malodourous wound dressing when it is being changed, and onto the stoma or wound itself, although the benefit of this is questionable.

Managing stomal complications

Following stoma formation > 1/3 of colostomists and > 1/2 of ileostomists and urostomists will experience problems with the management of their stoma.[84] Apart from impaction, management will generally require consultation with a stoma care nurse, and possibly the surgeon who fashioned the stoma (Box 11.1). However, in patients with a very poor prognosis simple supportive measures are all that is appropriate.

Box 11.1 Complications of a stoma		
Retraction	Bleeding	Granulation
Prolapse	Necrosis	Recurrent cancer
Herniation	Perforation	obstruction
Stenosis	Fistula	fungation

Rehabilitation/adaptation

Rehabilitation/adaptation includes addressing issues such as clothing, physical activity, sexual relationships and travel. Close relatives also need an opportunity to talk with nursing and/or medical staff about the stoma. This reduces misunderstandings and increases the likelihood of positive support for the patient from the family.

FISTULAS

A fistula is an abnormal communication between two hollow organs or between a hollow organ and the skin. Most fistulas in advanced cancer develop as a result of postoperative infection and/or radiotherapy. A few are caused solely by disease progression and necrosis.

Rectovaginal and rectovesical fistulas

Management is either conservative or surgical. A colostomy or ileostomy provides complete relief. On the other hand, stomas are not always trouble-free. Because of this or for psychological reasons, some patients prefer not to have surgery.

Enterocutaneous fistulas

Most enterocutaneous fistulas fall into one of three categories:
- simple: a single orifice in an otherwise intact abdominal wall around which the skin is flat and in reasonably good condition
- multiple: multiple orifices in the abdominal wall
- disrupted: a fistula caused by dehiscence of a surgical wound or scar.[85]

Management comprises:
- effluent collection
- monitoring plasma electrolytes
- skin protection
- odour control.

IV hyperalimentation should be considered in patients with a prognosis of >3 months. This prevents malnutrition through loss of nutrients in the effluent and promotes healing. About 50% of enterocutaneous fistulas will close spontaneously, particularly with a defunctioning ileostomy.[86]

Effluent collection
All types of fistula present a major nursing challenge. Management is time-consuming and frequent leakage demoralizes both nurses and patient. A stoma care or tissue viability nurse should be consulted. Acknowledgement by the doctors of the difficulties faced by the patient and the nurses is supportive.

A simple fistula is managed like a stoma. With more complicated fistulas, 1-piece appliances are necessary; 2-piece appliances with hard flanges are unsuitable because they will not lie flat. With multiple fistulas, it may be necessary to use two or more appliances, and/or encompass several openings into a suitable wound manager appliance.

High output fistulas are generally ileocutaneous. The effluent is caustic because of the presence of proteolytic and other enzymes; contact with the skin leads to erythema in <1h and excoriation in 3–4h. Effluent can be reduced by:
- loperamide ≤30mg/24h is useful in low ileal fistulas because it allows more ileal absorption as a result of a prolonged transit time and a pro-absorptive effect; should be taken as a divided dose, ideally about 1h before meals
- hyoscine butylbromide 60–120mg/24h by CSCI, reduces GI secretions[87]
- octreotide 100microgram SC t.d.s. or 250–500microgram/24h by CSCI; reduces GI secretions.[88]

Skin protection
Skin protection is essential. When the appliance is changed, it helps if the fistula can be plugged temporarily[89] or the flow of effluent removed by suctioning. The shape of the orifice is cut out of a sheet of hydrocolloid but, before application, crevices should be filled in with Stomahesive® paste (carmellose, gelatin, pectin, alcohol). If it is necessary to apply the paste in layers, wait for at least 30sec between applications.

The alcohol in Stomahesive® paste stings the raw areas transiently. After applying the paste, the appliance is attached. Alternatively, a Cohesive® seal can be used; this moulds to the contours of the body surface.

Special high output bags are available with an extension bag for use overnight. This enables a patient to sleep through the night without having to worry about overfilling and leakage.

Odour control
If the effluent is faecal there is the added problem of odour. This is embarrassing for the patient, the family and visitors, other patients and staff, and appropriate measures should be introduced (see p.339).

Buccal fistulas

Fistulas can occur between the mouth and the face or neck. In addition to the inevitable psychological distress associated with a visible deformity, buccal fistulas cause problems with leakage of saliva and of ingested fluids. If the fistula is of small diameter, a wad of gauze changed regularly may suffice. Neonatal stoma appliances can sometimes be used and are often acceptable to the patient. It may be helpful to reduce the volume of saliva with an antisecretory drug, e.g. hyoscine butylbromide, octreotide.

With a larger fistula, the use of a silicone foam casting should be considered. Silicone foam is available as Cavicare®. The use of plastic film results in a smoother surface to the casting. If a second casting is made, this can be inserted when the dressing is changed and the first one washed and dried. Silicone foam castings have also been used in the management of enterocutaneous fistulas.[90]

FUNGATING CANCER

Guidelines: Fungating cancer (India), p.344.

A proliferative or cavitating primary or secondary cancer in the skin can lead to ulceration and fungation, and may be associated with:

- stinging, soreness, pain
- pruritus, particularly in breast cancer
- exudate
- malodour (→ nausea)
- bleeding
- infection.

A fungating cancer is distressing to the patient and is repulsive to the carers, family and friends. Malodour can lead to social isolation and despair.

Management

The treatment of pain and bleeding are discussed in the Guidelines (see p.344). Topical morphine is a theoretical option but is not always feasible because of the extent of the ulceration (see p.43). Pruritus is probably caused by inflammatory substances, e.g. PGs, and may respond to an NSAID. Measures for dealing with exudate and infection are the same as those used with decubitus ulcers (see p.346).

However, in the UK, if a broader spectrum antibacterial is indicated because of deep infection or surrounding cellulitis, co-amoxiclav 625mg PO t.d.s. (or 1,200mg IV t.d.s. if severe) for 5–7 days is a good choice. The recommendation in the Guidelines (based on current palliative care practice in India) to use combined ampicillin and cloxacillin capsules is dictated by cost; co-amoxiclav is unaffordable by most of the population.

Malodour

Controlling malodour is often a major challenge. Malodour is caused partly by tumour necrosis and partly by deep anaerobic infection. Treatment options include:

- metronidazole, topical or systemic (see Guidelines, p.344)
- live yoghurt b.d. topically
- manuka honey b.d. topically (e.g. Activon®)

- an occlusive dressing:
  - ▷ film, e.g. Opsite® (totally occlusive)
  - ▷ hydrocolloid, e.g. Granuflex® (almost totally occlusive).

The benefit of charcoal-activated dressings, e.g. Actisorb Silver 220®, is questionable. Manuka honey impregnated dressings are also available, e.g. from Advancis Medical.

Domestic air fresheners are generally unsatisfactory. Even if these mask the malodour, it is often a case of replacing one disgusting odour with another. Fresh air through a wide-open window is the best option. Air filter systems are generally impractical and/or too costly for routine use. Most patients need to be nursed in a single-occupant room.

Oxidizing agents are no longer widely used because of concern for the surrounding healthy tissue. However, occasionally, they may have a part to play, e.g.:
- irrigation with 3% hydrogen peroxide
- packing a deep malignant ulcer with 10–20% benzoyl peroxide (Box 11.J).

Box 11.J   Use of benzoyl peroxide to reduce malodour in deep malignant ulcer

Benzoyl peroxide is a powerful organic oxidizing agent; it often causes an irritant dermatitis and may cause a contact allergic dermatitis.

Normal skin surrounding the ulcer must be protected with petroleum jelly or zinc oxide ointment, e.g. Morhulin®.

Surgical gauze soaked with 10–20% benzoyl peroxide should be firmly packed into large cavities and undercut margins.

A dressing is cut from sterile terry towelling to fit the ulcer exactly and saturated with benzoyl peroxide; the terry towelling must not overlap normal skin.

A plastic film is placed over the dressing, e.g. Clingfilm®, and allowed to adhere to the ointment or paste protecting the surrounding normal skin.

An abdominal pad dressing is taped over the plastic film with hypo-allergenic tape, e.g. Hypafix®, Micropore®.

Unless there is excessive exudate, the dressing need be changed only once daily.

The wound surface is cleaned with 0.9% saline at each change of dressing.

Occasionally a patient complains of burning in the ulcer when the new dressing is applied; this subsides within 30min.

Guidelines: Fungating cancer (India)

A proliferative or cavitating primary or secondary cancer in the skin can lead to ulceration and fungation. There may be associated pain, exudate, bleeding, infection and malodour. A fungating cancer generally has a major negative psychological impact on the patient and family. Malodour can cause or exacerbate nausea and anorexia.

Anticancer treatment

1 Discuss possibilities with oncologists (radiotherapy, chemotherapy, hormone therapy, debulking surgery, plastic surgery).

Correct the correctable

2 Antibacterials for anaerobic infection:
  - superficial infection:
    ▷ metronidazole 200mg tablet crushed and applied to the ulcerated area mixed in lubricating gel (e.g. KY jelly®) or 2% lidocaine gel; benefit often noticed within 12h *or*
    ▷ proprietary metronidazole gel 0.75% (75mg/10mL); is more expensive.
  - deep infection:
    ▷ metronidazole 400mg PO q8h for 5 days.
    ▷ the use of broader spectrum antibacterials should be considered when there is cellulitis, systemic upset, or a lack of response to metronidazole alone, e.g. combined ampicillin 250mg and cloxacillin 250mg capsules q6h for 5 days. [In the UK, co-amoxiclav (Augmentin®) would be a more appropriate choice.]

3 Maggots: after preliminary cleansing, use a syringe to sprinkle turpentine directly onto the ulcerated area. The turpentine may cause transient mild–moderate burning pain (<5 minutes). Maggots come up to the surface immediately and should be manually removed. Some maggots may remain, and turpentine should be applied once daily for 2 more days.

4 Mercurochrome 2–4% solution is used at some centres as an alternative to turpentine. However, it causes red discolouration which makes it less acceptable to some patients.

Topical treatment

5 Wound care can be done by doctor, nurse or family:
  - wash hands
  - cleanse ulcerated areas using boiled and cooled tap water
  - apply Gamgee pad or several layers of cotton pads (more if much exudate) and retain in position with a light bandage and/or adhesive tape.

Empowering the family in wound care can give a sense of control to the patient and family, and improve care as a bonus.

continued

6 Control of bleeding:
- apply cotton pads and *gentle* hand pressure (note: firm pressure over a friable tumour may exacerbate bleeding)
- if still bleeding after 10–15 minutes, pour diluted Hemolok® (feracrylum 1% w/w) onto pads and allow to soak in; use 1mL from 10mL ampoule diluted to 100mL; repeat after several hours if still bleeding
- subsequently once daily, apply sucralfate 1g tablet crushed and mixed in lubricating gel (e.g. KY jelly®), and cover with a cotton pad; soak pad with tap water before removing it. Continue indefinitely if bleeding persists.

7 Control of malodour (caused by necrosis and anaerobic infection):
- cleanse and debride the surface
- topical metronidazole (see above)
- counteract the malodour with strong pleasant odours in the patient's living area, e.g. camphor, herbs, incense, lavender.

Systemic treatment

8 If bleeding continues:
- step 1: discontinue any NSAID known to significantly impair platelet function, e.g. ibuprofen, naproxen; instead, prescribe paracetamol or an NSAID which does not exacerbate bleeding, e.g. celecoxib, diclofenac, nabumetone
- step 2: prescribe a haemostatic drug, e.g. etamsylate 500mg t.d.s. for 3 days; continue if helpful.

9 Relieve pain using the WHO 3-step analgesic ladder (but see comment above about NSAIDs). Note also:
- if feasible, apply bupivacaine 0.125% up to 40mL q2h p.r.n. (keep the ulcerated area covered with two layers of gauze, and soak the gauze with bupivacaine).
- if infected, the best analgesic may be metronidazole (see above).

Psychological support

10 Alteration of body image is a distressing association, and may exacerbate social alienation. Open discussion with the patient and the family is often helpful.

11 It is important to answer the question (spoken or unspoken): 'Will it heal, Doctor?' This is never easy, and requires tact and gentleness:

'Our short-term aims are to clean out the maggots and to reduce the smell. Unfortunately, it is unusual for an ulcer like yours to heal completely, if at all. In this respect, we have to wait and see.'

This could be the initial response; a more fundamental need is to address the 'question behind the question', and make use of the opportunity to discuss the diagnosis and prognosis.

DECUBITUS ULCERS

A decubitus ulcer is an ulcer of the skin ± subcutaneous tissue caused by ischaemia secondary to extrinsic pressure and/or shear.

Pathogenesis

Tissue ischaemia is caused by extrinsic pressure if it is greater than capillary pressure, i.e. >25mmHg. Pressure on the skin over the ischial tuberosities when sitting is about 300mmHg. The pressure on the skin when lying on a hospital foam mattress is about 160mm.[91] Pressure for periods as short as 1–2h may produce irreversible cellular changes leading to cell death. This occurs particularly over bony prominences (Box 11.K).

Box 11.K   Sites of decubitus ulcers in terminally ill patients

Major	**Minor**
Ear	Occiput
Spine	Mastoid
Sacrum	Acromion
Greater trochanter	Spine of scapula
Head of fibula	Lateral condyle of humerus
Malleolus	Ischial tuberosity
	Knees

Many other factors make tissue ischaemia more likely, e.g.:
- emaciation
- anaemia
- skin fragility
- incontinence
- immobility
- old age.

Chemotherapy, high-dose coticosteroids and NSAIDs are considered additional risk factors.[92]

Prevention

A scoring system, e.g. Hunter's Hill and Waterlow risk assessment cards, helps by reminding carers of the need to introduce specific preventive measures in high-risk patients.[92,93] However, some decubitus ulcers are inevitable in terminally ill patients. Further, patient comfort is paramount and there must be flexibility rather than rigid adherence to a nursing protocol.

Pressure redistribution

Mattresses vary in their pressure reducing properties (Table 11.6).

Feather pillows can reduce pressure considerably. In countries where airbeds are not readily available, consider using a camping mattress filled with water (Box 11.L); this reduces pressure more than a standard foam mattress. Carefully laundered natural sheepskin also helps but is now rarely used in the UK.

Table 11.6 Hospital mattresses in descending order of skin surface pressures

Type	Example
Foam (most skin pressure)	Standard hospital mattress (UK)
Profiled foam	Cyclone[®]
Foam + fibre overlay	Spenco[®]
Static pressure airbed	First Step[®], Roho[®], Vicair[®]
Alternating pressure airbed	Pegasus[®], Ripple[®]
Low loss airbed	Kinair[®], Mediscus[®a]
Air fluidized bed (least skin pressure)	Clinitron[®a]

a. pressure less than capillary pressure; patient need not be turned.

Box 11.L   Using a camping mattress as a makeshift water bed

Fill with warm water instead of air and cover with a sheet.

When the patient lies on the mattress, the top and bottom surfaces should not meet at any point, nor should the mattress present a hard surface because of overfilling.

The patient will maintain the water at body temperature. When the patient is out of bed in a temperate climate, heat is retained by an electric blanket or heating pad; this is not used when the patient is in bed.

A camping mattress weighs about 120kg when filled; it can be used at home where floors may not be able to stand the weight of a commercial water bed.

Mattresses are washed with soap and water before re-use.

Holes are mended with a bicycle puncture repair kit.

Sheets should not be tucked in tightly. For some patients, a bed cradle to raise the bedding off the body helps. Rolled towels or pillows can be used to 'fine-tune' the patient's position.

When sitting in a chair or wheelchair, a pressure-relieving cushion should be used for patients at risk of developing a decubitus ulcer, or with one, e.g.:
- profiled foam (Eggcrate[®])
- inflatable cushion (Roho[®]).

If strong enough, patients should be encouraged to raise themselves off the seat and shift their weight every 15–20min. Short walks should be encouraged if the patient is capable.

The tradition of repositioning very ill and unconscious patients q2h probably stems from the fact that this was the time it took the nurses to work their way round a Nightingale ward of 24–30 bedbound patients. Nowadays, the frequency of repositioning depends on various factors, including:
- distress when moved, e.g. pain or breathlessness
- discomfort when lying or sitting for long periods unmoved[94]

- presence of risk factors (see p.346)
- level of consciousness.

Skin care
- inspect the skin every time the patient's position is changed
- maintain optimal hygiene and hydration:
  ▷ dry skin (see p.329)
  ▷ wet skin (see p.330)
- avoid trauma:
  ▷ place pillows between the patient and bedrails
  ▷ patients lifted when repositioned, not dragged
  ▷ loose clothing and smooth bedding
  ▷ avoid overheating and sweating
  ▷ use loose bandaging instead of firmly adherent tape.

Nutrition
Nutritional goals can be modified in dying patients. It is not always possible to achieve the ideal of a plasma albumin concentration of $>$30g/L and Hb of $>$10g/dL.

Management

Most NHS Trusts in the UK have their own wound management guidelines. These will dictate the type of dressings to be used in specific circumstances.

An ulcer will not heal without an adequate blood supply. Local pressure must be avoided as much as possible. However, healing may be impossible and preventing further deterioration is often a more appropriate aim.

For the purposes of management, decubitus ulcers may be classified as follows:
- *necrotic*: covered with a hard dry black necrotic layer (Plate 1)
- *sloughy*: covered or filled with a soft yellow slough (Plate 2)
- *granulating*: red and clean with significant tissue loss (Plate 3)
- *epithelializing*: red and clean and superficial (Plate 4).

In addition, ulcers may be infected and malodourous. This classification reflects both the different types of wound and the various stages through which an ulcer passes as it heals.

Non-drug treatment
Growth of clean red granulation tissue will occur only after the elimination of local infection and necrotic tissue (eschar). Because it is normal for skin to be colonized with some bacteria, bacterial growth from a swab is not an indication for antibacterials unless there are clinical signs of infection. Systemic antibacterials should be used if there is surrounding cellulitis. Antiseptics are used less than in the past because they too may have undesirable effects. Cleanse with 0.9% saline or even tap water if it is safe to drink.

Granulation tissue must be protected from prolonged cooling, drying out and trauma when the dressing is changed (Box 11.M). Desloughing agents can cause maceration of normal skin and must be used with great care. The value of products containing dextranomer polysaccharide beads/paste and cadexomer iodine polysaccharide is questionable.[95] Further, in none of five trials of enzymatic agents was there a significant outcome in favour of the desloughing agent.[95]

As the condition of the wound changes, the type of dressing also changes (Table 11.7).

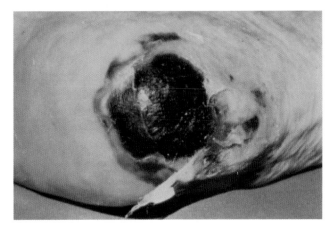

Plate 1   Black necrotic decubitus ulcer.

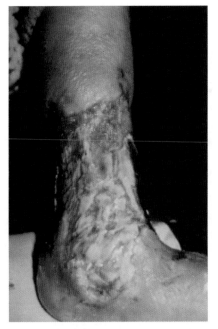

Plate 2   Yellow sloughy decubitus ulcer.

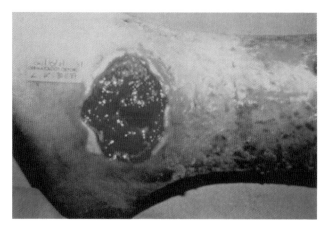

Plate 3   Deep red granulating decubitus ulcer.

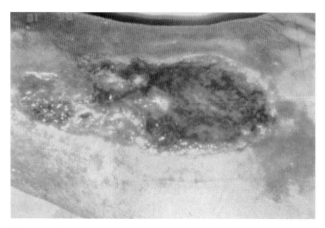

Plate 4   Superficial red epithelializing decubitus ulcer.

Box 11.M Commonly used wound dressings[96,97]

Films, e.g. Bioclusive®, Opsite®, Tegaderm®
Totally occlusive; maintain wound hydration and temperature, contain malodour but permeable to water vapour and oxygen.

Cannot absorb exudate but allow observation of the wound surface without removal.

Stretching the film eases removal but even so may be difficult to remove without causing trauma. Often used as an 'extra layer of skin' to help prevent ulceration, particularly on the elbows and spine.

Hydrocolloids, e.g. Aquacel®, Comfeel®, Granuflex®
Hydrocolloid dressings generally comprise an absorbent layer on a semi-permeable film or foam; also available as a paste for filling cavities. Maintain wound hydration and temperature. May be left in place for up to 1 week.

Suitable for softening eschars or for promoting granulation and as a preventive measure, particularly over the sacrum. The occlusive nature of their backing means that they are not suitable for heavily exuding wounds. Hydrocolloid dressings can be used on infected wounds (see manufacturer's literature).

When applied to non-flat surfaces, a warm hand placed on the dressing for 1–2min helps to mould them to the body shape and improves adherence.

Hydrogels, e.g. Granugel®, Intrasite® gel
Hydrogel dressings are generally supplied as an amorphous cohesive material which takes up the shape of a wound. They are easily inserted into and removed from cavities. However, because they can damage healing tissue if allowed to dry out, they must be covered with an occlusive film dressing to maintain wound hydration.

They facilitate autolysis of slough and eschar.

Alginates, e.g. Kaltostat®, Sorbsan®
These are highly absorbent and are suitable for moderately exuding wounds. They are also haemostatic but, if allowed to dry out, removal can cause tissue damage and bleeding.

Form a gel in contact with fluid but, if dried out, copious amounts of warm saline may be required to remove them without trauma. Not suitable for eschars or dry wounds.

Foams, e.g. Mepilex®, New Allevyn®
These are highly absorbent and also allow evaporation of the water content of the discharge. They are useful for desloughing.

Low adherent, e.g. Mepitel®
These protect the wound surface and absorb some exudate. If allowed to dry out, removal causes skin damage; if wet, they are easily removed.

Absorbent pads, e.g. Eclipse®, Mesorb®
These are both super-absorbent dressings, which can be placed over a low adherent layer, e.g. Mepitel® as a 2-layer dressing system.

Table 11.7 Choice of dressing for decubitus ulcers

Wound type	Aim	Dressing
Necrotic	Debride/remove eschar	Hydrogel or Hydrocolloid ± hydrocolloid paste
Sloughy	Remove slough; provide clean base for epithelialization	Hydrogel or Hydrocolloid ± hydrocolloid paste
Granulating	Promote granulation	Hydrogel or Hydrocolloid ± hydrocolloid paste or Foam or Alginate sheet ± rope
Epithelializing	Wound maturation	Hydrocolloid or Low-adherent dressing or Film
Infected	Treat infection and thereby reduce odour (note: infected ulcers produce considerable discharge)	*Infection* Antibacterials metronidazole PO or topical (for anaerobes) silver sulfadiazine (for *Pseudomonas*) *Dressing* Low-adherent dressing or Alginate sheet ± rope or Polyurethane foam or Eclipse® or Mesorb®

Drug treatment

Vitamin C 500mg–1g once daily aids healing in malnourished patients.[98] Zinc supplements help in zinc-deficient patients, and it may be worth checking the plasma concentration in a patient with a prognosis of several months.

1 Twycross RG et al. (2003) Itch: scratching more than the surface. Quarterly Journal of Medicine. **96**: 7–26.

2 Zylicz Z et al. (eds) (2004) Pruritus in Advanced Disease. Oxford University Press, Oxford.

3 Stander S et al. (2007) Clinical classification of itch: a position paper of the International Forum for the Study of Itch. Acta Dermato-Venereologica. **87**: 291–294.

4 Kimyai-Asadi A et al. (1999) Poststroke pruritus. Stroke. **30**: 692–693.

5 Dey DD et al. (2005) Central neuropathic itch from spinal-cord cavernous hemangioma: a human case, a possible animal model, and hypotheses about pathogenesis. Pain. **113**: 233–237.

6 Stander S and Schmelz M (2006) Chronic itch and pain – Similarities and differences. European Journal of Pain. **10**: 473–478.

7 Schmelz M et al. (1997) Specific C-receptors for itch in human skin. Journal of Neuroscience. **17**: 8003–8008.

8 Schmelz M et al. (2000) Which nerve fibers mediate the axon reflex flare in human skin? Neuroreport. **11**: 645–648.

9 Yao G et al. (1992) Histamine-caused itch induces Fos-like immunoreactivity in dorsal horn neurons: effect of morphine pretreatment. Brain Research. **599**: 333–337.

10 Hagermark O and Wahlgren C (1992) Some methods for evaluating clinical itch and their application for studying pathophysiological mechanisms. Journal of Dermatological Science. **4**: 55–62.

11 Lowitt M and Bernhard J (1992) Pruritus. Seminars in Neurology. **12**: 374–384.

12 Weisshaar E et al. (1997) Can a serotonin type 3 (5-HT3) receptor antagonist reduce experimentally-induced itch? Inflammation Research. **46**: 412–416.

13 Borgeat A and Stimemann H-R (1999) Ondansetron is effective to treat spinal or epidural morphine-induced pruritus. Anesthesiology. **90**: 432–436.

14 Browning J et al. (2003) Long-term efficacy of sertraline as a treatment for cholestatic pruritus in patients with primary biliary cirrhosis. American Journal of Gastroenterology. **98**: 2736–2741.

15 Mayo MJ et al. (2007) Sertraline as a first-line treatment for cholestatic pruritus. Hepatology. **45**: 666–674.

16 Zylicz Z et al. (2003) Paroxetine in the treatment of severe non-dermatological pruritus: a randomized, controlled trial. Journal of Pain and Symptom Management. **26**: 1105–1112.

17 Summerfield J (1980) Naloxone modulates the perception of itch in man. British Journal of Clinical Pharmacology. **10**: 180–183.

18 Szarvas S et al. (2003) Neuraxial opioid-induced pruritus: a review. Journal of Clinical Anesthesia. **15**: 234–239.

19 Suksompong S et al. (2008) Drugs for the prevention and treatment of pruritus in patients receiving neuraxial opioids (Protocol). The Cochrane Collaboration.

20 Jones E and Bergasa N (1996) Why do cholestatic patients itch? Gut. **38**: 644–645.

21 Yuan CS et al. (1998) Efficacy of orally administered methylnaltrexone in decreasing subjective effects after intravenous morphine. Drug and Alcohol Dependence. **52**: 161–165.

22 Tarkkila P et al. (1995) Premedication with promethazine and transdermal scopolamine reduces the incidence of nausea and vomiting after intrathecal morphine. Acta Anaesthesiologica Scandinavica. **39**: 983–986.

23 Yeh H et al. (2000) Prophylactic intravenous ondansetron reduces the incidence of intrathecal morphine-induced pruritus in patients undergoing cesarean delivery. Anesthesia and Analgesia. **91**: 172–175.

24 Chaplan SR et al. (1992) Morphine and hydromorphone epidural analgesia. Anesthesiology. **77**: 1090–1094.

25 Krajnik M (2004) Opioid-induced pruritus. In: Z Zylicz et al. (eds) Pruritus in Advanced Disease. Oxford University Press, London, pp. 84–96.

26 Kalso E and Vainio A (1990) Morphine and oxycodone in the management of cancer pain. Clinical Pharmacology and Therapeutics. **47**: 639–646.

27 Wood L et al. (1997) Barrier disruption increases gene expression of cytokines and the 55kD TNF receptor in murine skin. Experimental Dermatology. **6**: 98–104.

28 Man M-Q et al. (1999) Cutaneous barrier repair and pathophysiology following barrier disruption in IL-1 and TNF type I receptor deficient mice. Experimental Dermatology. **8**: 261–266.

29 Rubel DM et al. (1998) Tea tree oil allergy: what is the offending agent? Report of three cases of tea tree oil allergy and review of the literature. The Australasian Journal of Dermatology. **39**: 244–247.

30 Greaves M (1992) Itching-research has barely scratched the surface. New England Journal of Medicine. **326**: 1016–1017.

31 Guillet G et al. (2000) Increased histamine release and skin hypersensitivity to histamine in senile pruritus: study of 60 patients. European Academy of Dermatology and Venereology. **14**: 65–68.

32 Rajatanavin N et al. (1987) Baking soda and pruritus. Lancet. **2**: 977.

33 Anonymous (2005) Pharmacy information pointers. The preparation of menthol (1 per cent w/w) in aqueous cream BP. *Pharmaceutical Journal.* **274**: 469.

34 Smith E *et al.* (1984) Crotamiton lotion in pruritus. *International Journal of Dermatology.* **23**: 684–685.

35 Muston H *et al.* (1979) Differential effect of hypnotics and anxiolytics on itch and scratch. *Journal of Investigative Dermatology.* **72**: 283.

36 Twycross RG (1981) Pruritus and pain on en cuirass breast cancer. *Lancet.* **2**: 696.

37 Korfitis C and Trafalis DT (2008) Carbamazepine can be effective in alleviating tormenting pruritus in patients with hematologic malignancy. *Journal of Pain and Symptom Management.* **35**: 571–572.

38 Osterman PO (1976) Paroxysmal itching in multiple sclerosis. *The British Journal of Dermatology.* **95**: 555–558.

39 Closs S (1997) Pruritus and methotrimeprazine.

40 Figge J *et al.* (1979) Tricyclic antidepressants: potent blockade of histamine H_1 receptors of guinea pig ileum. *European Journal of Pharmacology.* **58**: 479–483.

41 Gilchrest B *et al.* (1997) Relief of uremic pruritus with ultraviolet phototherapy. *New England Journal of Medicine.* **297**: 136–138.

42 Breneman D *et al.* (1992) Topical capsaicin for treatment of hemodialysis-related pruritus. *Journal of the American Academy of Dermatology.* **26**: 91–94.

43 Peer G *et al.* (1996) Randomised crossover trial of naltrexone in uraemic pruritus. *Lancet.* **348**: 1552–1554.

44 Pauli-Magnus C *et al.* (2000) Naltrexone does not relieve uremic pruritus. *Journal of the American Society of Nephrology.* **11**: 514–519.

45 Silva S *et al.* (1994) Thalidomide for the treatment of uremic pruritus: a crossover randomized double-blind trial. *Nephron.* **67**: 270–273.

46 Wolfhagen F *et al.* (1997) Oral naltrexone treatment for cholestatic pruritus: A double-blind, placebo-controlled study. *Gastroenterology.* **113**: 1264–1269.

47 Ghent C and Carruthers S (1988) Treatment of pruritus in primary biliary cirrhosis with rifampin. Results of a double-blind crossover randomized trial. *Gastroenterology.* **94**: 488–493.

48 Ahrens E *et al.* (1950) Primary biliary cirrhosis. *Medicine.* **29**: 299–364.

49 Lloyd-Thomas H and Sherlock S (1952) Testosterone therapy for the pruritus of obstructive jaundice. *British Medical Journal.* **ii**: 1289–1291.

50 Aymard J *et al.* (1980) Cimetidine for pruritus in Hodgkin's disease. *British Medical Journal.* **280**: 151–152.

51 Fjellner B and Hagermark O (1979) Pruritus in polycythemia vera: treatment with aspirin and possibility of platelet involvement. *Acta Dermato-Venereologica (Stockh).* **59**: 505–512.

52 Tefferi A and Fonseca R (2002) Selective serotonin reuptake inhibitors are effective in the treatment of polycythemia vera-associated pruritus. *Blood.* **99**: 2627.

53 Asokumar B *et al.* (1998) Intrathecal bupivacaine reduces pruritus and prolongs duration of fentanyl analgesia during labor: a prospective, randomized, controlled trial. *Anaesthesia and Analgesia.* **87**: 1309–1315.

54 Charuluxananan S *et al.* (2000) Ondansetron for treatment of intrathecal morphine-induced pruritus after cesarean delivery. *Regional Anesthesia and Pain Medicine.* **25**: 535–539.

55 Tarcatu D *et al.* (2007) Are we still scratching the surface? A case of intractable pruritus following systemic opioid analgesia. *Journal of Opioid Management.* **3**: 167–170.

56 Colbert S *et al.* (1999) The effect of rectal diclofenac on pruritus in patients receiving intrathecal morphine. *Anaesthesia.* **54**: 948–952.

57 Colbert S *et al.* (1999) The effect of intravenous tenoxicam on pruritus in patients receiving epidural fentanyl. *Anaesthesia.* **54**: 76–80.

58 Cork M (1998) Complete emollient therapy. In: *The National Association of Fundholding Practices Official Yearbook.* BPC Waterlow, Dunstable, pp. 159–168.

59 Cork MJ *et al.* (2003) An audit of adverse drug reactions to aqueous cream in children with atopic eczema. *Pharmaceutical Journal.* **271**: 747–748.

60 Quigley C and Baines M (1997) Descriptive epidemiology of sweating in a hospice population. *Journal of Palliative Care.* **13 (1)**: 22–26.

61 Kirby K (1990) Dermatology. In: P Kumar and M Clarke (eds) *Clinical Medicine.* Baillière Tindall, London, pp. 1000–1001.

62 Ganong WF (1979) *Review of Medical Physiology* (9e). Lange Medical Publications, pp. 177–181.

63 Ryan T (1996) Diseases of the skin. In: DJ Weatherall (ed) *Oxford Textbook of Medicine* (thirde). Oxford University Press, Oxford, pp. 3765–3767.

64 Tabibzadeh S *et al.* (1989) Interleukin-6 immunoreativity in human tumours. *American Journal of Pathology.* **135**: 427–433.

65 Tsavaris N *et al.* (1990) A randomized trial of the effect of three nonsteroidal anti-inflammatory agents in ameliorating cancer-induced fever. *Journal of Internal Medicine.* **228**: 451–455.

66 Hargrove J and Eisenberg E (1995) Menopause. *Medical Clinics of North America.* **79**: 1337–1356.

67 Quella S *et al.* (1998) Long term use of megestrol acetate by cancer survivors for the treatment of hot flashes. *Cancer.* **82**: 1784–1788.

68 Miller J and Ahmann F (1992) Treatment of castration-induced menopausal symptoms with low dose diethylstilbestrol in men with advanced cancer. *Urology.* **40**: 499–502.

69 Pandya K *et al.* (2000) Oral clonidine in postmenopausal patients with breast cancer experiencing tamoxifen-induced hot flashes: a university of Rochester Cancer Centre community clinical oncology program study. *Annals of internal medicine.* **132**: 788–793.

70 Simpson N (1988) Treating hyperhidrosis. *British Medical Journal.* **296**: 1345.

71 Murphy R and Harrington C (2000) Iontophoresis should be tried before other treatments. *British Medical Journal.* **321**: 702–703.

72 Collin J and Whatling P (2000) Treating hyperhidrosis: surgery and botulinum toxin are treatments of choice in severe cases. *British Medical Journal.* **320**: 1221–1222.

73 Atkins J and Butler P (2000) Treating phyperhidrosis: excision of axillary tissue may be more effective. *British Medical Journal.* **321**: 702.

74 Mercadante S (1998) Hyoscine in opioid-induced sweating. *Journal of Pain and Symptom Management.* **15**: 214–215.

75 Pittelkow M and Loprinzi C (2003) Pruritus and sweating in palliative medicine. In: D Doyle *et al.* (eds) *Oxford Textbook of Palliative Medicine* (3e). Oxford University Press, Oxford, pp. 573–587.

76 Zylicz Z and Krajnik M (2003) Flushing and sweating in an advanced breast cancer patient relieved by olanzapine. *Journal of Pain and Symptom Management.* **25**: 494–495.

77 Calder K and Bruera E (2000) Thalidomide for night sweats in patients with advanced cancer. *Palliative Medicine.* **14**: 77–78.

78 Deaner P (2000) The use of thalidomide in the management of severe sweating in patients with advanced malignancy: trial report. *Palliative Medicine.* **14**: 429–431.

79 McGrath A and Porrett T (eds) (2005) *Stoma Care – Essential Clinical Skills for Nurses.* Blackwell Publishing, Oxford.

80 Breckman B (ed) (2006) *Stoma Care and Rehabilitation.* Churchill Livingston, Edinburgh.

81 Burch J (2008) *Stoma Care.* Wiley Blackwell, West Sussex.

82 Williams J (2008) Selecting stoma care appliances and accessories. *Nursing and Residential Care.* **10**: 130–133.

83 Williams J (2008) Flatus, odour and the ostomist: coping strategies and interventions. *The British Journal of Nursing.* **17**: S10, S12–14.

84 Lyon C and Smith A (eds) (2001) *Abdominal Stomas and their Skin Disorders – an Atlas of Diagnosis and Management.* Martin Dunitz, London.

85 Forbes A (2001) *Clinicians Guide to Inflammatory Bowel Disease* (2e). Chapman and Hall, London.

86 Lange M *et al.* (1989) Management of multiple enterocutaneous fistulas. *Heart and Lung.* **18**: 386–391.

87 De-Conno F *et al.* (1991) Continuous subcutaneous infusion of hyoscine butylbromide reduces secretions in patients with gastrointestinal obstruction. *Journal of Pain and Symptom Management.* **6**: 484–486.

88 Fallon M (1994) The physiology of somatostatin and its synthetic analogue, octreotide. *European Journal of Palliative Care.* **1**: 20–22.

89 Walls A *et al.* (1994) The closure of an abdominal fistula using self-polymerizing silicone rubbers – case study. *Palliative Medicine.* **8**: 59–62.

90 Streza G *et al.* (1977) Management of enterocutaneous fistulas and problem stomas with silicone casting of the abdominal wall defect. *American Journal of Surgery.* **134**: 772–776.

91 Hatz R *et al.* (1994) *Wound Healing and Wound Management.* Springer-Verlag, London.

92 Waterlow J (1998) The history and use of the waterlow card. *Nursing Times.* **94**: 63–67.

93 Chaplin J (2000) Pressure sore risk assessment in palliative care. *Journal of Tissue Viability.* **10**: 27–31.

94 Gebhardt K (1994) Preventing pressure sores. *Elder Care.* **6**: 23–28.

95 Bradley M *et al.* (1999) The debridement of chronic wounds: systematic review. *Health Technology Assessment.* **3**: Part 1.

96 Chaby G *et al.* (2007) Dressings for acute and chronic wounds: a systematic review. *Archives of Dermatology.* **143**: 1297–1304.

97 Cowley S and Grocott P (2007) Research design for the development and evaluation of complex technologies. *Evaluation.* **13**: 285–305.

98 Breslow R (1991) Nutritional status and dietary intake of patients with pressure ulcers: review of the research literature 1943–1989. *Decubitus.* **4**: 16–21.

12: EMERGENCIES

This chapter deals with the list of emergencies in the UK Palliative Medicine Specialty Training Curriculum.[1] A sense of urgency is important in symptom management. This is helped by setting goals with and for patients, with regular reviews at appropriate intervals. However, there are circumstances when one is faced with an emergency which demands an even greater sense of urgency and speed of action (Box 12.A).

Box 12.A Emergencies in palliative care

Haematological
  severe haemorrhage (see p.243)
  pulmonary embolism (see p.244)
Anaphylaxis
Respiratory
  choking
  SVC obstruction
  stridor
  acute tracheal compression
  bronchospasm
  pneumothorax
Cardiac
  cardiac tamponade
  acute heart failure
  cardiac arrest
Neurological
  spinal cord compression
    (see p.264)
  generalized convulsive seizures
    (see p.279)
  multifocal myoclonus in the
    moribund (see p.279)
Acute renal failure
  hyperkalaemia
Acute urinary retention
Hypoglycaemia

Pain
  biliary and ureteric colic
  intrahepatic haemorrhage
  bladder spasm (see p.293)
  acute vertebral collapse
  spinal instability
  fracture of long bone
Psychiatric
  suicidal ideas
  panic (see p.189)
  delirium (see p.207 and p.429)
  violent patient
Overdose
  opioid overdose
  benzodiazepine overdose
Substance withdrawal
  drug withdrawal
  alcohol withdrawal
Adverse drug reactions
  acute dystonia and oculogyric crisis
  neuroleptic (antipsychotic) malignant syndrome
  serotonin toxicity
Complications of therapeutic procedures
  blood transfusion
  paracentesis
  chest aspiration

ANAPHYLAXIS

Anaphylaxis is a life-threatening systemic allergic reaction.[2] It manifests as a constellation of features but there is disagreement over which are essential. The confusion about definition arises partly because systemic allergic reactions can be mild, moderate or severe. In practice, the term 'anaphylaxis' should be reserved for cases where there is:
• respiratory difficulty (related to laryngeal oedema or bronchoconstriction) *or*
• hypotension (presenting as fainting, collapse or loss of consciousness) *or*
• both.

Urticaria, angioedema or rhinitis alone are best not described as anaphylaxis because neither respiratory difficulty nor hypotension is present.[2]

Causes

In anaphylaxis, an allergic reaction results from the interaction of an allergen with specific IgE antibodies bound to mast cells and basophils. This leads to activation of the mast cell with release of chemical mediators stored in granules (including histamine) as well as rapidly synthesized additional mediators. A rapid major systemic release of these mediators causes capillary leakage and mucosal oedema, resulting in shock and respiratory difficulty.[2]

In contrast, anaphylactoid reactions are caused by activation of mast cells and release of the same mediators, but without the involvement of IgE antibodies. For example, certain drugs act directly on mast cells. In terms of management it is not necessary to distinguish anaphylaxis from an anaphylactoid reaction. This difference is relevant only when investigations are being considered.

Anaphylaxis is rare in palliative care and is generally associated with an antibacterial or an NSAID (including aspirin). A possible case has been recorded in a woman with known peanut allergy who received an arachis (peanut) oil enema.[3] Anaphylaxis is:
• specific to a given drug or chemically-related class of drugs
• more likely after parenteral administration
• more frequent in patients with aspirin-induced asthma or systemic lupus erythematosus.

Clinical features

No single set of criteria will identify all anaphylactic reactions, but anaphylaxis is likely when all three of the following criteria are met:
• sudden onset and rapid progression of symptoms
• life-threatening respiratory or circulatory problems
• skin and/or mucosal changes.

Anaphylaxis causes a range of signs and symptoms (Box 12.B).[4] Bronchospasm occurs in only 10% of patients (see p.364). Skin and mucosal changes occur in 80% of patients, but may be subtle. Angioedema may develop anywhere in the body but often involves the lips, eyes, hands or feet. Oedema of the larynx may lead to stridor and acute airway obstruction.[5]

Management

Anaphylaxis requires urgent treatment with adrenaline (epinephrine) followed by an antihistamine and hydrocortisone (Box 12.C). However, corticosteroids are only of secondary value because their impact is not immediate.

Box 12.B   Clinical features of anaphylaxis

Essential
Sudden onset of life-threatening circulatory and/or respiratory problems, e.g.

Circulatory problems
Tachycardia
Hypotension
Shock
Decreased consciousness
Cardiac arrest

Respiratory problems
Airway
    pharyngeal/laryngeal oedema
    hoarse voice
    stridor
Breathing
    breathlessness
    wheeze/bronchospasm
    cyanosis
    respiratory arrest

Possible
Skin/mucosal changes
Flushing or pallor
Erythema of skin
Urticaria
Angioedema[a]

Other
Agitation
Confusion
Abdominal pain
Vomiting
Diarrhoea
Incontinence
Tingling of the extremities
Rhinitis
Conjunctivitis

a. angioedema is swelling in the dermis, subcutaneous and submucosal tissues.

Box 12.C   Management of anaphylaxis in adults[4,6]

1 Stop causal agent, e.g. IV antibacterial.

2 Oxygen is of primary importance ($>$ 10L/min).

3 Adrenaline (epinephrine) 1mg/1mL (1 in 1,000), 500microgram (0.5mL) IM; repeat every 5min until blood pressure, pulse and breathing are satisfactory.

4 If an adrenaline (epinephrine) auto-injector is used, 300microgram (0.3mL) is generally sufficient.

5 Chlorphenamine to counter histamine-induced vasodilation:
   • 10mg IM or IV over 1min
   • if necessary, repeat up to a maximum of 40mg/24h
   • 4–8mg PO q.d.s. for 24–72h to prevent relapse.

6 Hydrocortisone sodium succinate or phosphate[a] 200mg IM or slow IV for patients with bronchospasm, and for all severe or recurrent reactions to prevent further deterioration. Note: may take up to 6h to act. Also prescribe prednisolone 40–50mg PO once daily for 3 days to prevent a relapse.[7]

7 If still shocked, give 1–2L of IV fluid (a crystalloid, e.g. normal saline, may be safer than a colloid).[8]

8 If bronchospasm has not responded to the above, give a nebulized β_2-agonist, e.g. salbutamol 5mg.

a. the phosphate may cause paraesthesia and pain after IV use; the acetate is unsuitable because its microcrystalline structure precludes IV use.

If there is doubt about the adequacy of the circulation, adrenaline (epinephrine) can be given as a dilute IV solution, i.e. 1mg/10mL (1 in 10,000), *using 50microgram (0.5mL) boluses, titrated to response.* However, because injecting adrenaline (epinephrine) IV too rapidly can cause ventricular arrhythmias, IV administration is discouraged unless given by a specialist, and intensive care facilities are available.[4,6] Occasionally, emergency tracheotomy and assisted respiration are necessary.

RESPIRATORY

Choking

Choking is the sudden inability to breathe because of an acute obstruction of the pharynx, larynx or trachea.

Causes

Choking is relatively rare, and generally occurs when food is not chewed properly and enters the upper airway. Risk factors include:

- talking or laughing while eating
- poorly fitting dentures
- impaired swallowing as a result of sedative drugs or alcohol
- neurological impairment, e.g.:
  ▷ Parkinson's disease
  ▷ pseudobulbar palsy (dysfunction of the lower cranial nerves), e.g. caused by MND/ALS, base of skull metastases, head and neck cancers
  ▷ brain tumour (primary or secondaries)
  ▷ post-stroke.

Clinical features

- generally occurs while eating
- coughing or gagging
- panic
- sudden inability to talk
- hand signals, e.g. clutching or pointing to the throat
- wheezing
- cyanosis
- loss of consciousness
- death.

Management

Call for help and commence first aid. Determine if it is a partial (mild) or complete (severe) airway obstruction by asking 'Are you choking?' and proceed accordingly:[9]

Partial
- able to speak, breathe, cough forcefully, not cyanosed
- encourage coughing to clear obstruction but do nothing else.

Complete
- unable to speak, breathe or cough, cyanosed

- give up to 5 back blows:
  - ▷ stand to side and slightly behind person
  - ▷ support chest with one hand and lean the person well forward to facilitate clearance of the obstructing object out of the mouth
  - ▷ with the heel of your other hand give a sharp blow between the shoulder blades
  - ▷ check after each blow for success; if 5 blows fail, proceed to abdominal thrusts
- give up to 5 abdominal thrusts (Heimlich manoeuvre):
  - ▷ stand behind the person and lean them forward
  - ▷ make a fist with one hand; put your arms around the person and grasp your fist with your other hand in the midline, halfway between the lower sternum and the umbilicus
  - ▷ make a quick, hard movement inward and upward
  - ▷ check after each thrust for success; if 5 thrusts fail, return to back blows
- continue alternating back blows and abdominal thrusts until:
  - ▷ the obstruction is cleared
  - ▷ the person can breathe and cough forcefully
- if the person loses consciousness and if appropriate, e.g. the person was not already close to their anticipated death before choking:
  - ▷ call for an ambulance/cardiac arrest team
  - ▷ begin CPR.

Superior vena caval obstruction

Superior vena caval (SVC) obstruction is generally caused by extrinsic compression by metastases in the upper mediastinal lymph nodes. However, intravascular extension of tumour or thrombosis may contribute. Venous thrombosis can cause an acute onset of obstructive symptoms (Box 12.D). Lung cancer is responsible for 80% of cases. SVC obstruction occurs in about 15% of patients with lung cancer, particularly SCLC. It is also associated with other malignancies such as lymphoma, breast cancer and testicular seminoma.[10,11] Non-cancer causes of SVC obstruction include central venous catheters, post-radiotherapy fibrosis or goitre and thrombosis.[12]

Management

SVC obstruction with severe symptoms is an emergency. The usual treatment consists of high-dose corticosteroids (e.g. dexamethasone 16mg once daily/8mg b.d. PO/IV) and radiotherapy to the mediastinum. Corticosteroids reduce peritumour oedema and thereby reduce extrinsic compression.

Particularly if insertion was recent and traumatic, consider removing a central venous catheter. Chemotherapy may be of benefit in patients with lymphoma or SCLC.

Alternatively, or in addition, a self-expanding metal stent can be introduced into the SVC via a brachiocephalic or femoral vein under radiological guidance, and positioned across the narrowed area of the SVC.[13-15] Patients are anticoagulated with heparin before stent insertion. If there is associated thrombosis, thrombolytic treatment, e.g. streptokinase, may also be necessary.[16] However, the possibility of massive haemorrhage from occult cerebral or endobronchial metastases must be taken into account before thrombolysis is carried out.[17]

Few adverse events are reported but include stent misplacement, stent migration, pulmonary oedema, and transient chest pain. Stent insertion provides more rapid symptom relief in a greater proportion of patients than radiotherapy or chemotherapy.[15,18] Long-term anticoagulation may be advisable, particularly in those

---

Box 12.D   Clinical features of SVC obstruction

Common symptoms
Breathlessness (50%)
Neck and facial swelling (40%)
Trunk and arm swelling (40%)
A sensation of choking
A feeling of fullness in the head
Headache

Other potential symptoms
Chest pain
Cough
Dysphagia
Cognitive impairment
Hallucinations
Seizures

Common physical signs
Thoracic vein distension (65%)
Neck vein distension (55%)
Facial oedema (55%)
Tachypnoea (40%)
Plethora of face (15%)
Cyanosis (15%)
Arm oedema (10%)
Vocal cord paresis (3%)
Horner's syndrome (3%)

If severe
Laryngeal stridor
Coma
Death

---

who required thrombolysis[17,19] but this is debatable.[18] After stenting, >90% of patients die without recurrence of the obstruction.

Stridor

Stridor is a harsh high-pitched sound produced during breathing; it is generated by vibration of the walls of critically narrowed airways:[20,21]

- inspiratory stridor generally indicates extrathoracic airways obstruction, i.e. obstruction in trachea, larynx or pharynx
- expiratory stridor generally indicates intrathoracic airway obstruction, i.e. obstruction in the lower part of the trachea, carina or bronchus. It may occur with severe upper airways obstruction
- biphasic stridor may indicate glottic or subglottic obstruction.

Stridor is a symptom and not a diagnosis. The cause must always be sought and treated appropriately.

Causes

Stridor may be caused by conditions involving the respiratory, cardiovascular, GI, and central nervous systems (Box 12.E). Onset may be acute or chronic. Chronic stridor may deteriorate rapidly if a mucous plug or haemorrhage into a cancer occludes an already narrowed airway. Stridor is more common in children and is generally associated with infection.

Evaluation

Where appropriate, a careful history should help to elicit the cause of stridor. Examination may show the level of obstruction. Look for signs of imminent complete airway obstruction (Box 12.F). The following investigations may be helpful but, in a terminally ill patient close to death, few (if any) will be appropriate:[21]

- pulse oximetry
- arterial blood gases

- imaging:
    - ▷ AP and lateral chest radiographs
    - ▷ CT or MRI
- laryngoscopy and bronchoscopy
- pulmonary function tests.

Box 12.E Causes of stridor in adults[20]

Narrowing above the larynx
Anaphylaxis (see p.358)
Retropharyngeal abscess
Pharyngeal tumour
Acute epiglottitis

**Narrowing inside larynx
or trachea**
Aspiration of foreign body
  (see Choking, p.360)
Mucous plug
Infection
  acute laryngitis
  tuberculosis
  diptheria
Inflammation
  sarcoidosis
  Wegener's granulomatosis
Trauma
  neck surgery
  prolonged intubation
  bronchoscopy
Laryngeal cancer
Laryngospasm
  hypocalcaemia
  inhalation injury, e.g. from smoke

**External compression of larynx
or trachea**
Mediastinal tumours or metastases
Hodgkin's lymphoma
SVC obstruction (see p.361)
Retrosternal goitre
  haemorrhage into adenomatous goitre
Thoracic aortic aneurysm
Infection
  cellulitis of neck
  fungal infection, e.g. histoplasmosis

Laryngeal nerve palsies
Bulbar or pseudobulbar palsy
Bilateral recurrent laryngeal nerve damage

Narrowing of both main bronchi
Lung cancer
Mediastinal tumours
Tuberculous strictures of main bronchi

Box 12.F Signs of incipient complete airway obstruction

Inability to talk
Drooling
Violent respiratory effort
Chest wall movement but no breath sounds
Cyanosis
Coma

Management

This will depend on the cause of stridor and the patient's overall condition. Where appropriate, emergency management includes:

- back blows (hit between the scapulas with the heel of your hand) or abdominal thrusts if inhalation of a foreign body suspected (see Choking, p.360)
- maintain airway
- administer oxygen
- cricothyroidotomy or tracheostomy

Acute airway obstruction may be the terminal event for some patients, e.g. haemorrhage from an advanced laryngeal cancer. It should be responded to in the same way as severe haemorrhage (see p.243):

- IV diazepam/midazolam until the patient is unconscious (5–20mg)
- PR diazepam or SC/buccal midazolam 10–20mg if IV administration is not possible
- continuous company.

Bronchospasm

Bronchospasm is caused by acute contraction of bronchial smooth muscles which leads to constriction of the bronchi and thus to airflow limitation. This may be associated with inflammation and oedema of bronchial mucosa and increased mucus production from bronchial glands.

Causes

The most common causes of bronchospasm are asthma and COPD. However, other causes must be considered and treated appropriately (Box 12.G).

Box 12.G Causes of bronchospasm in adults	
Asthma	Drugs
COPD	aspirin
Chest infection	NSAIDs
Exercise	paracetamol
Anaphylaxis	β-blockers
Allergy	Irritants
pets	cigarette smoke
house dust mite	aerosol spray

Clinical features

Clinical features of bronchospasm vary according to the intensity (Box 12.H).

Evaluation

May include:

- pulse oximetry
- arterial blood gases
- peak expiratory flow rate
- chest radiograph
- if sepsis suspected, consider sputum and blood cultures.

Box 12.H   Clinical features of bronchospasm

Common symptoms
Breathlessness
Wheeze
Hoarse voice
Cough
Chest tightness
Inability to complete sentences in
   single breath

Common physical signs
Tachypnoea
Tachycardia
Polyphonic wheeze

Life-threatening symptoms
Inability to talk
Exhaustion
Confusion
Coma

Life-threatening signs
Poor respiratory effort
Cyanosis
Bradycardia
Hypotension
Silent chest

Management
Whatever the cause of bronchospasm, emergency management necessitates:
- administration of oxygen to maintain SaO_2 > 92%
- salbutamol 5mg via (oxygen driven) nebulizer, repeated every 15–30min *or*
- salbutamol 100microgram/metered inhalation, 4–10 puffs inhaled separately via spacer, repeated every 10–20min
- if necessary, add ipratropium 500microgram q.d.s. via (oxygen driven) nebulizer
- if the patient is a known asthmatic, follow specific treatment guidelines
- if the patient has recently started an NSAID (or paracetamol), discontinue the drug, and review.

Pneumothorax
Pneumothorax is air in the pleural space, i.e. between the lung and chest wall. A pneumothorax may be:
- *primary*: without underlying lung disease (although most patients have subpleural blebs and bullae)
- *secondary*: with underlying lung disease.

A plain PA chest radiograph gives a misleading impression of the size of a pneumothorax. A pneumothorax of 1cm on the PA chest radiograph occupies about 25% of the hemithorax volume, and a 2cm pneumothorax occupies 50%. A pneumothorax <2cm is regarded as 'small' and one ⩾2cm as 'large'.

A tension pneumothorax arises when air is drawn into the pleural space during inspiration but cannot escape during expiration because of a pathological one-way valve. When sufficient air has been drawn into the pleural space so that intrapleural pressure exceeds atmospheric pressure throughout inspiration and expiration, a tension pneumothorax results. This is a life-threatening emergency (see below).[22]

Causes
Most pneumothoraces in palliative care patients are secondary (Box 12.I).

Box 12.I Causes of secondary pneumothorax

Infective
Pneumonia
Lung abscess
TB
Pneumocystis carinii pneumonia

Iatrogenic
Pleural aspiration or biopsy
Central line insertion
Percutaneous liver biopsy
Positive pressure ventilation

Cancer
Lung (primary or secondary)

Other
Asthma
COPD
Connective tissue disorders
Lung fibrosis
Sarcoidosis
Trauma

Clinical features

Because of underlying chest disease and associated reduced respiratory reserve, patients with a secondary pneumothorax often experience breathlessness disproportionate to the size of the pneumothorax (Box 12.J).

Box 12.J Clinical features of pneumothorax

Symptoms
Breathlessness (may be of sudden onset)
Chest tightness or pain
Anxiety

Physical signs
Tachypnoea
Tachycardia
Examination of the affected lung:
   reduced expansion
   hyperresonance to percussion
   increased vocal resonance
   reduced breath sounds

Evaluation
- pulse oximetry
- arterial blood gases
- chest radiograph
- lateral chest or lateral decubitus radiograph if high clinical suspicion of pneumothorax but normal PA radiograph
- CT may be required to differentiate pneumothorax from a complex bullous lesion.

Management

Management depends on whether the pneumothorax is primary or secondary, its size, the patient's age, symptoms and overall clinical condition. Given the proximity of the lung surface to the chest wall in a pneumothorax <1cm, aspiration is not recommended but can be safely carried out in a pneumothorax ≥2cm. A secondary pneumothorax should be managed as follows:[22]
- patient not breathless, with very small pneumothorax (<1cm) or isolated apical pneumothorax:
  ▷ observe for ≥24h

- patient minimally breathless, <50 years old, small pneumothorax (<2cm):
  - ▹ administer high flow oxygen 10L/min (aids absorption of air from pleural cavity)
  - ▹ perform simple aspiration with a 16G cannula connected to a 3-way tap and 50mL syringe
  - ▹ observe for ≥24h after aspiration
- moderate–severely breathless patient, pneumothorax >1cm:
  - ▹ administer high flow oxygen 10L/min
  - ▹ insert small bore (10–14Fr) intercostal tube chest drain.

It is advisable to perform aspiration or intercostal tube chest drain insertion in sites where radiography facilities are available. Failure of the pneumothorax to expand within 24h, presence of a persistent air leak, or worsening symptoms should prompt referral to a chest physician for consideration of suction, insertion of a large bore drainage tube, or referral to a thoracic surgeon.

In cases of persistent air leak or failure of the lung to re-expand, a thoracic surgical opinion should be sought within 5 days. Patients with a recurrent pneumothorax should also be referred to a thoracic surgeon. Open thoracotomy and pleurectomy has the lowest recurrence rate for pneumothoraces. However, pleurodesis by minimally invasive procedures, e.g. video-assisted thoracoscopic surgery (VATS) with talc pleurodesis, are acceptable alternatives and more likely to be appropriate in palliative care patients. This procedure should be covered with adequate analgesia, e.g. 1% lidocaine 25mL into the intrapleural space.

AIDS-related pneumothoraces are generally secondary to *Pneumocystis carinii* infection and have a high recurrence rate. Thus, if possible, they should be managed with tube drainage followed by 'blind' talc pleurodesis, VATS-assisted talc pleurodesis or pleurectomy.[22]

Tension pneumothorax
This is a life-threatening emergency which requires immediate treatment. The clinical features are shown in Box 12.K.

Box 12.K   Clinical features of tension pneumothorax

Symptoms	**Examination**
Severe breathlessness	Tracheal deviation (trachea pushed away
Chest tightness or pain	from side of pneumothorax)
Marked anxiety	Affected lung
	reduced expansion
Physical signs	hyperresonance to percussion
Tachypnoea	increased vocal resonance
Tachycardia	reduced breath sounds
Cyanosis	
Sweating	
Hypotension	
Cardiac arrest	

If tension pneumothorax is clearly identified on clinical grounds, do not wait for a chest radiograph but treat immediately:
- administer high flow oxygen 10L/min
- *initial emergency procedure*:
  - ▷ insert large bore (16G) IV cannula into 2nd intercostal space in mid-clavicular line (insert the cannula into the lower part of the intercostal space to avoid the neurovascular bundle which lies under the lower edge of the second rib)
  - ▷ withdraw the needle from the cannula, and listen for hiss of air
  - ▷ tape cannula to chest wall
- *definitive procedure*:
  - ▷ insert axillary chest drain on the affected side.

CARDIAC

Cardiac tamponade
Accumulation of fluid within the pericardium raises intrapericardial pressure. When this becomes high enough, it reduces ventricular filling, causing cardiac output to fall; this is called cardiac tamponade.

The volume of pericardial fluid required to cause tamponade varies. If the fluid has accumulated slowly, 1–2L may be present; if the fluid has accumulated rapidly or the pericardium is rigid, smaller volumes may cause tamponade.

Causes
A pericardial effusion severe enough to cause tamponade may develop from any cause of pericarditis (Box 12.L). Malignant effusions are generally caused by metastases to the parietal pericardium, e.g. from breast or lung cancers. Malignant pericardial effusions from primary cardiac tumours are rare.

Box 12.L   Causes of pericardial effusion and cardiac tamponade

Cancer	**Debility**

Metastases to
    parietal pericardium
    myocardium
Mediastinal lymphadenopathy
	Uraemia
	
	Concurrent
	Myocardial infarction

Treatment	Viral or bacterial pericarditis
Radiotherapy to the chest or mediastinum	Tuberculosis Dissecting aorta Following thoracic surgery

---

Clinical features
A high index of suspicion is needed to diagnose cardiac tamponade because its clinical features are not specific (Box 12.M). The presence of a raised JVP is essential for diagnosis, and Beck's triad may be present, namely:
- falling blood pressure
- raised JVP
- quiet heart sounds.

Box 12.M   Clinical features of cardiac tamponade

Symptoms	**Signs**
Breathlessness	Tachycardia
Chest pain	Tachypnoea
Dizziness on standing	Postural hypotension
Anorexia	Hypotension
Cough	Raised JVP[a]
Dysphagia	Distended veins on head and neck
	Quiet heart sounds on auscultation
If severe	Pulsus paradoxus[b]
Cyanosis	
Reduced level of consciousness	
Cardiogenic shock	

a. Kussmaul's sign may be elicited, i.e. a rise in JVP with inspiration
b. pulsus paradoxus is an accentuation of the normal fall in arterial pressure on inspiration. In severe tamponade, a large fall in arterial pressure can be palpated at the radial artery; on inspiration the pulse fades or becomes impalpable. In mild cases, pulsus paradoxus is detected by a fall of > 10mmHg in arterial pressure on inspiration.

The differential diagnosis of cardiac tamponade includes any cause of low cardiac output:
- massive pulmonary embolism
- severe ventricular disease; pulmonary congestion likely to be present – this is *not* a feature of cardiac tamponade
- septic shock or hypovolaemic shock; JVP will be low.[23]

Evaluation
- ECG may show low voltage QRS complexes and, if severe, electrical alternans (i.e. alternate QRS complexes have different patterns)
- chest radiograph may show a large, globular heart *without* evidence of pulmonary oedema
- echocardiography is generally diagnostic.

Management
Where emergency treatment of tamponade is appropriate:
- insert large bore (16G) IV cannula into a peripheral vein
- check FBC, urea and electrolytes, coagulation status (PT, APTT), and blood group
- stop anticoagulant medication
- arrange immediate transfer to a coronary care unit for pericardial aspiration (under echocardiographic guidance).

Ninety percent of malignant pericardial effusions re-accumulate within 3 months of pericardiocentesis.[24] Greater control is achieved by catheter drainage ± instillation of a sclerosing or chemotherapy agent (e.g. bleomycin). Surgical options include percutaneous balloon pericardiotomy or, for those which recur, more invasive surgery to create a pericardial window or to undertake pericardiotomy.[25,26]

When definitive management is not feasible, i.e. the patient is in the last days of life, cardiac tamponade should be managed symptomatically with opioids and anxiolytics.

Acute heart failure

Heart failure means a cardiac output insufficient to meet the metabolic demands of the body. Heart failure may be divided into:

- right ventricular failure (RVF)
- left ventricular failure (LVF)
- LVF with preserved ejection fraction (diastolic failure).[27]

'Biventricular' failure occurs when both ventricles are failing, and generally refers to RVF resulting from LVF. Biventricular heart failure may lead to 'congestion' (congestive heart failure/CHF), i.e. peripheral and/or pulmonary oedema.

Clinical manifestations of heart failure depend on whether the patient presents with RVF or LVF (or both). Symptoms of heart failure may be of rapid and severe onset (acute failure) or take a more insidious course (chronic failure). Acute LVF presenting with pulmonary oedema is a life-threatening emergency.

Causes

Acute LVF is generally a low output state; the failing left ventricle is unable to meet the demands of the body. There are a number of causes of acute LVF (Box 12.N). Other factors, e.g. arrhythmias or infection, may exacerbate LVF or precipitate acute decompensation in an already failing heart. High-output failure is rare. This occurs when cardiac output is normal or even increased but the metabolic needs of the body are very high, e.g. in thyrotoxicosis, Gram-negative septicaemia, anaemia of pregnancy.

Patients who have received mediastinal radiotherapy and/or cardiotoxic chemotherapy (e.g. anthracyclines, high-dose cyclophosphamide or trastuzumab) are predisposed to developing heart failure. Heart failure caused by chemotherapy should be managed as for other causes of heart failure. However, anthracycline-induced cardiomyopathy is frequently associated with tachycardia, so β-blockers may have an important role here.[28]

Box 12.N   Causes of acute LVF

Myocardial disorders
Myocardial infarction
Ischaemic heart disease
Cardiomyopathy

Valvular disorders
Aortic stenosis/regurgitation
Mitral stenosis/regurgitation[a]
Mitral valve rupture

Pericardial disorders
Constrictive pericarditis
Cardiac tamponade (see above)

Conduction disturbances
Complete heart block

Extra-cardiac causes
Malignant hypertension
IV fluid overload

Undesirable drug effects
Negative inotropes, e.g. calcium-channel blockers
Bradycardia, e.g. β-blockers, amiodarone, digoxin

a. mitral stenosis does not cause LVF, but it does cause left atrial hypertension and the signs of LVF.

Clinical features

Acute LVF often presents with rapid-onset severe breathlessness and distress (Box 12.O). Blood pressure may initially be normal or rise as LVF progresses; hypotension develops when LVF becomes severe.

Box 12.O   Clinical features of acute LVF

Symptoms
Severe breathlessness
Orthopnoea
Paroxysmal nocturnal dyspnoea
Wheeze
Cough
Pink frothy sputum
Distress

Signs
Tachypnoea
Tachycardia
Hypertension
Pulsus alternans[a]
Raised JVP
Auscultation of heart
　　third heart sound (gallop rhythm)
　　murmurs of aortic or mitral disease
Auscultation of chest
　　bi-basal end-inspiratory crackles
　　wheeze
　　pleural effusions

If severe
Reduced level of consciousness
Hypotension
Cardiogenic shock

a. alternating weak and strong pulse.

Evaluation
- pulse oximetry and blood pressure
- blood tests for urea and electrolytes, cardiac enzymes (troponin, CK, AST)
- ECG
- chest radiograph
- consider echocardiography.

Management
Treatment should be started before detailed investigations are undertaken to elucidate the cause of LVF (Box 12.P). The extent of investigations will depend on the patient's performance status, prognosis and wishes.

Box 12.P   Initial management of acute LVF[29]

Sit patient upright.

Administer oxygen to maintain SaO_2 > 92%.

Morphine 5–10mg slow IV.

Furosemide 40–80mg slow IV.[a,b]

Glyceryl trinitrate tablet 600microgram SL (or 2 puffs of 400microgram spray SL).

If no response after 30min, repeat furosemide 40–80mg slow IV.

If no response, consider transfer to a high dependency unit for diuretic infusion, nitrate infusion or inotropic support.

---

a. higher doses may be required if the patient is already taking an oral loop diuretic or if patient in renal failure

b. SC furosemide may be given but is likely to be of limited effectiveness if the patient is peripherally vasoconstricted.

Once the patient has been stabilized and, if appropriate, the underlying cause of the LVF should be sought, and the patient managed as for chronic heart failure.

Cardiac arrest

Most patients in specialist palliative care units are in the final stages of an illness where death is imminent and unavoidable. CPR is inappropriate in such patients.[30] However, it could be appropriate to provide CPR for a patient with a DNAR decision who develops a condition that is easily reversible, e.g. choking, blocked tracheostomy tube, anaphylaxis. If the patient is at high risk of this, it should be discussed with the patient to ascertain their wishes (see p.409).

If a patient has an implantable cardiac defibrillator (ICD), a discussion should be held with the patient and their cardiologist about the most appropriate time to de-activate it. Magnets are available from the manufacturers to de-activate the ICD in an emergency.

Causes

Ischaemic heart disease is the most common cause of cardiac arrest in adults (Box 12.Q). The arrest is usually triggered by an acutely ischaemic or infarcted myocardium causing ventricular fibrillation.[31]

Box 12.Q   Causes of cardiac arrest

Cardiac
Myocardial infarction
Electrophysiological disorders,
    e.g. long QT syndrome
Valvular heart disorders
Cardiac tamponade
Cardiomyopathy

Circulatory
Hypovolaemic shock
Septic shock
Pulmonary embolism
Tension pneumothorax

Other
Anaphylaxis
Drowning
Electrocution

Respiratory
Hypoxia
Hypercapnia

Metabolic
Hyper/hypokalaemia
Hypoglycaemia
Hypothermia

Drug overdose, e.g.
β-Blockers
Cocaine
Digoxin
TCAs

Clinical features

- unresponsive, unconscious patient
- abnormal or absent breathing pattern; 40% of patients suffering sudden cardiac arrest have agonal breathing (slow, laboured or noisy breathing with occasional gasps). This should not be mistaken for a sign of life
- absent carotid pulse; this should be checked only by those experienced in doing so, but is not strictly necessary because absent or abnormal breathing in an unresponsive patient is the main sign of cardiac arrest.[32]

Management

Where CPR is appropriate, early defibrillation maximizes the chance of survival.[33] Basic life support should be started immediately and carried out until a defibrillator arrives (Box 12.R). The correct hand position for chest compression is the middle of the lower half of the sternum. Chest compression should be carried out at a rate of 100 compressions/min, to a depth of 4–5cm, with 2 rescue breaths every 30 compressions with an inspiratory time of 1sec. Once the airway has been secured, ventilate the patient's lungs at 10 breaths/min.

If the patient is not breathing but has a pulse, ventilate the patient's lungs at a rate of 10 breaths/min, and check for a pulse every minute.

Box 12.R Basic life support for cardiac arrest[34]

Collapsed and apparently unconscious patient.

Shout for help or press bedside emergency call bell.

Check for response by gently shaking patient and asking loudly, 'Are you all right?'

If patient does not respond, turn patient onto their back and open airway by tilting the head back and lifting the chin. Clear mouth of foreign body using suction or forceps.

Check for signs of normal breathing for no more than 10sec. Check for carotid pulse for no more than 10sec.

If no signs of life, ask a staff member to bring the automated external defibrillator, if available.

Ask a staff member to phone for an emergency ambulance (999 or, if using a mobile/cell phone, 112), or the cardiac arrest team if in hospital.

Give 100 chest compressions/min, with 2 rescue breaths every 30 compressions, using pocket mask and oral airway, if available.

Continue at a ratio of compressions to ventilation of 30:2 until defibrillator or ambulance/cardiac arrest team arrive.

Some specialist palliative care units will be equipped with an automated external defibrillator. Staff should ensure that they are familiar with the equipment and drugs available to them, and attend regular training sessions on CPR.

ACUTE RENAL FAILURE

Acute renal failure (ARF) describes a significant deterioration in renal excretory function (glomerular filtration rate/GFR) occurring over hours–days. This leads to accumulation of nitrogenous waste products, measured by rising plasma urea and creatinine.[35]

Causes

Most cases of ARF are caused by renal hypoperfusion or acute tubular necrosis. These are potentially reversible, depending on the severity of the underlying cause, co-morbidities and the patient's age. ARF may have more than one cause or occur on a

background of chronic renal failure (decompensated chronic renal failure). Causes of ARF may be divided into:
- pre-renal (renal hypoperfusion)
- renal (intrinsic damage to kidney)
- post-renal (urinary tract obstruction at any point between the kidney and urethral meatus).

Obstructing lesions may lie within the lumen, wall or outside the urinary tract and cause dilation of the tract above the level of obstruction (Box 12.S).

Box12.S Causes of acute renal failure.

Pre-renal
Hypovolaemia, e.g.
  septic shock, haemorrhage,
  pancreatitis
Reduced cardiac output
  acute LVF
Defective renal autoregulation and
  reduced renal blood flow, e.g.
  ACE inhibitors, NSAIDs

Post-renal
Within lumen of urinary tract, e.g.
  blood clot, calculus, tumour of
  renal pelvis or ureter or bladder
Within wall of urinary tract, e.g.
  ureteric/urethral stricture,
  neuropathic bladder
Outside lumen, e.g.
  retroperitoneal or pelvic tumour,
  colon or prostate cancer, aortic
  aneurysm, diverticulitis

Renal
Renal vasculature
  artery stenosis
  artery/vein embolism
  vasculitis, e.g. polyarteritis nodosa,
    Wegener's granulomatosis
  Goodpasture's syndrome
  accelerated hypertension
Glomeruli
  glomerulonephritis
Tubules
  interstital nephritis
  acute tubular necrosis
  haemorrhage
  severe hypovolaemia
  heart failure
  septic shock
  hepatorenal syndrome
  drugs, e.g. NSAIDs, gentamicin,
    tetracycline, cisplatin, ciclosporin

Clinical features
Patients with ARF may present with few non-specific symptoms or with life-threatening complications:
- nausea, malaise, fatigue
- oliguria (urine output <400mL/24h)
- symptoms and signs consistent with underlying cause of ARF
- pulmonary oedema, bruising, haemorrhage, cardiac arrest from hyperkalaemia, uraemic encephalopathy, pericarditis.

Evaluation
Examine every patient for signs of urinary tract obstruction:
- palpable bladder
- ballotable kidneys or abdominal mass
- consider PR examination for enlarged prostate.

Further, look for signs of causes of ARF, e.g. sepsis, acute LVF.

Investigation will depend upon the patient's overall condition, and the aims of care. If the patient was not close to death prior to developing ARF, consider:
- temperature, blood pressure, oxygen saturation
- FBC (anaemia), PT, APTT
- plasma electrolytes (raised urea and creatinine); compare with previous results where available to confirm diagnosis of ARF
- plasma calcium, phosphate, LFTs, glucose, creatine kinase, LDH (for rhabdomyolysis)
- arterial blood gases (metabolic acidosis)
- ECG (hyperkalaemia) and chest radiograph
- urine dipstick test for WBC, nitrites, protein, blood, ketones
- urine microscopy for RBC, WBC, crystals and casts
- urgent renal tract ultrasound to exclude obstruction
- if sepsis suspected, consider blood and urine cultures
- if the cause remains unclear, consider serum and urine electrophoresis, serum immunoglobulins, complement level, ESR.

Management

Renal failure will be the anticipated terminal event for some patients, for example in those with bilateral ureteric obstruction from a large pelvic tumour for whom ureteric stenting is not possible or not desired by the patient.

If the patient is close to death before diagnosis of ARF, it may not be appropriate to manage the complications of ARF (e.g. hyperkalaemia) if the patient will be unable to tolerate treatment of the cause of ARF (e.g. cardiogenic shock from a massive pulmonary embolus). In such cases, treatment should be directed towards the relief of distressing symptoms such as breathlessness and agitation (see p.426).

Where active management of ARF is appropriate, consider seeking specialist advice from a renal physician, and transferring the patient to a high dependency unit if life-threatening complications of ARF ensue. Initial measures include:
- review drug chart, stop all nephrotoxic drugs, and stop or reduce the dose of all renally excreted drugs
- treat hyperkalaemia (Box 12.T)
- treat pulmonary oedema (see p.370)

Box 12.T   Management of hyperkalaemia

When ECG abnormalities are present, first give calcium gluconate 10% 10ml IV to protect against arrhythmia; this is important because initially β_2-agonists may transiently increase the plasma potassium concentration.[36,37]

Administer salbutamol:
- 1,200microgram (12 puffs) inhaled over 2min via a spacer device *or*
- 10–20mg nebulized (use 5mg/ml formulation) over 10–30min; effective within 5–30min; duration of effect $\geqslant$1–2h *or*
- 2.5mg nebulized every 20min as tolerated.

Repeat salbutamol if necessary.[38]

If above ineffective, or hyperkalaemia is $\geqslant$6mmol/L, also give insulin and dextrose.[37]

- control bleeding; uraemia impairs haemostasis and may exacerbate a haemorrhagic cause of ARF
- monitor fluid balance; insert urinary catheter and keep strict fluid balance charts
- correct hypovolaemia with IV fluids, and consider inserting a central venous line
- treat sepsis with antibacterials targeted at probable cause.

Dialysis is indicated for persistent hyperkalaemia ($K^+ > 7$mmol/L), worsening metabolic acidosis, worsening pulmonary oedema, uraemic pericarditis, uraemic encephalopathy. However, it is unlikely that most patients with advanced cancer will be able to tolerate the physiological demands of dialysis. If there is any uncertainty, a time-limited trial of dialysis could be considered.

ACUTE URINARY RETENTION

Acute urinary retention is defined as sudden inability to pass urine. It occurs in 10% of men in their 70s and ≤30% in their 80s.[39] Acute urinary retention is uncommon in women.

Causes
There are many possible causes of acute urinary retention (Box 12.U). Functionally, these fall into several categories:
- factors that increase the resistance to flow of urine
- bladder overdistension
- interruption of sensory innervation of the bladder wall or motor supply of detrusor (through nerve damage or as undesirable drug effect).

Box 12.U   Causes of acute urinary retention

Cancer
Malignant enlargement of prostate
Infiltration of bladder neck
Blood clot in bladder
Peripheral nerve damage
   cauda equina compression
   sacral nerve root compression
   presacral plexopathy
   spinal shock

Treatment
Drugs
   antimuscarinics
   morphine (occasionally)
   spinal analgesia (particularly
   with bupivacaine)
Intrathecal nerve block
   (e.g. with phenol)

Debility
Loaded rectum
Inability to stand to void
Generalized weakness
Pain

Concurrent
Central neurological damage
   encephalitis
   multiple sclerosis
   Parkinson's disease
   stroke
Lower urinary tract instrumentation
Alcohol toxicity
Prostatitis, acute or chronic
Benign prostatic hypertrophy
Urethral stricture/stone

The most common cause in men >50 years is benign prostatic hyperplasia with bladder neck outflow obstruction (Box 12.U).

Clinical features

Patients present with great distress and suprapubic discomfort or pain. Examination may reveal:

- hypertension
- distended bladder that is palpable and/or dull to percussion
- tender bladder.

In an unconscious or delirious patient urinary retention must always be considered as a possible cause of their distress.

Evaluation

If urinary retention occurs during the final hours or days of life, detailed investigation is unlikely to be appropriate and patient comfort should be maintained.

Generally, detailed examination and investigation should be postponed until the patient has voided:

- neurological examination for spinal cord compression (see p.264)
- digital rectal examination to determine the size of the prostate, and to exclude loaded/impacted rectum
- plasma electrolytes (renal failure)
- plasma prostate specific antigen (PSA); if possible, before rectal examination and catheterization because both these can raise the PSA level
- urine dipstick test and culture
- renal ultrasound scan.

Management

If urinary retention occurs during the final hours or days of life, proceed directly to catheterization to achieve and maintain comfort.

If the patient is not in great distress and is well enough, the following may aid voiding:

- privacy on ward
- ambulation
- standing to void
- voiding to sound of running water
- voiding in warm bath
- analgesia for pain.

If the above fail or are impracticable, insert a urethral catheter under aseptic technique. Residual urine volume should be recorded. If there is evidence of a UTI or the patient is immunocompromised, catheter insertion should be covered with antibacterials, e.g. ciprofloxacin 250mg PO stat. If it is not possible to insert a urethral catheter, e.g. because of urethral strictures or a large prostate, a supra-pubic catheter should be placed.

Rapid bladder decompression may cause mucosal haemorrhage. This is generally mild and self-limiting but some authorities recommend that a maximum of 500mL/hour of urine is drained to reduce the chances of this occurring. Post-obstruction diuresis is a rare complication of catheterization. Because it may lead to dehydration, hypotension and collapse (rare), urine output and blood pressure should be monitored. Some patients may require treatment with IV fluids.

HYPOGLYCAEMIA

Hypoglycaemia is defined as a blood glucose of <2.5mmol/L. The threshold for symptoms varies between patients. Those with long-standing diabetes may develop autonomic neuropathy and lose both the adrenergic warning symptoms of hypoglycaemia and adrenaline (epinephrine)-induced increase in blood glucose (Box 12.V).

Box 12.V   Signs and symptoms of hypoglycaemia

Adrenergic	**Neuroglycopenic**
Hunger	Pallor
Tremor	Mental detachment
Sweating	Clumsiness
Pounding heart	Mannerisms
Tachycardia	Personality change
	Confusion
	Mutism
	Drowsiness
	Seizures
	Transient hemiplegia (rare)
	Coma

Causes

Causes of hypoglycaemia can be divided into two types:
- fasting hypoglycaemia; the commonest cause of which is excess insulin or sulphonylurea treatment in a known diabetic (Box 12.W)
- post-prandial hypoglycaemia; may be caused by 'dumping syndrome' following gastric surgery, or reactive hypoglycaemia particularly after ingestion of alcohol.

Box 12.W   Causes of fasting hypoglycaemia[40]

Drugs	**Endocrine**
Drugs used to treat diabetes	Pituitary insufficiency
sulphonylureas	Addison's disease
meglitinides	
insulin	**Cancer**
Other drugs	Islet cell tumours
alcohol	insulinoma
quinine sulphate	Non-islet cell tumours
pentamidine	mesenchymal tumours
aminoglutethimide	any advanced cancer
	Auto-immune
Organ damage	Hodgkin's disease
Hepatic failure	
Pancreatitis	

Non-islet cell tumours cause hypoglycaemia by production of an abnormally large form of insulin-like growth factor 2 (big IGF-2). This has insulin-like activity, suppresses growth hormone secretion and in addition increases normal free IGF-2 by preventing it from binding to its binding proteins. Hypoglycaemia in Hodgkin's disease may be caused by anti-insulin receptor antibodies.

Evaluation

In the majority of cases, measurement of blood glucose using a fingerstick test will be sufficient to establish hypoglycaemia. If the cause of hypoglycaemia is not clear, further investigation may be necessary:
- fasting venous blood glucose
- fasting pro-insulin, insulin, C-peptide, IGF-1, IGF-2, big IGF-2
- anti-insulin receptor antibodies.

Management

Oral glucose is the first-line treatment (Box 12.X). Glucagon is of limited value in malnourished and cachectic patients with advanced cancer because their liver glycogen stores are likely to be depleted. IV glucose is more effective in such patients. When the blood glucose level has improved, the patient should, if possible, be given a starch-based meal, e.g. toast, to prevent further falls in blood glucose.

Box 12.X Treatment of hypoglycaemia

If conscious, give glucose 10–20g PO. About 10g of glucose is contained in:
- 3 glucose tablets
- GlucoGel® oral ampoule
- 2 teaspoons or 3 lumps of sugar
- 60mL of Lucozade® (not diet version)
- 90mL of Coca-Cola® (not diet version)
- 120–180mL of fruit juice.

If drowsy/unconscious and swallowing unsafe, but is not malnourished or cachectic, give glucagon 1mg IM/IV (can be given SC but acts more slowly).

If no response in 10min, give glucose 20% 50mL IV.

If definitive treatment of non-islet cell tumour hypoglycaemia is not possible (surgery, radiotherapy or chemotherapy), hypoglycaemia can be treated with a glucocorticoid, e.g. dexamethasone 4–8mg PO once daily.[41] Patients should also be given small, regular starch-based meals. If hypoglycaemia is persistent, diazoxide may be given. Recombinant human growth hormone has been tried in resistant cases.[42]

PAIN

Biliary and ureteric colic

The treatment of choice for biliary colic is an IM or IV injection of an NSAID, e.g. diclofenac 75mg.[43] If this fails to provide relief in 20–30min, it should be supplemented by diamorphine 5mg SC/IV or morphine 10mg SC/IV.

Alternatively, if already receiving PO morphine for cancer pain give:
- a double dose of morphine PO *or*
- an injection of diamorphine/morphine equal in mg to the previous regular PO dose; this will have 2–3 times the effect of the oral dose.

Intrahepatic haemorrhage

Occasionally with liver metastases, the patient experiences increasingly severe right upper quadrant pain. Unless associated features suggest an alternative diagnosis, e.g. perforated peptic ulcer or cholecystitis, the most likely diagnosis is an intrahepatic haemorrhage causing acute distension of the hepatic capsule. When this is the case:
- explain the cause to the patient
- give double the previous oral analgesic morphine requirement *or*
- if the patient has already taken an extra rescue dose of morphine with inadequate relief, *treble* the previous oral morphine dose; the presence of severe pain despite an additional dose of morphine indicates that the dose can be safely increased to this level.[44]

This is an acute phenomenon which resolves as the hepatic capsule adapts and the haematoma is resorbed. Advise the patient that, in about a week, analgesic requirements are likely to be similar to that needed before the haemorrhage. Tentative dose reductions can be made after 3 days or sooner if the patient is comfortable but complaining of drowsiness. Failure to reduce the dose may result in increased undesirable opioid effects, e.g.:
- nausea and vomiting
- drowsiness
- delirium.

Acute vertebral collapse

Typically the patient is already taking regular analgesics for bone pain and, before being seen by a doctor, will already have taken one or more rescue doses of oral morphine. If these have failed to give adequate relief, it may be necessary to *treble* the previous satisfactory dose of morphine for several weeks (after which it is generally possible to reduce the dose again over several days/weeks to its pre-collapse level).

Palliative radiotherapy is generally beneficial but it may take 4–6 weeks to achieve maximal relief. In patients with secondary muscle spasm, diazepam 5mg stat and 5–10mg at bedtime may help.

For those with associated nerve compression pain, dexamethasone 4–8mg once daily may also help. Alternatively, some patients benefit by epidural depot methylprednisolone 80mg in 2mL. This can be repeated once or twice at daily or weekly intervals.

Some patients experience excruciating back pain even with slight movement (incident pain) which may well be overwhelming. This is more likely in patients with radiologically confirmed spinal instability (see p.268). Spinal cord compression (SCC), suggested by radicular pain, motor weakness, sensory symptoms and bladder dysfunction, should be excluded (see p.264).

Management options for incident pain associated with acute vertebral collapse include:
- nitrous oxide (50% with oxygen) before and during movement
- epidural analgesia with morphine and bupivacaine
- percutaneous vertebroplasty in highly selected cases, i.e. injection of bone cement containing polymethylmethacrylate into the fractured vertebral body under fluoroscopic guidance[45,46]
- orthopaedic surgery in patients with a prognosis of >3 months and neurological impairment, particularly if SCC is suspected.[47–49]

Depending on the primary site, surgery may be followed by radiotherapy, chemotherapy or hormone therapy. These should also be considered for patients unable to undergo surgery.

Pathological fracture of a long bone
Conservative management of pathological fractures of a long bone may well be unsatisfactory, with pain and reduced mobility continuing for many weeks if the fracture does not heal. Surgery should be considered for impending or established fractures in all patients because it offers the most reliable and rapid means of relieving pain and restoring function. Surgery requires the patient to be willing and generally fit enough to undergo an operation and the presence of enough bone for stable fixation. Radiotherapy should be considered after surgical stabilization.[50] Even in cases of non-union of the fracture, the inserted device (e.g. an intramedullary nail) can give sufficient stability for pain relief and satisfactory function.

While awaiting surgery, it is important to ensure that sufficient analgesia is provided together with night sedation. If surgery is planned, ensure that pre-fracture analgesics are continued and that additional p.r.n. postoperative medication is prescribed at an appropriate level (see *PCF3*, Chapter 16, Management of postoperative pain in opioid-dependent patients).

Humerus
Immediate care is generally conservative, using a loosely fitting sling to part-immobilize the limb. The sling should allow the arm to hang down freely, which will improve bone alignment and reduce muscle spasm.

The patient should be encouraged to keep the arm in this position as much as possible, and to sleep in a semi-upright position. To prevent joint stiffening, the patient should be encouraged to use their fingers as much as possible and, at least twice a day, the arm should be removed from the sling and the elbow completely straightened.

Alternative measures include:
- splint arm to trunk with Netelast® and/or Velcro® *or*
- fracture braces (humeral shaft).

It is important to provide adequate analgesia (see *PCF3*, Chapter 16). If pain remains a major problem, consider a nerve block. In some patients, surgery may be appropriate. If the patient is expected to live for more than a few weeks, arrange for radiotherapy.

Femur
Immediate care (or if surgery inappropriate):
- immobilize leg with pillows or skin traction
- use appropriate nursing techniques for turning the patient in bed, e.g. 'logrolling'

- administer a local anaesthetic femoral nerve block with 10mL of 0.5% bupivacaine before obtaining a radiograph
- use a Thomas splint or bandage the legs together if transferring to orthopaedic/accident service (plus local anaesthetic block)
- if treating conservatively, consider epidural analgesia
- consider radiotherapy.

PSYCHIATRIC

Nearly 1/2 of patients with cancer have a psychiatric disorder as judged by criteria in the *Diagnostic and Statistical Manual of Mental Disorders*.[51] However, in 2/3 of these it is a transient adjustment disorder with depressed, anxious or mixed mood rather than a florid psychiatric illness. The other 1/3 comprise, in order of occurrence, depression, delirium, anxiety disorders, personality disorders or psychoses. Unrelieved pain is particularly associated with depression and delirium.

The suicidal patient

Suicidal statements range from comments which merely reflect the 'heat of the moment' to ones which are an expression of despair. Suicidal ideas are relatively common in patients with cancer, and the risk of suicide is increased compared with the general population.[52,53] However, in patients supported by a specialist palliative care service suicide is rare, less than 1 in 3,000.[54,55]

Suicidal cancer patients are likely to be suffering from:
- an adjustment disorder with anxious and depressed features (50%)
- major depression (30%)
- delirium (20%).

Depression, a sense of hopelessness and exhaustion (physical, psychological, social, spiritual or financial) greatly increase the risk of suicide. There are also many other risk factors[56] (Box 12.Y).

Exploring suicidal thoughts is imperative; find out if definite plans to commit suicide have been made and take note of any risk factors. Obtain help from a psychiatrist in evaluation and in formulating a management plan (Box 12.Z).

The violent patient

Isolated episodes of violent behaviour are uncommon in palliative care patients. They are most likely to occur as part of delirium (p.207), terminal agitation (p.430) and in patients with a psychiatric history. Such episodes should be anticipated, and appropriate care plans drawn up by the multiprofessional team.

Causes

A frightened and/or angry patient may resort to violence. This is more likely in delirium (p.207). Numerous other disorders may also precipitate violence (Box 12.AA).

Evaluation

If possible, check blood glucose levels. Further evaluation is unlikely to be possible until the patient has calmed down.

Box 12.Y Risk factors for suicide[53,57,58]

Historical
Family history of suicide
Previous attempt
Pre-existing psychiatric disorder
Experience of domestic violence
Experience of abuse as a child

Diagnostic
Cancer
    particularly head and neck
    recent diagnosis
AIDS
Spinal cord injury
Multiple sclerosis
Substance abuse
Huntington's chorea
Systemic lupus erythematosus
Visual impairment

Psychological
Depression
Frequent suicidal thoughts
Other psychiatric disorder
Recent bereavement
Social isolation
Fear of serious physical deformity
    or suffering
A sense of helplessness associated with
    physical dependency and loss of control

Physical
Severe pain
Multiple physical symptoms

Box 12.Z Dealing with suicidal cancer patients[52]

Preliminaries
Establish *rapport*.

Explore the patient's understanding of their illness and present symptoms.

Evaluation
Mental status, e.g. cognitive function, mood, fears.

Uncontrolled pain or other distressing symptoms?

Any past major psychiatric disorders (patient or family), suicide threats, suicide attempts?

Seriousness of suicidal thoughts/intent/plans.

Presence of other risk factors?

Management
If the patient is actively suicidal, constant supervision is required.

Explore possible alternatives to death and indicate what can be done to improve the quality of life by relieving pain, other physical symptoms, delirium, anxiety, depression, etc.

As far as possible, give the patient some degree of control.

Make use of the patient's social network.

Box 12.AA   Causes of violence in patients

Biochemical disturbance
Hypercalcaemia
Hypoglycaemia
Thiamine deficiency

Intoxication/withdrawal
Alcohol

Neurological
Brain tumour(s) or metastases
Paraneoplastic syndrome
Post-ictal confusion
Non-convulsive status epilepticus

Substance of abuse
Amphetamines, e.g.
  methylenedioxymethamfetamine
  (MDMA, Ecstasy)
Cocaine
Lysergic acid diethylamide (LSD)

Drug-induced
Antimuscarinics
Chemotherapy, e.g. cisplatin, 5-FU,
  ifosfamide, methotrexate
Corticosteroid-induced psychosis
Immunomodulators, e.g. interferon,
  interleukin

Psychiatric disorder
Mania
Paranoid disorders
Personality disorder
Schizophrenia

Organ failure
Hepatic encephalopathy

Management
Prevent the preventable
Health professionals should be aware of their own trigger factors and vulnerabilities which may contribute to the development of a violent encounter. Aim to prevent violent behaviour developing in a patient by being aware of and acting on warning signs (Box 12.BB).[59]

It is important to maintain the safety of the staff and other patients when managing a potentially violent encounter:
• never manage the situation alone; obtain help from another health professional, e.g. a nurse who knows the patient well
• move towards a safe place and avoid being trapped without an exit
• move other patients from the immediate area
• if possible, remove potential weapons and ask the patient to move to a designated safe area, if one exists.

It is not realistic to expect a patient exhibiting disturbed behaviour simply to calm down. De-escalation techniques should be used before physical or pharmacological restraint:[59]
• one staff member should take control of a violent situation
• allow greater body space than normal between staff member and patient
• avoid excessive eye contact
• maintain a relaxed but attentive posture
• use a re-assuring and non-judgemental tone
• attempt to establish a *rapport* with the patient and emphasise co-operation
• listen carefully, show empathy and acknowledge any grievances or frustrations
• allow the patient to vent anger

> **Box 12.BB** Warning signs of a violent patient[59]
>
> **Communication**
> Discontentment
> Fear
> Refusal to communicate
> Withdrawal
> Irritation
> Reporting angry or violent feelings
> Verbal threats
> Increased speech volume
> Shouting or chanting
>
> **Arousal**
> Tachypnoea
> Dilated pupils
> Muscle tension
> Muscle twitching
>
> **Physical**
> Facial expressions tense and angry
> Prolonged eye contact
> Restlessness
> Erratic movements
> Angry gestures
> Pacing
>
> **Psychiatric**
> Poor concentration
> Thought processes unclear
> Confusion
> Paranoid ideas
> Delusions or hallucinations with violent content

- ask open questions about reasons for the patient's anger
- negotiate realistic options and avoid threats
- develop a mutually acceptable action plan.

Non-drug treatment
Should de-escalation techniques fail, it may be necessary to call security or the police. Physical or pharmacological restraint may be required to prevent the patient from harming himself, other patients or staff. Any such action is a step of last resort and should be proportionate to the level of threat posed by the patient and used for the shortest time possible. These actions are permitted under English common law and the Mental Capacity Act 2005.[60]

Ideally, physical restraint should be carried out only by trained staff, if there are sufficient numbers of such staff present. Where possible, items of clothing should be held. If limbs have to be restrained, they should be held near large joints to prevent fracture or dislocation. Pressure should never be applied to the patient's neck, throat, chest or abdomen.

Drug treatment
If hypoglycaemic, give 10% dextrose 200mL IV; glucagon 1mg IM/IV may be given as an alternative (see Box 12.X, p.379).

Pharmacological restraint may be carried out with antipsychotics or benzodiazepines:
- haloperidol 2.5mg–10mg IM; occasionally, higher doses may be needed
- lorazepam 1–4mg IM
- midazolam 5mg IM/IV in 2.5mg–5mg boluses until patient sedated.

The patient's airway should be maintained and respiratory function monitored at all times.

Depending on the patient's overall condition and the cause of violent behaviour, a management plan should be written on managing the patient once the initial sedation wears off. Advice from a psychiatrist or crisis mental health team may be sought.

OVERDOSE

Overdose of prescription drugs or self-poisoning with other substances by a patient may be deliberate or accidental. Deliberate overdose may be a genuine suicide attempt or an episode of self-harm (parasuicide). Because the approach to management is the same, they can be considered together.[58]

Overdose by a patient is unlikely to occur in an inpatient palliative care setting because the patient should not have access to drugs. However, most palliative care patients are at home for much of the time. If a patient takes an overdose at home, the palliative care team may be asked about the patient's mental capacity, and the applicability of an Advance Decision to Refuse Treatment (ADRT). Further, the team may be involved in a decision about whether to admit the patient to the local palliative care unit/hospice if they have competently declined admission to hospital.

In the general population, drugs commonly used to overdose are:
- analgesics, including paracetamol
- psychotropics, mostly antidepressants and benzodiazepines.

Together these classes of drugs account for >75% of overdoses.[58] Alcohol will also have been consumed by about 50% of those who overdose. Palliative care patients collectively have ready access to such drugs.

Evaluation
Medication and/or empty containers should be collected and examined.

It is important to identify:
- the time the overdose was taken
- the drugs ingested (often more than one)
- quantities taken
- whether consumed with alcohol, or by a patient with a history of alcohol misuse.

If there is time, and the patient is willing and able to answer questions, sensitively explore the reason's for the patient's action, the patient's mental status and risk of a further overdose attempt (see Box 12.Z, p.383). Such a discussion should not delay treatment of severe or life-threatening symptoms, and in many cases will need to be deferred until after medical management of the overdose.

Consent for treatment
Mental capacity in a patient who has self-harmed must be presumed unless there is evidence to the contrary.[61] Patients should be provided with full information on treatment options, and meaningful and informed consent sought. If a patient declines treatment, mental capacity must be evaluated.[61] If the patient is deemed to have capacity their decision must be respected, even if there is a risk of permanent injury or death.

The fact that a patient has a mental disorder is not sufficient to override the assumption of capacity. However, if a patient is detained under Section 2 or 3 of the Mental Health Act 2005, compulsory treatment may sometimes include medical treatment for the effects of overdose.

If a patient is considered to lack mental capacity, they must be treated in their best interests, taking account of any stated wishes, ADRT, etc. (see p.407).[61] However, it may be difficult for the treating doctor rapidly to establish whether an ADRT is applicable or valid, particularly if the doctor has not met the patient before. Validity may be compromised if the patient had depression severe enough to render them mentally incompetent when making the ADRT, or was experiencing undue pressure or coercion. When such concerns exist about the validity or applicability of the ADRT, life-saving treatment or treatment to prevent severe deterioration may be provided until these concerns are answered.[61]

Management

For most patients, management of an overdose should be carried out in hospital. Immediate action may include:

- maintain airway
- administration of oxygen to maintain SaO_2 > 95%
- monitor blood pressure
- determine and monitor level of consciousness
- check temperature
- check blood glucose level (fingerstick test)
- obtain IV access
- check ECG.

In the UK, those working within the NHS can obtain information about the management of specific drug overdoses from:

- TOXBASE website (www.toxbase.org)
- National Poisons Information Service telephone advice line.

Medicinal opioid overdose

Medicinal opioid overdose, because of, for example, drug accumulation, drug interaction, or excessive ingestion, is a distinct problem from an accidental or deliberate overdose in an addict. In the latter, the aim is to reverse the full effect of the opioid and it is treated vigorously with IV naloxone, e.g. 400microgram–2mg IV every 2–3min p.r.n., up to a total of 10mg, in order to fully reverse respiratory depression and drowsiness/coma.

However, when a patient is taking medicinal opioids for pain relief, it is important to titrate the dose of naloxone carefully against respiratory function and *not* the level of consciousness. Total opioid antagonism will cause a return of severe, possibly excruciating, pain with hyperalgesia and, if the patient is physically dependent, severe physical withdrawal symptoms, and marked agitation.[62] It is obviously important to avoid this. Thus, *there should be a reluctance to use naloxone in palliative care patients, and it should never be used just to reverse a reduced level of consciousness.* On the rare occasions when naloxone can be justified, very small doses are indicated (Box 12.CC).

The only exception to this cautious approach is buprenorphine. Because buprenorphine has very strong receptor affinity (reflected in its high relative potency with morphine), naloxone in standard doses does not reverse the effects of buprenorphine and, if naloxone is indicated, much higher doses must be used (Box 12.DD).[64–67]

However, significant respiratory depression is rarely seen with clinically recommended doses of buprenorphine, although in addicts the concurrent use of a benzodiazepine appears to increase the risk of serious or fatal respiratory depression.[68]

The non-specific respiratory stimulant doxapram can also be used, 1–1.5mg/kg IV over 30sec, repeated if necessary at hourly intervals, or 1.5–4mg/min CIVI.[69,70]

Benzodiazepine overdose

Overdose of benzodiazepines alone is rarely fatal. However, if taken with other psychotropics, opioids or alcohol, benzodiazepines can potentiate the central depressant effects of these drugs, inducing coma and death.[71,72]

Box 12.CC Naloxone for iatrogenic opioid overdose (based on the recommendations of the American Pain Society)[63]

If respiratory rate ≥8 breaths/min, and the patient easily rousable and not cyanosed, adopt a policy of 'wait and see'; consider reducing by 50% (or omitting totally) the next regular dose of morphine.

If respiratory rate <8 breaths/min, and the patient comatose/unconscious and/or cyanosed:
- dilute a standard ampoule containing naloxone 400microgram to 10mL with 0.9% saline for injection
- administer 0.5mL (20microgram) IV every 2min until the patient's respiratory status is satisfactory
- further boluses may be necessary because naloxone is shorter-acting than morphine and other opioids, particularly when a m/r formulation has been taken
- occasionally, and particularly with methadone, a carefully monitored IV infusion of naloxone may be indicated for ≤24h.

Box 12.DD Reversal of buprenorphine-induced respiratory depression

---

Discontinue buprenorphine (stop CSCI/CIVI, remove TD patch).

Give oxygen by mask.

Give IV naloxone *2mg* stat over 90sec.

Commence naloxone *4mg/h* by CIVI.

Continue CIVI until the patient's condition is satisfactory (probably <90min).

Monitor the patient frequently for the next 24h, and restart CIVI if respiratory depression recurs.

If the patient's condition remains satisfactory, restart buprenorphine at a reduced dose, e.g. 1/2 the previous dose.

Flumazenil is a competitive antagonist of benzodiazepines. It is *not* licensed in the UK for the diagnosis and treatment of benzodiazepine overdose. Flumazenil has a shorter duration of action than most benzodiazepines, so may need to be given in repeated doses or as an infusion to prevent the recurrence of sedation.[73] It must be administered slowly and in small doses to reduce the chance of patients becoming agitated or developing seizures.

Flumazenil should *not* be used in patients:
- suspected of taking a mixed overdose including TCAs or other pro-convulsants (lower seizure threshold)[74]
- with a history of epilepsy because seizures may be induced
- who are dependent on benzodiazepines.

It should only be given under expert advice and, ideally, where resuscitation facilities are available:[58,75]
- 200microgram IV over 15sec, then 100microgram at 1min intervals p.r.n.
- normal dose range 300–600microgram; maximum total dose 1mg.

Sedation or respiratory depression caused by medicinal use or intentional overdose of opioids or benzodiazepines does not preclude the future use of these drugs with appropriate caution, e.g. dose reduction, close monitoring.

SUBSTANCE WITHDRAWAL

Substance withdrawal is a substance-specific syndrome which causes significant distress or impairment in social, occupational or other important areas of functioning. It is associated with physiological and cognitive symptoms. Substance withdrawal is generally associated with substance dependence. Specific substance withdrawal syndromes are recognized for:
- alcohol (see below)
- amphetamines
- cocaine
- nicotine
- opioids
- anxiolytic-sedatives and hypnotics.[76]

Drugs most commonly misused in the UK are cannabis, cocaine and stimulants such as amphetamines. Many patients who misuse drugs misuse more than one simultaneously or sequentially. Opioids are misused less commonly, although they present the most significant health problems.[77] Help in managing such patients should be sought from a psychiatrist specializing in drug misuse. Managing pain in opioid-dependent patients requires particular care (for more information, see PCF3, Chapter 16, Management of postoperative pain in opioid-dependent patients).

Substance abuse and dependence can cause significant distress to patient and family, so should be addressed even if the patient has a limited prognosis. When time is short, therapy goals may be different, e.g. maintenance rather than abstinence-oriented.[78]

Features of withdrawal depend upon the substance used, but most are the opposite of symptoms caused by intoxication with that substance. Onset of a withdrawal syndrome depends upon the duration of action of the substance. The withdrawal syndrome associated with long-acting drugs generally takes longer to develop, lasts longer, but has less intense symptoms than that associated with a short-acting drug. For example, heroin (diamorphine) withdrawal is of more acute onset and lasts a shorter time than methadone withdrawal.

If a patient misuses more than one substance, it may be difficult to differentiate symptoms of withdrawal from one substance from those of intoxication with another, e.g. intoxication with amphetamines may mimic withdrawal symptoms of alcohol or anxiolytic-sedatives. Other differential diagnoses must also be considered (see Delirium, p.207).[76]

Drug treatment can help in the management of acute withdrawal symptoms for alcohol, nicotine and opioids. This should be followed up with psychosocial interventions, e.g. self-help groups and contingency management plans.[77]

Alcohol withdrawal

Alcohol dependence is found in 10–20% of the general hospital population.[79] In an inpatient palliative care unit in Canada, the incidence was found to be as high as 30%.[80] The syndrome of alcohol withdrawal occurs on cessation or reduction of alcohol consumption in patients who have become alcohol-dependent through heavy and prolonged alcohol use. Alcohol withdrawal must always be considered as a cause of delirium or terminal agitation (see p.207).

Pathophysiology

Alcohol is a depressant of the CNS. It decreases GABA-receptor activity in the ventral tegmental area, thereby disinhibiting GABA-mediated inhibition of ventral tegmental dopamine neurones. This results in increased dopamine neurotransmission. Chronic alcohol users also have more glutamate binding sites in the midbrain; these also inhibit GABA activity.[81]

Chronic exposure to alcohol leads to upregulation of CNS neural mechanisms to counteract this. Abrupt reduction or cessation of alcohol leaves these adaptive mechanisms unopposed, resulting in the hyperexcitable state of alcohol withdrawal syndrome.

Clinical features

Alcohol withdrawal syndrome varies from mild–severe in its presentation (Box 12.EE). Delirium tremens is the most severe form of withdrawal. It is characterized by agitation, disorientation, marked tremor and visual hallucinations. Patients often feel terrified and may become violent. Signs of delirium tremens include marked sympathetic hyperactivity with sweating, tachycardia, tachypnoea, mydriasis and pyrexia. If delirium tremens develops, it is likely that other clinically relevant medical conditions will be present, e.g. hypoglycaemia, pneumonia, hepatic failure, electrolyte imbalance. Severe withdrawal symptoms, including delirium tremens, occur in <10% of patients, and <3% develop generalized seizures.[76,82]

Box 12.EE Diagnostic criteria for alcohol withdrawal[76]

A Cessation of (or reduction in) alcohol use which has been heavy and prolonged.

B Two (or more) of the following, developing within several hours or a few days after criterion A:
- autonomic hyperactivity (e.g. sweating or pulse rate >100)
- increased hand tremor
- insomnia
- nausea or vomiting
- transient visual, tactile or auditory hallucinations or illusions
- psychomotor agitation
- anxiety
- generalized convulsive seizures.

C The symptoms in criterion B cause clinically significant distress or impairment in social, occupational, or other important areas of functioning.

D The symptoms are not caused by a general medical condition and are not better accounted for by another mental disorder.

Withdrawal symptoms generally develop acutely, within 4–12h after reducing or stopping alcohol intake. These symptoms generally peak after 2 days of abstinence and improve markedly within 5 days. The onset of delirium tremens is 2–4 days after alcohol cessation and may last 1–3 days, although some patients have a remitting course over several days or weeks. A chronic withdrawal syndrome may also develop, with symptoms such as anxiety, insomnia and autonomic dysfunction persisting for 6 months.[76]

Evaluation

Examine patient for signs of related illnesses that will worsen symptoms of withdrawal, e.g. pneumonia, hepatic failure, hypoglycaemia.

Investigation will depend upon the patient's overall condition, and the aims of care. If the patient is not close to death, consider:

- FBC (macrocytosis, anaemia)
- plasma electrolytes (hyponatraemia), LFTs, PT
- plasma glucose and regular glucose monitoring with blood fingerstick test
- blood, urine, sputum cultures if evidence of infection
- temperature
- blood pressure
- pulse oximetry.

Management

If a dying patient has chronic alcohol dependence and does not want to stop drinking alcoholic beverages, a plan could be negotiated with the patient, relatives and nurses to decide:

- mutually acceptable levels and times of alcohol consumption
- who is to supply the alcoholic beverages
- whether friends and relatives are to be permitted to drink with the patient.

Such an option may assure alcohol-dependent patients who might otherwise decline admission to a palliative care unit.

Prevent the preventable

If there is any concern about possible alcohol dependence in a patient, a screening test should be used to identify it to prevent acute, unmanaged withdrawal. The 10-item AUDIT (Alcohol Use Disorders Identification Test) questionnaire,[83] and its derivatives, are superior to the CAGE questionnaire[84] and have been validated in many settings.

Drug treatment

Uncomplicated alcohol withdrawal can be managed without medication.[85] When medication is required, benzodiazepines should be used.[86] Chlordiazepoxide is the benzodiazepine of choice.[87] The symptom-triggered, front-loading technique (where a benzodiazepine is initially administered at 2h intervals until the patient is asymptomatic, and then only when the patient develops sufficiently severe symptoms) results in lower doses of benzodiazepines being used but requires close and regular monitoring by staff.[88] A tapered regimen is generally more practical (Table 12.1).

Table 12.1 Chlordiazepoxide PO regimen for alcohol withdrawal

Day	Dose
1–2	20–30mg q.d.s.
3–4	15mg q.d.s.
5	10mg q.d.s.
6	10mg b.d.
7	10mg at bedtime

The initial dose of chlordiazepoxide will depend upon the severity of alcohol dependence, the patient's liver function and their weight. A loading dose of 100mg chlordiazepoxide can be given if early signs of delirium appear. If symptoms are very severe, p.r.n. doses of chlodiazepoxide 10–20mg PO q.d.s. may be required.[89] Diazepam is an acceptable alternative to chlordiazepoxide, and can similarly be given as a tapered regimen (chlordiazepoxide 15mg is approximately equivalent to diazepam 5mg).

If the patient is at risk of Wernicke's encephalopathy, prophylactic treatment should be given:[90]
- Pabrinex® IV/IM 1 pair of ampoules once daily for 3–5 days
- maintain with thiamine 100mg PO b.d.–t.d.s.

If acute alcohol withdrawal presents in the last few days of life and when the oral route is unreliable, it should be managed as for terminal agitation (see p.430) with midazolam by CSCI. Thiamine replacement is unlikely to be appropriate.

ADVERSE DRUG REACTIONS

Serotonin toxicity
Serotonin toxicity is caused by the excessive ingestion of drugs which increase central and peripheral concentrations of serotonin. Individuals vary in their susceptibility, but a continued increase in serotonin levels inevitably leads to toxicity (cf. digoxin toxicity). The incidence of serotonin toxicity is difficult to estimate because, when mild, it may not be recognized. Severe life-threatening toxicity is rare.[91]

Pathophysiology
Drugs increase central serotonin concentrations by:
- increasing serotonin synthesis and release *or*
- inhibiting serotonin breakdown and re-uptake *or*
- stimulating serotonin receptors.[92]

Of the seven families of serotonin (5HT) receptors, no single receptor appears responsible for the development of toxicity. However, stimulation of $5HT_{2A}$ receptors may contribute substantially.[93,94] Dopaminergic receptors and other neurotransmitters including GABA- and NMDA-receptor antagonists have been implicated.[91]

Causes
Serotonin toxicity is caused by many antidepressants, several other psychotropics, some opioids, various other prescription drugs, certain illicit drugs, and some OTC drugs and herbal products (Box 12.FF). Severe toxicity is more likely to result from a combination of two or more serotoninergic drugs which elevate serotonin levels by different mechanisms.

Clinical features
Serotonin toxicity is characterized by a triad of neuro-excitatory symptoms (Box 12.GG). Spontaneous, inducible or ocular clonus is the most reliable indicator of toxicity. Sweating, tremor, altered mental state and leg hyperreflexia are also essential for making a firm diagnosis.

Box 12.FF   Drugs with clinically relevant serotoninergic potency[91,94–96]

Antidepressants
Mono-amine oxidase inhibitors (MAOIs)
All types (non-selective or selective type A/type B; reversible or irreversible)
Clorgyline, iproniazid, isocarboxazid, moclobemide, nialamid, pargyline, phenelzine, toloxatone, tranylcypromine

Selective serotonin re-uptake inhibitors (SSRIs)
Citalopram, fluoxetine, fluvoxamine, paroxetine, sertraline

Serotonin and norepinephrine re-uptake inhibitors (SNRIs)
Clomipramine, duloxetine, imipramine, milnacipran, venlafaxine (but not other TCAs)

Psychostimulants (serotonin releasers)
Dexamfetamine, methylenedioxymethamfetamine (MDMA, Ecstasy) (but not methylphenidate)

Other drugs
H₁-antihistamines (serotonin re-uptake inhibitors)
Chlorphenamine, bromphenamine (but not other H₁-antihistamines)

Opioids (serotonin re-uptake inhibitors)
Dextromethorphan, dextropropoxyphene, fentanils, methadone, pentazocine, pethidine, tramadol (but not other opioids)

Miscellaneous
Furazolidone, linezolid (antibacterials) ⎤
Methylene blue   ⎬ **MAOIs**
Procarbazine (antineoplastic)   ⎟
Selegiline (antiparkinsonian)   ⎦
Sibutramine (anorectic) **SNRI**

Box 12.GG   Clinical features of serotonin toxicity

Neuromuscular hyperactivity
Tremor
Clonus   ⎤
Hyperreflexia   ⎬ marked in legs
Spasticity   ⎦

Altered mental state
Agitation
Hypomania
Delirium

Autonomic hyperactivity
Sweating
Fever (→ hyperthermia)
Tachycardia
Hypertension
Tachypnoea
Sialorrhoea
Diarrhoea

Patients may present with mild, moderate or severe cases of toxicity:[91,97]

- *mild*: tachycardia, anxiety, shivering, sweating, mydriasis with lower-limb hyperreflexia and intermittent tremor or myoclonus
- *moderate*: hyperthermia, overactive bowel sounds, diarrhoea, sustained clonus and ocular clonus. Mental state changes are more marked with agitation and hypomania
- *severe*: delirium, hyperthermia (core temperature $>38.5°C$), shock, and spasticity/hypertonicity severe enough to impair respiration and mask clonus and hyperreflexia.

Symptom onset is generally rapid, occurring in minutes–hours after starting the causal drug, or increasing the drug dose. In severe cases, symptoms may progress rapidly towards death. Occasionally, mild toxicity may occur for several weeks before the development of severe toxicity.

Serotonin toxicity should be differentiated from neuroleptic (antipsychotic) malignant syndrome (NMS). NMS is caused by antipsychotics and has a much slower onset, generally over several days (see p.395). Like serotonin toxicity, symptoms include hyperthermia, tachycardia and hypertension. However, NMS can be identified by the presence of bradykinesia and extrapyramidal (lead-pipe) rigidity in all muscle groups, muteness and possible stupor.

Evaluation
Diagnosis is based on drug history and recognition of clinical signs. It is important to inquire about the use of herbal medications, e.g. St John's Wort, OTC drugs (e.g. cough remedies containing dextromethorphan), and illicit drugs (e.g. methylenedioxy-methamfetamine/MDMA, Ecstasy) as these can cause or contribute to toxicity.

There are no diagnostic tests for serotonin toxicity. If severe, blood tests may show metabolic acidosis, rhabdomyolysis, renal failure and DIC.

Management
Correct the correctable
Recognition of mild forms of toxicity is crucial so that the doses of the causal drugs are not increased, and new serotoninergic drugs are not started. Such actions may lead to a dramatic decline in the patient's condition.

Drug treatment
Discontinue the causal medication. Symptoms will resolve in most patients within 24h. In severe toxicity it may be necessary to administer a benzodiazepine, e.g. midazolam 5–10mg SC p.r.n., to control agitation, and to prevent seizures (Box 12.HH).

Acute dystonias and oculogyric crisis
For more information, see *PCF3*.

Acute dystonias are extrapyramidal drug-induced movement disorders (Box 12.II). They are caused by drugs which block dopamine receptors in the CNS; these include all antipsychotics and metoclopramide (Box 12.JJ).[98]

Treatment
If possible, discontinue or reduce the dose of the causal drug; if metoclopramide, substitute domperidone. For immediate relief, give one of the following:
- an antimuscarinic antiparkinsonian drug, e.g.:
  ▷ benzatropine 1–2mg IV/IM *or*
  ▷ procyclidine 5–10mg IV/IM *or*
  ▷ diazepam 5mg IV[103]

Box 12.HH   Treatment of serotonin toxicity[91]

Severe cases should be managed in an intensive care unit.

Discontinue causal medication (toxicity generally resolves within 24h).

Provide supportive care, e.g. IV fluids.

Symptomatic measures:
- benzodiazepines for agitation, myoclonus and seizures, e.g. midazolam 5–10mg SC p.r.n.
- $5HT_{2A}$ antagonists, e.g.:
  ▷ chlorpromazine 50–100mg IM
  ▷ olanzapine 10mg IM
  ▷ cyproheptadine 12mg PO stat followed by 8mg q6h and 2mg q2h p.r.n. until symptoms resolve; tablets can be crushed and given by nasogastric tube
- stabilization of blood pressure:
  ▷ hypotension from MAOI interactions, give low doses of a sympathomimetic, e.g. adrenaline (epinephrine), noradrenaline (norepinephrine)
  ▷ hypertension, give short-acting agents, e.g. nitroprusside (a vasodilator), esmolol (β-adrenergic receptor antagonist).

If severe hyperthermia (>41°C), consider immediate:
- sedation
- neuromuscular paralysis with a non-depolarizing agent, e.g. vecuronium
- ventilation.

- some centres use an antihistaminic antimuscarinic, e.g. diphenhydramine 20–50mg IV/IM (not UK)
- with the antimuscarinics, benefit is typically seen in 10–20min, but:
  ▷ if necessary, repeat the injection after 30min
  ▷ continue treatment PO for 1 week with orphenadrine 50mg b.d.–t.d.s. *or* diphenhydramine 25–50mg b.d.–q.d.s. (not UK).[104]

Neuroleptic (antipsychotic) malignant syndrome

Neuroleptic (antipsychotic) malignant syndrome (NMS) is an idiosyncratic adverse drug reaction associated with both typical and atypical antipsychotics.[93] It occurs in <1% of those prescribed an antipsychotic.[105,106] Symptoms of NMS range from mild to potentially life-threatening; death occurs in up to 20% of cases, mostly as a result of respiratory failure.

Pathogenesis

NMS is caused by dopamine-receptor antagonism in the hypothalamus, nigrostriatal and mesocortical areas. It leads to disruption of inhibitory inputs to the sympathetic nervous system and a cascade of dysregulation which culminates in a hypermetabolic state.[107,108]

Symptoms indistinguishable from NMS have been reported in patients with Parkinson's disease when long-term treatment with levodopa and bromocriptine has been abruptly discontinued.[109–111] This has led to the suggestion that the syndrome would be better called 'acute dopamine depletion syndrome'.[111]

Box 12.II Movement disorders associated with dopamine-receptor antagonists[99]

Parkinsonism
Coarse resting tremor of limbs, head, mouth and/or tongue
Muscular rigidity (cogwheel or lead-pipe)
Bradykinesia, notably of face
Sialorrhoea (drooling)
Shuffling gait

Acute dystonias
one or more of:
- abnormal positioning of head and neck (retrocollis, torticollis)
- spasms of jaw muscles (trismus, gaping, grimacing)
- tongue dysfunction (dysarthria, protrusion)
- dysphagia
- laryngopharyngeal spasm
- dysphonia
- eyes deviated up, down or sideways (oculogyric crisis)
- abnormal positioning of limbs or trunk

Acute akathisia
one or more of:
- fidgety movements or swinging of legs
- rocking from foot to foot when standing
- pacing to relieve restlessness
- inability to sit or stand still for several minutes

Tardive dyskinesia
Exposure to antipsychotic medication for >3 months (>1 month if >60 years old)
Involuntary movement of tongue, jaw, trunk or limbs:
- choreiform (rapid, jerky, non-repetitive)
- athetoid (slow, sinuous, continual)
- rhythmic (stereotypic)

Box 12.JJ Drugs which may cause extrapyramidal effects[100-102]

Palliative care	General
Antidepressants[a]	Diltiazem
TCAs	Fenfluramine
venlafaxine	5-Hydroxytryptophan
SSRIs	Levodopa, methyldopa
Antipsychotics	Lithium
Carbamazepine	Methysergide
Metoclopramide	Reserpine
Ondansetron	
Valproate	

a. all classes of antidepressants have been implicated except Reversible Inhibitors of Mono-amine oxidase type A (RIMAs), e.g. moclobemide.

Clinical features

NMS is a hypodopaminergic state, where progressive bradykinesia results in a state of immobilization, akinesia and stupor, accompanied by extrapyramidal (lead-pipe) rigidity, fever, and autonomic instability (Box 12.KK). Symptoms generally develop over a few days but in some cases NMS may follow a fulminant course. Two thirds of cases of NMS develop within 1 week of starting neuroleptics, and virtually all cases occur within 1 month.[107,112]

Box 12.KK   Clinical features of NMS (DSM IV-TR)

Essential
Severe muscle rigidity
Pyrexia $\pm$ sweating

Additional
Muteness, drowsiness, coma
Tremor
Tachycardia and elevated/labile blood pressure
Urinary incontinence
Leucocytosis
Raised plasma CPK $\pm$ other evidence of muscle injury, e.g. myoglobinuria

---

Risk factors for the development of NMS include: dehydration; agitation; physical restraint; iron deficiency; high dose, rapid titration and parenteral administration of neuroleptic medication.[107] NMS is a diagnosis of exclusion. Other causes of hyperthermia, rigidity, rhabdomyolysis and altered mental state must be ruled out. (Box 12.LL)

Box 12.LL   Differential diagnosis of NMS[107]

Infection
Meningitis or encephalitis
Brain abscess
Sepsis

Neurological
Midbrain lesion, e.g.
   infarction, tumour
Non-convulsive status epilepticus

Psychiatric
Agitated delirium
Benign extrapyramidal undesirable effects
Idiopathic malignant catatonia

Endocrine
Thyrotoxicosis
Phaeochromocytoma

Toxic
Serotonin toxicity (see p.392)
Malignant hyperthermia
Antimuscarinic toxicity
Salicylate poisoning
Substances of abuse, e.g.
   amphetamines
   methylenedioxymethamfetamine
   (MDMA, Ecstasy)
Withdrawal
   dopamine agonists
   baclofen
   sedative hypnotics
   alcohol

Other
Heat stroke
Acute intermittent porphyria

Evaluation

There is no diagnostic test for NMS. Investigations include:
- FBC for leucocytosis
- measurement of serum electrolytes, urea, creatinine, CPK
- urine dipstick and microscopy for myoglobinuria
- CT or MRI to exclude midbrain lesion
- lumbar puncture.

Management

Discontinue the causal drug. Resolution of NMS generally occurs in 1–2 weeks, unless caused by a depot antipsychotic when resolution may take 4–6 weeks (Box 12.MM). There is a 30% risk of recurrent NMS if treatment with an antipsychotic is restarted; seek specialist advice from a toxicologist or psychiatrist before doing so.

Box 12.MM Treatment of NMS[107,113]

Severe cases should be managed in an intensive care unit.

Discontinue causal medication (toxicity generally resolves within 2 weeks).

Symptomatic measures:
- supportive care, e.g. IV fluids, cooling
- benzodiazepines for agitation and myoclonus, e.g.:
  - lorazepam 1–2mg IM/IV every 4–6h
- dopaminergic agent, e.g.:
  - bromocriptine 2.5mg PO b.d.–t.d.s.
- dantrolene for extremes of hyperthermia and muscle rigidity
- ECT.

Phenytoin neurotoxicity

Phenytoin has a narrow therapeutic window. It is about 90% bound to plasma albumin and its pharmacological effect is limited to the free, unbound portion. This will be a greater proportion of the total if the patient is hypo-albuminaemic (cf. hypercalcaemia in the presence of hypo-albuminaemia). Those at risk include elderly patients and those with chronic renal failure; they may develop neurotoxicity even when plasma concentrations are reported as being in the therapeutic range.

Elimination follows zero-order kinetics (i.e. a constant amount is eliminated per unit of time), and clearance does *not* increase with increasing plasma concentrations of phenytoin. Thus, what seems like a small increase (e.g. 300mg → 350mg) may lead to a large increase in plasma levels and toxicity.

Clinical features

Phenytoin toxicity generally manifests as a syndrome of cerebellar, vestibular and ocular effects, including some or all of the following:
- nystagmus:
  - on lateral gaze only (early sign)
  - spontaneous (more severe toxicity)
- blurred vision/diplopia
- slurred speech
- ataxia.

These may be accompanied by lethargy and/or delirium. Some patients experience break-through seizures (or an increase in the frequency of seizures) when the free phenytoin plasma concentration increases to toxic levels.

Evaluation
If phenytoin toxicity is suspected, check the plasma phenytoin concentration just before the next dose is due to obtain a trough level, and the plasma albumin concentration. The normal therapeutic range with a normal plasma albumin is 40–80micromol/L (10–20microgram/mL). However, one should be prepared to make the diagnosis clinically (e.g. if nystagmus ± other classical symptoms develop), and act accordingly.

Management
There is no specific antidote to phenytoin. If the patient has clinical features suggestive of toxicity, reduce the dose of phenytoin to a known previous non-toxic level. Generally, symptoms resolve when the plasma phenytoin concentration falls.[114]

Treat break-through seizures with benzodiazepines (see p.279) because other anti-epileptics may exacerbate the toxicity. If the frequency of seizures increases as the phenytoin toxicity resolves, seek the advice of a neurologist.

COMPLICATIONS OF THERAPEUTIC PROCEDURES

Blood transfusion[115]
Serious adverse reactions to transfused blood products are rare but may be life-threatening. Adverse reactions may develop within minutes of starting an infusion (acute complications) or up to 2 weeks after an infusion (delayed complications). New symptoms or signs that develop during a transfusion must be taken seriously because they may herald a serious reaction.

Acute life-threatening transfusion reactions:
- acute haemolytic transfusion reaction occurs with ABO incompatible RBC but may also occur following infusion of platelets or fresh frozen plasma (FFP) because these may contain high titres of anti-red cell antibodies. Infusion of even a few mL of ABO incompatible blood may cause symptoms within minutes
- reaction to infusion of bacterially contaminated blood products is rare but is more likely to occur with platelets than RBC. Contaminating organisms include *Staphylococcus epidermidis, Staphylococcus aureus, Bacillus cereus*, Group B *Streptococci, Escherischa coli, Pseudomonas* species
- transfusion-related acute lung injury (TRALI) typically develops within 6h of transfusion. The patient develops breathlessness, non-productive cough, hypotension and possibly monocytopenia or neutropenia. A chest radiograph shows bilateral nodular infiltrates in a batwing pattern, typical of acute respiratory distress syndrome
- acute fluid overload; symptoms and signs are the same as those of acute LVF; stop transfusion and manage as for acute LVF (see p.370)
- anaphylaxis generally occurs in the early part of a transfusion. Stop transfusion, take down unit and giving set and manage as for anaphylaxis of any cause (see p.358).

Less severe reactions to blood transfusion:
- mild urticarial reaction and/or itching occurring within minutes of starting an infusion are quite common
- febrile non-haemolytic transfusion reaction; fever (>1.5°C above baseline) or rigors during infusion of RBC or platelets affect 1–2% of patients, mainly

multi-transfused or previously pregnant patients. These features tend to occur towards the end of the transfusion or up to 2h after it has been completed.

Clinical features
The early symptoms and signs of these adverse reactions may be very similar, making it difficult initially to determine the cause of the reaction (Box 12.NN).

Box 12.NN   Clinical features of transfusion reactions

Mild	**Severe**
Itch	Tachycardia
Urticarial rash	Hypo/hypertension
Shivering	Bone/muscle/chest/abdominal pain
Rigors	Breathlessness
Temperature rise >1.5°C	Blood oozing from venepuncture sites
General discomfort	

Evaluation and management
If any of the features of transfusion reaction develop, *stop the transfusion*, call a doctor and check:
- temperature
- pulse and blood pressure
- respiratory rate and oxygen saturation
- details on the blood product and compatibility label to confirm that they match those in the patient's notes.

Should a suspected life-threatening complication occur:
- take down unit and giving set and return intact to the blood bank
- check FBC, PT, APTT, D-dimers, fibrinogen
- blood culture
- sample from blood product unit for culture.

Further management depends on the cause of the transfusion reaction. Severe transfusion reactions are likely to be terminal events for most palliative care patients, for whom symptomatic management may be most appropriate.

Acute haemolytic reaction
- IV fluids and monitor urine output
- manage DIC (see p.250)
- discuss with consultant haematologist and, if appropriate, consider transfer to high dependency unit for inotropic support.

Reaction to infusion of bacterially contaminated blood product unit
Manage as for acute haemolytic transfusion reaction. In addition, after obtaining specialist advice from a microbiologist, administer the appropriate combination of antibacterials. In the absence of specialist advice, follow the local protocol for the management of neutropenic sepsis. Otherwise, give antibacterials active against both Gram-positive and Gram-negative bacteria (Box 12.OO).

Transfusion-related acute lung injury
This may be difficult to distinguish from acute LVF or other non-cardiogenic causes of pulmonary oedema. Give 100% oxygen, but diuretics are not helpful. Urgent advice

---

Box 12.OO Antibacterials for management of sepsis from bacterially contaminated blood product

Gram-negative bacteria
Piperacillin/tazobactam 4.5g IV t.d.s. *or*
Ceftriaxone 1g IV once daily
    (2g if severe infection) *or*
Meropenem 1g IV t.d.s

Gram-positive bacteria including most MRSA
Teicoplanin 400mg IV b.d. for
    two doses then once daily *or*
Vancomycin 1g IV b.d. then adjust
    according to levels (may add to any
    renal impairment)

should be sought from a consultant haematologist and critical care team and, if appropriate, the patient should be transferred to an intensive care unit and managed as for acute respiratory distress syndrome.

Febrile non-haemolytic transfusion reaction
If the temperature rises <1.5°C, observations are stable and the patient is otherwise well, give paracetamol 1g PO. Then restart the infusion at a slower rate, and perform observations every 15min for the first hour.

Mild urticarial reaction
Give chlorphenamine 10mg IV. If there is no progression of symptoms after 30min, restart the infusion at a slower rate, and perform observations every 15min for the first hour.

Delayed complications of transfusion
- *haemolytic transfusion reaction*: occurs 1–14 days after transfusion, in a patient immunized to a red cell antigen by previous transfusion or pregnancy. Features include an unexpectedly small rise in Hb, falling Hb concentration, jaundice, fever and rarely haemoglobinuria or renal failure. Check Hb, blood film, direct antiglobulin test, LDH, urea and creatinine, LFTs, haptoglobin and perform urinalysis. Specific treatment is rarely required but advice from a haematologist should be sought
- *purpura*: rare but potentially fatal complication presenting 5–10 days following transfusion, with bleeding and an extremely low platelet count. Treatment is with high-dose IV immunoglobulin, under the supervision of a haematologist
- *graft-versus-host disease (GVHD)*: a rare and generally fatal complication caused by engraftment and proliferation of transfused donor lymphocytes. Patients at risk are those who are immunocompromised and those who have received a transfusion from a first- or second-degree relative. The condition presents 1–2 weeks following transfusion with fever, rash, diarrhoea and hepatitis
- *infections, e.g. HIV, hepatitis B*: rare but remain a risk.

Pleural aspiration
Pleural aspiration and intercostal tube drainage without instillation of a sclerosing substance are associated with a high recurrence rate of malignant pleural effusion but a small risk of iatrogenic pneumothorax and empyema.[116] Most iatrogenic pneumothoraces are small and resolve with observation alone. If the patient is breathless, treatment of the pneumothorax is required. Simple aspiration is sufficient in most cases (see p.365).[117]

Empyema should be suspected if the patient develops a fever following pleural instrumentation. A chest radiograph will show a pleural effusion. Pleural fluid should be aspirated and sent for:

- microscopy and culture
- pH (<7.2), glucose (reduced, <3.3mmol/L), LDH (increased, pleural:serum ratio >0.6).

Once the diagnosis has been confirmed, an intercostal chest tube drain should be inserted. After obtaining the advice of a microbiologist, broad-spectrum antibacterials should be commenced until the results of the culture are available, e.g. a third-generation cephalosporin such as ceftriaxone 1g IV once daily, and metronidazole 500mg IV t.d.s.[118]

Abdominal paracentesis
Complications of paracentesis include hypotension, bleeding and peritonitis.

Hypotension
Large volume paracentesis can lead to haemodynamic changes resulting in hypovolaemia, hypotension and, in severe cases, collapse and pre-renal renal failure, which is fatal is about 2% of patients.[119] Risk is minimized by limiting paracentesis to ≤5L in patients with cirrhosis receiving diuretics, and any patient with serum creatinine >250micromol/L (indicative of renal failure), albumin <30g/L or sodium <125mmol/L (see p.132).

If the patient develops a significant fall in blood pressure ± symptoms such as dizziness, light-headedness or 'wooziness':

- clamp the paracentesis drain
- monitor blood pressure every 30min–1h
- if persistent hypotension, give IV fluid, e.g. 5% dextrose 1L IV over 6–8h
- restart paracentesis only if symptoms resolve and the blood pressure improves, draining fluid more slowly, e.g. 2L over 4h
- monitor urea and electrolytes daily as appropriate.[120]

Bleeding
The reported incidence of haematoperitoneum or clinically significant bleeding at the paracentesis drain puncture site is very low. This may be because most clinical trials exclude patients with coagulopathy (PT >21sec, INR >1.6, platelet count <50×10^9/L).

If bleeding occurs at the drain site, apply direct pressure. Check FBC, PT, APTT, D-dimers, fibrinogen; correct coagulopathy if possible and appropriate. Significant drain site bleeding or haematoperitoneum is likely to be a terminal event in most palliative care patients.

Peritonitis
Also see p.136.

Peritonitis from infection or intestinal perforation is rare.[121] Because the intestines may have become tethered to the parietal peritoneum, perforation is more likely to occur in patients who have had abdominal radiotherapy, intra-abdominal chemotherapy, or repeated paracentesis. Ultrasound guided paracentesis should be considered in these patients.[119]

If a patient develops unexplained fever ± abdominal pain during or following paracentesis, the diagnosis of peritonitis should be considered. Peritonitis may be caused by the introduction of bacterial contaminants at the time of drain insertion, or by perforation of the GI tract (faeculent peritonitis). Peritonitis is likely to be a terminal event for most palliative care patients. If investigation and treatment are appropriate, ascitic fluid should be sent for microscopy and culture. If the paracentesis drain is no longer in place, consider performing an ascitic tap to obtain fluid. Start treatment with a third-generation cephalosporin such as ceftriaxone 2g IV once daily, and metronidazole 500mg IV t.d.s. until the results of the culture are available. Appropriate analgesia should also be prescribed.

1 Joint Royal Colleges of Physicians Training Board (2007) Specialty Training Curriculum for Palliative Medicine. Available from: http://www.jrcptb.org.uk/Specialty/Pages/default.aspx

2 Soar J (2009) Emergency treatment of anaphylaxis in adults: concise guidance. *Clinical Medicine.* **9**: 181–185.

3 Pharmax (1998) *Data on file.*

4 Resuscitation Council (UK) (2008) Emergency treatment of anaphylactic reactions: Guidelines for healthcare providers. Available from: http://www.resus.org.uk/pages/reaction.pdf

5 CKS (2007) Angio-oedema and Anaphylaxis (Topic Review). In: *Clinical Knowledge Summary Service.* Available from: http://www.cks.library.nhs.uk/angio_oedema_and_anaphylaxis

6 BNF (2008) Section 3.4.3 Anaphylaxis. In: *British National Formulary* (No. 55). British Medical Association and the Royal Pharmaceutical Society of Great Britain, London. Current BNF available from: www.bnf.org/bnf/bnf/current/

7 Poon M and Reid C (2004) Best evidence topic reports. Oral corticosteroids in acute urticaria. *Emergency Medicine Journal.* **21**: 76–77.

8 Schierhout G and Roberts I (1998) Fluid resuscitation with colloid or crystalloid solutions in critically ill patients: a systematic review of randomised trials. *British Medical Journal.* **316**: 961–964.

9 Resuscitation Council (UK) (2005) The Resuscitation Guidelines. Available from: www.resus.org.uk

10 Tabbarah H (1988) Intrathoracic complications. In: D Casciato and B Lowitz (eds) *Manual of Clinical Oncology* (2e). Little Brown, Boston, Mass, pp. 435–452.

11 Kee S et al. (1998) Superior vena cava syndrome: treatment with catheter-directed thrombolysis and endovascular stent placement. *Radiology.* **206**: 187–193.

12 Rice TW et al. (2006) The superior vena cava syndrome: clinical characteristics and evolving etiology. *Medicine (Baltimore).* **85**: 37–42.

13 Nicholson A et al. (1997) Treatment of malignant superior vena cava obstruction: metal stents or radiation therapy. *Journal of Vascular and Interventional Radiology.* **8**: 781–788.

14 Renwick I (1999) Metallic stents in palliative care. *CME Bulletin of Palliative Medicine.* **1**: 41–44.

15 NICE (2004) Interventional procedure overview of stent placement for vena cava obstruction. Available from: http://www.nice.org.uk/guidance/index.jsp?action=byID&o=11137

16 Jackson J and Brooks D (1995) Stenting of superior vena caval obstruction. *Thorax.* **50**: 531–536.

17 Marcy PY et al. (2001) Superior vena cava obstruction: is stenting necessary? *Support Care Cancer.* **9**: 103–107.

18 Rowell NP and Gleeson FV (2001) Steroids, radiotherapy, chemotherapy and stents for superior vena caval obstruction in carcinoma of the bronchus. *Cochrane Database of Systematic Reviews.* CD001316.

19 Stock K et al. (1995) Treatment of malignant obstruction of the superior vena cava with the self-expanding wallstent. *Thorax.* **50**: 1151–1156.

20 Studdy PR (1996) Stridor. In: IAD Boucher et al. (eds) *French's Index of Differential Diagnosis* (13e). Butterworth Heinemann.

21 Draper R (2007) Stridor. In: *PatientPlus.* Available from: http://www.patient.co.uk/

22 Henry M et al. (2003) BTS guidelines for the management of spontaneous pneumothorax. *Thorax.* **58 Suppl 2**: ii39–52.

23 Warrell D et al. (eds) (2004) Ch. 15:38. Pericardial disease. In: *Oxford Textbook of Medicine* (4e). Oxford University Press, Oxford.

24 Vaitkus PT et al. (1994) Treatment of malignant pericardial effusion. *Jama.* **272**: 59–64.

25 Cullinane CA et al. (2004) Prognostic factors in the surgical management of pericardial effusion in the patient with concurrent malignancy. *Chest.* **125**: 1328–1334.

26 Gasper WJ et al. (2007) Palliation of thoracic malignancies. *Surg Oncol.*

27 Kopecky S et al. (2007) Heart Failure in Adults. 10th Ed. ICSI (Institute for Clinical Systems Improvement). Available from: www.icsi.org

28 Hunt SA et al. (2005) Guideline Update for the Diagnosis and Management of Chronic Heart Failure in the Adult. ACC/AHA. Available from: http://circ.ahajournals.org/cgi/content/full/112/12/e154

29 Kopecky S et al. (2007) Heart Failure in Adults. Institute for Clinical Systems Improvement. Available from: www.icsi.org

30 BMA (2007) Decisions relating to cardiopulmonary resuscitation. British Medical Association, The Resuscitation Council (UK) and the Royal College of Nursing. Available from: www.bma.org.uk/ap.nsf/Content/CPRDecisions07

31 Eisenberg MS and Mengert TJ (2001) Cardiac resuscitation. *The New England Journal of Medicine.* **344**: 1304–1313.

32 Resuscitation Council (UK) (2005) Adult Basic Life Support. Available from: www.resus.org.uk

33 Resuscitation Council (UK) (2005) The use of Automated External Defibrillators. Available from: www.resus.org.uk

34 Resuscitation Council (UK) (2005) In-hospital Resuscitation. Available from: www.resus.org.uk

35 Warrell D et al. (eds) (2004) Chapter 20:6. Acute renal failure. In: *Oxford Textbook of Medicine* (4e). Oxford University Press, Oxford.

36 Mandelberg A et al. (1999) Salbutamol metered-dose inhaler with spacer for hyperkalemia: how fast? How safe? *Chest.* **115**: 617–622.

37 Evans KJ and Greenberg A (2005) Hyperkalemia: a review. *Journal of Intensive Care Medicine.* **20**: 272–290.

38 Mahoney BA et al. (2005) Emergency interventions for hyperkalaemia. *Cochrane Database of Systematic Reviews.* **2**: CD003235.

39 Emberton M and Anson K (1999) Acute urinary retention in men: an age old problem. *British Medical Journal.* **318**: 921–925.

40 Marks V (2004) Section 12:19. Hypoglycaemia. In: D Warrell et al. (eds) *Oxford Textbook of Medicine* (4e). Oxford University Press, Oxford.

41 Ford-Dunn S et al. (2002) Tumour-induced hypoglycaemia. *Palliative Medicine.* **16**: 357–358.

42 Teale JD and Marks V (1998) Glucocorticoid therapy suppresses abnormal secretion of big IGF-II by non-islet cell tumours inducing hypoglycaemia (NICTH). *Clinical Endocrinology.* **49**: 491–498.

43 DTB (1987) NSAIDs for renal and biliary colic: intramuscular diclofenac. *Drug and Therapeutics Bulletin* **25**: 85–86.

44 Hagen N et al. (1997) Cancer pain emergencies: a protocol for management. *Journal of Pain and Symptom Management.* **14**: 45–50.

45 NICE (2003) Guidance on Percutaneous Vertebroplasty. National Institute for Clinical Excellence. Available from: http://www.nice.org.uk/IPG012guidance

46 Hide IG and Gangi A (2004) Percutaneous vertebroplasty: history, technique and current perspectives. *Clinical Radiology.* **59**: 461–467.

47 Fallon M and O'Neill W (1993) Spinal surgery in the treatment of metastatic back pain: three case reports. *Palliative Medicine.* **7**: 235–238.

48 Klekamp J and Samii H (1998) Surgical results for spinal metastases. *Acta Neurochirurgica (Wein).* **140**: 957–967.

49 Patchell RA et al. (2005) Direct decompressive surgical resection in the treatment of spinal cord compression caused by metastatic cancer: a randomised trial. *Lancet.* **366**: 643–648.

50 Townsend P et al. (1995) Role of postoperative radiation therapy after stabilization of fractures caused by metastatic disease. *International Journal of Radiation Oncology, Biology and Physics.* **31**: 43–49.

51 APA (1994) *Diagnostic and Statistical Manual of Mental Disorders.* (4e). American Psychiatric Association, New York.

52 Roth A and Breitbart W (1996) Psychiatric emergencies in terminally ill cancer patients. *Haematology and Oncology Clinics of North America.* **10**: 235–259.

53 Hem E et al. (2004) Suicide risk in cancer patients from 1960 to 1999. *Journal of Clinical Oncology.* **22**: 4209–4216.

54 Grzybowska P and Finlay I (1997) The incidence of suicide in palliative care patients. *Palliative Medicine.* **11**: 313–316.

55 Ripamonti C et al. (1999) Suicide among patients with cancer cared for at home by palliative-care teams. *Lancet.* **354**: 1877–1878.

56 O'Connell H et al. (2004) Recent developments: suicide in older people. *British Medical Journal.* **329**: 895–899.

57 Waern M et al. (2003) Predictors of suicide in the old elderly. *Gerontology.* **49**: 328–334.

58 National Collaborating Centre for Mental Health (2004) The short-term physical and psychological management and secondary prevention of self-harm in primary and secondary care. National Institute for Clinical Excellence.

59 NICE (2005) Violence: the short-term management of disturbed/violent behaviour in psychiatric inpatient settings and emergency departments. In: *National Institute for Clinical Excellence Clinical Guideline 25.* Available from: www.nice.org.uk/CG025NICEguideline

60 Anonymous (2005) Mental Capacity Act 2005: Elizabeth II. Chapter 9 Reprinted May and December 2006; May 2007. Available from: www.opsi.gov.uk/acts/acts2005/20050009.htm

61 Department for Constitutional Affairs (2005) Mental Capacity Act. Available from: www.dca.gov.uk/menincap/legis.htm

62 Cleary J (2000) Incidence and characteristics of naloxone administration in medical oncology patients with cancer pain. *Journal of Pharmaceutical Care in Pain and Symptom Control.* **8**: 65–73.

63 Max MB et al. (1992) Principles of Analgesic Use in the Treatment of Acute Pain and Cancer Pain (3e). American Pain Society, Skokie, Illinois, p. 12.

64 van Dorp E et al. (2006) Naloxone reversal of buprenorphine-induced respiratory depression. Anesthesiology. 105: 51–57.

65 Budd K and Raffa R (eds) (2005) Buprenorphine – the Unique Opioid Analgesic. Georg Thieme Verlag, Stuttgart, Germany, p. 134.

66 Knape J (1986) Early respiratory depression resistant to naloxone following epidural buprenorphine. Anesthesiology. 64: 382–384.

67 Gal T (1989) Naloxone reversal of buprenorphine-induced respiratory depression. Clinical Pharmacology and Therapeutics. 45: 66–71.

68 Reynaud M et al. (1998) Six deaths linked to concomitant use of buprenorphine and benzodiazepines. Addiction. 93: 1385–1392.

69 Orwin JM (1977) The effect of doxapram on buprenorphine induced respiratory depression. Acta Anaesthesiologica Belgica. 28: 93–106.

70 BNF (2008) Section 3.5.1 Respiratory stimulants. In: British National Formulary (No. 55). British Medical Association and Royal Pharmaceutical Society of Great Britain, London. Current BNF available from: www.bnf.org/bnf/bnf/current/.

71 Bayer MJ et al. (1992) Treatment of benzodiazepine overdose with flumazenil. Clinical Therapeutics. 14: 978–995.

72 Litovitz TL et al. (1991) 1990 Annual report of the American Association of Poison Control Centers national data collection system. American Journal of Emergency Medicine. 9: 461–509.

73 Weinbroum A et al. (1991) The use of flumazenil in the management of acute drug poisoning – a review. Intensive Care Medicine. 17 Suppl 1: S32–38.

74 Spivey WH (1992) Flumazenil and seizures: analysis of 43 cases. Clinical Therapeutics. 14: 292–305.

75 BNF (2008) Emergency treatment of poisoning. In: British National Formulary (No. 55). British Medical Association and Royal Pharmaceutical Society of Great Britain, London. Current BNF available from: www.bnf.org/bnf/bnf/current/.

76 APA (American Psychiatric Association) (2000) Diagnostic and Statistical Manual of Mental Disorders. (Text revision). (4e). American Psychiatric Association, New York.

77 NICE (2007) Drug misuse. Psychosocial interventions. In: NICE Clinical Guideline 51. Available from: www.nice.org.uk/CG051

78 Passik SD and Theobald DE (2000) Managing addiction in advanced cancer patients: why bother? Journal of Pain and Symptom Management. 19: 229–234.

79 Mayo-Smith MF (1997) Pharmacological management of alcohol withdrawal. A meta-analysis and evidence-based practice guideline. American society of addiction medicine working group on pharmacological management of alcohol withdrawal. The Journal of American Medical Association. 278: 144–151.

80 Bruera E et al. (1995) The frequency of alcoholism among patients with pain due to terminal cancer. Journal of Pain and Symptom Management. 10: 599–603.

81 Johnson BA et al. (2003) Oral topiramate for treatment of alcohol dependence: a randomised controlled trial. Lancet. 361: 1677–1685.

82 Huff CA (2004) Section 26:18. Problems of alcohol and drug users in the hospital. In: DA Warrell et al. (eds) Oxford Textbook of Medicine (5e). Oxford University Press, Oxford.

83 Saunders JB et al. (1993) Development of the Alcohol Use Disorders Identification Test (AUDIT): WHO Collaborative Project on Early Detection of Persons with Harmful Alcohol Consumption-II. Addiction; 88(6): 791–804.

84 Mayfield D et al. (1974) The CAGE questionnaire: Validation of a new alcoholism screening instrument. American Journal of Psychiatry. 131: 1121–1123.

85 Parker AJ et al. (2008) Diagnosis and management of alcohol use disorders. British Medical Journal. 336: 496–501.

86 Ntais C et al. (2005) Benzodiazepines for alcohol withdrawal. Cochrane Database of Systematic Reviews. CD005063.

87 Raistrick D et al. (2006) Review of the Effectiveness of Treatment for Alcohol Problems. National Treatment Agency for Substance Misuse (NHS:UK). Available from: www.nta.nhs.uk

88 Day E et al. (2004) Evaluation of a symptom-triggered front-loading detoxification technique for alcohol dependence: a pilot study Psychiatric Bulletin. 28: 407–410.

89 CKS (2007) Alcohol – problem drinking (Topic Review). In: Clinical Knowledge Summaries Service. Available from: www.cks.library.nhs.uk/hypothyroidism

90 Lingford-Hughes AR et al. (2004) Evidence-based guidelines for the pharmacological management of substance misuse, addiction and comorbidity: recommendations from the British Association for Psychopharmacology. Journal of Psychopharmacology. 18: 293–335.

91 Boyer EW and Shannon M (2005) The serotonin syndrome. The New England Journal of Medicine. 352: 1112–1120.

92 Anderson T et al. (2005) Serotonin syndrome: a hidden danger in palliative care. European Journal of Palliative Care. 12(3): 97–100.

93 Isbister GK et al. (2002) Comment: neuroleptic malignant syndrome associated with risperidone and fluvoxamine. The Annals of Pharmacotherapy. **36**: 1293; author reply 1294.

94 Gillman P (2006) Serotonin toxicity, serotonin syndrome: 2006 update, overview and analysis. Available from: www.psychotropical.com

95 Gillman PK (2005) Monoamine oxidase inhibitors, opioid analgesics and serotonin toxicity. British Journal of Anaesthesia. **95**: 434–441.

96 Gillman PK (2006) A review of serotonin toxicity data: implications for the mechanisms of antidepressant drug action. Biological Psychiatry. **59**: 1046–1051.

97 Dunkley EJ et al. (2003) The hunter serotonin toxicity criteria: simple and accurate diagnostic decision rules for serotonin toxicity. QJM: Montly Journal of the Association of Physicians. **96**: 635–642.

98 Tonda M and Guthrie S (1994) Treatment of acute neuroleptic-induced movement disorders. Pharmacotherapy. **14**: 543–560.

99 APA (American Psychiatric Association) (1994) Neuroleptic-induced movement disorders. In: Diagnostic and Statistical Manual of Mental Disorders (4e). American Psychiatric Association, New York, pp. 736–751.

100 Zubenko G et al. (1987) Antidepressant-related akathisia. Journal of Clinical Psychopharmacology. **7**: 254–257.

101 Anonymous (1994) Drug-induced extrapyramidal reactions. Current Problems in Pharmacovigilance. **20**: 15–16.

102 Tarsy D and Simon DK (2006) Dystonia. The New England Journal of Medicine. **355**: 818–829.

103 Gagrat D et al. (1978) Intravenous diazepam in the treatment of neuroleptic-induced acute dystonia and akathisia. The American Journal of Psychiatry. **135**: 1232–1233.

104 Caligiuri MR et al. (2000) Antipsychotic-Induced movement disorders in the elderly: epidemiology and treatment recommendations. Drugs Aging. **17**: 363–384.

105 Caroff S and Mann S (1993) Neuroleptic malignant syndrome. Medical Clinics of North America. **77**: 185–202.

106 Adnet P et al. (2000) Neuroleptic malignant syndrome. British Journal of Anaesthesia. **85**: 129–135.

107 Strawn JR et al. (2007) Neuroleptic malignant syndrome. The American Journal of Psychiatry. **164**: 870–876.

108 Gurrera RJ (1999) Sympathoadrenal hyperactivity and the etiology of neuroleptic malignant syndrome. The American Journal of Psychiatry. **156**: 169–180.

109 Mann S et al. (1991) Pathogenesis of neuroleptic malignant syndrome. Psychiatry Annals. **21**: 175–180.

110 Ong K et al. (2001) Neuroleptic malignant syndrome without neuroleptics. Singapore Medical Journal. **42**: 85–88.

111 Keyser DL and Rodnitzky RL (1991) Neuroleptic malignant syndrome in Parkinson's disease after withdrawal or alteration of dopaminergic therapy. Archives of Internal Medicine. **151**: 794–796.

112 Stanley N and Caroff MD (2003) Neurolpetic malignant syndrome. Still a risk, but which patients may be in danger? Current Psychiatry. **2**: 36–42.

113 Dressler D and Benecke R (2005) Diagnosis and management of acute movement disorders. Journal of Neurology. **252**: 1299–1306.

114 Perkin GD (2004) Ch. 24:53. Epilepsy in later childhood and adults. In: DA Warrell et al. (eds) Oxford Textbook of Medicine (5e). Oxford University Press, Oxford.

115 McClelland DBL (2007) Handbook of Transfusion Medicine. United Kingdom Blood Transfusion Services. Available from: http://www.transfusionguidelines.org.uk

116 Antunes G et al. (2003) BTS guidelines for the management of malignant pleural effusions. Thorax. **58 (Suppl ii)**: ii29–ii38.

117 Henry M et al. (2003) BTS guidelines for the management of spontaneous pneumothorax. Thorax. **58 (Suppl ii)**: ii39–ii52.

118 British Society for Antimicrobial Chemotherapy (2005) Management of Hospital Infection: web based teaching resource. Available from: www.bsac.org.uk

119 Ross GJ et al. (1989) Sonographically guided paracentesis for palliation of symptomatic malignant ascites. AJR American Journal of Roentgenology. **153**: 1309–1311.

120 Becker G et al. (2006) Malignant ascites: systematic review and guideline for treatment. European Journal of Cancer. **42**: 589–597.

121 Gines P et al. (2004) Management of cirrhosis and ascites. New England Journal of Medicine. **350**: 1636–1654.

13: LAST DAYS

ADVANCE PLANNING

'In this world nothing is certain but taxes and death.' Benjamin Franklin

Despite this certainty, many people live their lives without really considering their own mortality. However, the diagnosis of a life-limiting illness, and particularly the awareness of physical deterioration as the illness progresses, will prompt the patient (and those close to them) to face their impending death. This is generally psychologically and spiritually demanding, and the extent to which a person is able to do this, and discuss it with others, varies.

Certain coping styles (e.g. 'Must think positive' or 'Must put on a brave face') can impede communication and reflection. It is a challenging area for health professionals, and it is easier to re-inforce the positive thinking ('Perhaps the next cycle of chemotherapy will help') rather than help the patient plan for all eventualities ('Hope for the best, but plan for the worst').

Patients may come to terms with the fact that their life is drawing to a close but see no need to make specific arrangements. However, pro-active 'Advance Care Planning' is now recommended.[1,2] In the UK, national guidelines provide advice about how, when, and where to discuss this with patients.[3]

A health professional should introduce the topic sensitively when they consider it likely to benefit the care of the patient. This should be done before the terminal phase, such as at the time of:
- diagnosis of a life-limiting illness
- disease progression, leading to multiple hospital admissions
- increased risk of cardiorespiratory arrest
- admission to a care home.

However, it can be done at any time by anyone, e.g. a well person prompted to do so by the death of a relative or friend. It is a voluntary process and there should be no pressure to take part. The choice not to confront future issues should be respected.

Advance care planning involves discussion between health professionals and the patient, and (if the patient wishes) relatives/informal carers, in order to identify:
- their concerns
- their understanding of their illness and prognosis
- important values or personal goals for care
- preferences for the types of care or treatment that may be beneficial in the future and the availability of these.

The discussion should be:
- documented
- regularly reviewed
- communicated to key persons involved in their care.

Possible outcomes arising from such a discussion include completion of:
- an informal statement of wishes and preferences (Box 13.A)
- a formal Advance Decision to Refuse Treatment (ADRT, see p.409)
- a Lasting Power of Attorney, to appoint a welfare attorney who would take decisions on a person's behalf should they subsequently lose capacity.

An example of advance care planning is the Preferred Place of Care (PPC) Plan, a nationally recommended tool to support high quality terminal care.[4,5] This comprises a patient-held record documenting the patient's wishes, the socio-economic circumstances of the family, the services being accessed, reasons for change in the care, and a needs assessment which documents care on an ongoing basis. It aims to facilitate:
- greater choice for patients in where they wish to live and die
- fewer emergency admissions of patients who wish to die at home
- fewer older people being transferred from a care home to hospital in the last week of life.

Box 13.A   Statement of wishes and preferences[6]

This is a statement recorded in the patient's clinical notes to convey their:
- wishes and preferences about future treatment and care, e.g.:
  - ▷ personal preferences
  - ▷ who they want involved in future decision-making
  - ▷ types of medical treatment which may or may not be wanted
  - ▷ place of care
- beliefs or values that govern how they make decisions in order to guide future decision-making.

Acts which are illegal cannot be included, e.g. assisted suicide.

They are not legally binding.

When a person lacks mental capacity, a professional carer formulating a decision about care or treatment must take any statement of wishes and preferences into account when trying to determine the patient's best interests.

If not documented in the clinical notes, relatives or other carers should be contacted to determine whether any statement of wishes or preferences exists, or for help in determining the patient's probable wishes.

Advance Decision to Refuse Treatment

An Advance Decision to Refuse Treatment (ADRT) is a set of instructions that a person aged over 18 years with mental capacity can make to refuse treatment should they lose capacity in the future. It is covered by statute law in England and Wales (Mental Capacity Act 2005), and by common law in Scotland and Northern Ireland. A valid and applicable ADRT is as legally binding as a contemporary refusal of treatment made by a person with capacity (Box 13.B).

Box 13.B   The law and an Advance Decision to Refuse Treatment (ADRT)[7]

Legal requirements for an ADRT which refuses life-sustaining treatment are:
- it must be in writing (this includes being recorded in the clinical notes or being written on behalf of the patient)
- it must contain a specific statement that the person wishes the ADRT to apply even though treatment refusal may result in earlier death
- it must be signed by the person (or on their behalf in their presence) and by a witness.

An ADRT is valid if:
- the person had mental capacity when they made the ADRT (Box 13.C)
- the ADRT was made voluntarily, i.e. the person was not put under undue pressure or coerced into making it
- the person was informed as to the broad nature and purpose of the treatment they are refusing.

An ADRT is applicable if:
- there is a refusal of a specific treatment, e.g. CPR, chemotherapy
- the treatment in question is that specified by the ADRT
- the circumstances in which the refusal is to apply are specified and exist at the time the decision needs to be made.

An ADRT may not be valid or applicable if:
- there have been changes in circumstances which give reasonable grounds for believing these would have affected the person's refusal, e.g. a new treatment has been discovered for the person's illness
- since making the ADRT, the person has done anything clearly inconsistent with the ADRT remaining their fixed decision
- since making the ADRT, the person has subsequently withdrawn their decision (verbally or in writing)
- the person has subsequently conferred power to make that decision on an attorney.[8]

On the other hand, a *request for treatment* is *not* legally binding, although it will provide the clinical team with insight into the person's wishes and preferences. A person may not make a request for their life to be ended. A person with a Living Will or Advance Directive written before October 2007 needs to ensure that it complies with the standards for an ADRT, particularly if they wish to refuse life-sustaining treatment. Life-sustaining treatment is defined as a treatment which the healthcare provider regards as necessary to sustain life.

Box 13.C Mental capacity[7]

Persons over the age of 16 years are presumed to have mental capacity until shown otherwise.

Any evaluation of capacity has to be made in relation to a particular decision (e.g. choice of treatment) at a particular time.

An evaluation of capacity will normally involve discussion with the person's family, friends or carers, or an Independent Mental Capacity Advocate (IMCA) if one has been appointed.

An individual's capacity can vary over time, so health and social care professionals should identify the time and manner most suitable to the patient to discuss treatment options. It may be necessary to call upon expert evaluation of the person's capacity, e.g. psychiatrist, clinical psychologist.

Loss of capacity may be temporary, e.g. due to a reversible concurrent illness or complication. If the patient who lacks capacity may regain it soon, e.g. after receiving medical treatment, defer decision making until then, if possible.

The two stage test of capacity

1 *Diagnostic*: does the patient have an impairment of the mind or brain, which means that they are unable to make the decision for themselves?
2 *Functional*: the patient is unable to:
   • understand the information relevant to the decision, including the likely consequences of making or not making the decision
   • retain that information for as long as is necessary to make and communicate the decision
   • use that information as part of the process of making the decision
   • communicate the decision by some means.

All evaluations of a person's capacity should be documented in the patient's clinical notes. Determining capacity should be conducted using a multi-professional approach. However, the final responsibility remains with the senior professional involved.

A person may refuse any treatment but can never refuse basic care, e.g. shelter, warmth, hygiene measures, the offer of oral food and fluids. Artificial nutrition and hydration are regarded as treatment and may thus be refused. It is essential this is pointed out to people at the time the ADRT is created.

An ADRT may be verbal or written. However, if a person wishes to refuse life-sustaining treatment, this part of the ADRT must be written and follow a specific format (Box 13.B). Although it is recommended that people talk to their GP, consultant or solicitor before formulating an ADRT, this is not a legal requirement. If a person gives a verbal ADRT, it should if possible be documented in the clinical notes and signed by the person. However, people should be encouraged to produce a formal written ADRT.

There is no official format for a written ADRT, unless life-sustaining treatment is refused (Box 13.B). There is no set review period for an ADRT. Decisions made a long time in advance are not automatically invalid or inapplicable, but a regularly reviewed ADRT is more likely to be valid and applicable to current circumstances.

An ADRT may be withdrawn in full or in part either in writing or verbally at any time while the person has capacity. If a verbal withdrawal is made, it should be documented in the clinical notes.

Health professionals must take practical and reasonable steps to determine whether a patient has made an ADRT. It is good practice for the clinical team to ask the patient, family member or GP if an ADRT exists. However, the onus is on the patient to ensure that clinical teams involved in their care know about the ADRT. Patients should be advised to provide a copy of the ADRT for their GP, clinical notes, solicitor and family members.

An ADRT only comes into effect if a person loses mental capacity. All patients are assumed to have mental capacity unless they fail the test for capacity (Box 13.C). Once the clinical team has been given an ADRT belonging to a patient who has lost mental capacity, they must establish if it is valid and applicable (Box 13.B). If it is found to be so, the ADRT must be complied with or they could be liable to criminal or civil proceedings.

If an ADRT is not valid or applicable to current circumstances, it may still provide the clinical team with insight into the person's wishes and preferences. A retrospective evaluation of the validity of an ADRT may be difficult to make. If a health professional or family member has reasonable doubts or there are disagreements over the validity or applicability of an ADRT, the senior clinician in charge of the patient should consult with all parties involved in the patient's care to seek evidence concerning the validity and scope of the ADRT (not to try to overrule it). Details of these discussions should be recorded in the patient's clinical notes. If the senior clinician comes to the view that the ADRT is valid and applicable, it must be complied with.[8]

If serious doubt or disagreement persist, apply to the Court of Protection for a ruling. The court can rule if the ADRT exists, is valid and is applicable, but cannot overturn a valid and applicable ADRT.

While court proceedings are being undertaken, or in an emergency where there may not be sufficient time to evaluate the validity and applicability of an ADRT, health professionals may provide life-sustaining treatment, or any treatment necessary to prevent a serious deterioration in the patient's condition.

If a health professional has a conscientious objection to complying with an ADRT, this should be discussed with the multiprofessional team. If necessary, care of the patient should be transferred to another health professional who is able to comply with the ADRT. This must be done without affecting the patient's care.

An ADRT for a mental disorder may not apply if the person is, or is liable, to be detained under the Mental Health Act 1983. If necessary, clarification should be sought from a psychiatrist.[8]

Lasting Power of Attorney (LPA)
Different statutes cover proxy decision-making in England and Wales, and Scotland.

England and Wales
LPA is covered by statute law in England and Wales (Mental Capacity Act 2005). A person aged over 18 years who has capacity may make an LPA to appoint one or more persons as attorney(s) to take decisions on their behalf if they subsequently lose capacity. An LPA can cover decisions relating to healthcare and/or personal welfare (a personal welfare attorney), and/or property and financial affairs (a property and financial affairs attorney). A personal welfare attorney can refuse treatment on behalf

of an incapacitated person, but can only refuse life-sustaining treatment if the LPA specifies this. A personal welfare attorney cannot demand inappropriate medical treatment. The LPA replaces the previous role of Enduring Power of Attorney.

An ADRT overrules a personal welfare attorney, unless the LPA was made after the ADRT and specifies that the personal welfare attorney has authority to make decisions about the same treatment. Before relying on the authority of a personal welfare attorney, the clinical team must be satisfied that:

- the patient lacks capacity to make the decision
- the LPA has been registered with the Office of the Public Guardian
- a statement has been included in the LPA specifically authorizing the welfare attorney to make decisions relevant to the current situation
- the decision being made by the attorney is in the patent's best interests.

Scotland

A different statute covers the appointment of welfare attorneys in Scotland (Adults with Incapacity (Scotland) Act 2000).[9] In Scotland, a person aged over 16 years may appoint one person as welfare attorney to take decisions on their behalf if they subsequently lose capacity. The Sheriff may appoint a welfare guardian with similar powers. As in England and Wales, the welfare attorney or guardian cannot demand inappropriate medical treatment. Before relying on the authority of a welfare attorney, the clinical team must be satisfied that:

- the patient lacks capacity to make the decision
- the welfare attorney or guardian has specific power to consent to treatment
- the decision being made by the attorney would benefit the patient
- the attorney has taken account of the patient's past and present wishes as far as they can be ascertained.

Where there is disagreement between the healthcare team and welfare attorney or guardian (e.g. the healthcare team believe it would benefit the patient to attempt CPR in the event of cardiorespiratory arrest but the welfare attorney disagrees), the clinical team should apply to the Mental Welfare Commission of Scotland to appoint a 'nominated medical practitioner' to give an opinion. This opinion is final unless appealed by either party to the Court of Sessions.

Northern Ireland

In Northern Ireland, there is currently no provision for the appointment of proxy decision-makers for patients who lack capacity. However, those close to the patient should be consulted by the clinical team when determining the patient's best interests.

Independent Mental Capacity Advocate (IMCA)

Most adults who lack capacity, and who have not written an ADRT or appointed a welfare attorney, will have family, friends or carers who can and should be consulted about their views if a decision needs to be made on their behalf. In England and Wales, statute law stipulates that if there is no-one appropriate to consult, an IMCA should be appointed for the person when decisions have to be made about:[10]

- serious medical treatment e.g. chemotherapy, major surgery, withholding or withdrawing artificial nutrition and hydration:
  - ▷ when the likely benefits and possible burdens are finely balanced
  - ▷ when a decision between choice of treatment is finely balanced
  - ▷ when what is proposed is likely to have serious consequences, e.g. potentially shortening the person's life, serious and prolonged pain or other major distress

- moving the person into long-term care ($>$ 4 weeks in a hospital or 8 weeks in a care home)
- a long-term move ($\geqslant$ 8 weeks) to a different hospital or care home
- adult protection (in England).

The role of the IMCA is to support the person for whom the decision is being made by obtaining as much information as possible from that person and other sources about their wishes, feelings, beliefs and values. The IMCA will then prepare a written report for the healthcare team. The IMCA will not be the final decision-maker, but the decision-maker must take into account the information provided by the IMCA.

If a patient is known to be 'friendless', i.e. there is no one who could be consulted about their wishes should they lose capacity, they should be encouraged to partake in some form of advanced care planning, e.g. write an ADRT or appoint a welfare attorney.

Best interests

In England and Wales, decisions which are made on behalf of mentally incapacitated persons by health professionals or welfare attorneys must be in their best interests. Best interests are not limited to medical ones but encompass all of a person's interests, including psychological and social ones (Box 13.D). In Scotland, decisions made on behalf of mentally incapacitated persons by health professionals or welfare attorneys must be made for their benefit, taking into account their past and present wishes, as far as they can be ascertained.

Box 13.D   Checklist for determining best interests[7]

Involve the person as much as possible in making the decision.

Find out the person's views, including past and present wishes and feelings that have been expressed verbally, in writing (i.e. a statement of wishes and preferences; see Box 13.A, p.408), through behaviour or habits; any religious, cultural or moral beliefs or values which might be likely to influence the decision.

Identify all relevant circumstances which the person who lacks capacity would take into account if they were making the decision themselves.

Avoid discrimination, e.g. age, appearance, condition or behaviour.

Consult and take into account the views of any welfare attorney, IMCA or court-appointed deputy, and as far as possible and where appropriate, anyone previously named by the person, e.g. carers, close family and friends.

If the decision concerns life-sustaining treatment, it must not be motivated by a desire to bring about the person's death.

When everyone appropriate has been consulted, create a 'balance sheet', listing the advantages and disadvantages of the various options, before making a final decision.

Any concerns or disputes regarding ADRTs, LPAs, decisions made by welfare attorneys, IMCAs or determination of best interests should be discussed with a senior colleague or reviewed in a case conference. If necessary, an application can be made to the Court of Protection (England and Wales) for a ruling. In certain circumstances, the

Court of Protection can appoint a deputy to undertake the role of welfare attorney, for example, where a person has ongoing lack of capacity, is undergoing complex medical treatment and is subject to dispute between family members.

CARDIOPULMONARY RESUSCITATION

General principles
National guidelines outline the general principles and provide a decision-making framework (Figure 13.1) on which local cardiopulmonary resuscitation (CPR) policies should be based. Written information about CPR policies should be readily available to patients and those close to them.[11]

DNAR, Do Not Attempt Cardiopulmonary Resuscitation
When making decisions about CPR:[11]
- it must be tailored to the patient's individual circumstances
- patients should be given opportunities to talk about CPR, but should not be forced to discuss the subject if they do not want to
- the responsibility rests with the senior clinician involved in the patient's care; this is generally a doctor, but can be a senior nurse in nurse-led services, or can be delegated to another competent person
- if possible, the decision should be agreed with the whole clinical team
- if there is doubt or disagreement about whether CPR would be appropriate, a further senior clinical opinion should be sought.

Elucidating the balance of the likely burdens, risks and benefits of CPR for an individual patient is important (Box 13.E). It must not be assumed that the same decision will be appropriate for all patients with a particular condition. The guidance highlights that a blanket policy which denies CPR to groups of patients, e.g. to all patients in a hospice, is unethical and probably unlawful.

Clinicians should familiarize themselves with their local guidelines. The following points in the BMA guidelines contain information of particular relevance to palliative care.[11] Subtle differences exist between England and Wales and other areas of the UK.

Presumption in favour of CPR when there is no DNAR decision
Although the presumption is that health professionals will attempt CPR in the event of cardiorespiratory arrest, the guidelines state that this is clearly inappropriate in patients in the final stages of a terminal illness where death is imminent and unavoidable and CPR would not be successful. Thus, clinicians can make a considered decision not to commence CPR in such circumstances even when no formal DNAR decision has been made.[11]

Clinical decisions not to attempt CPR
If the clinical team believes that CPR will not restart the heart and maintain breathing, it should not be offered or attempted, and a DNAR decision documented in the clinical notes. CPR is unlikely to be successful in patients with a life-limiting illness in their terminal phase.[11]

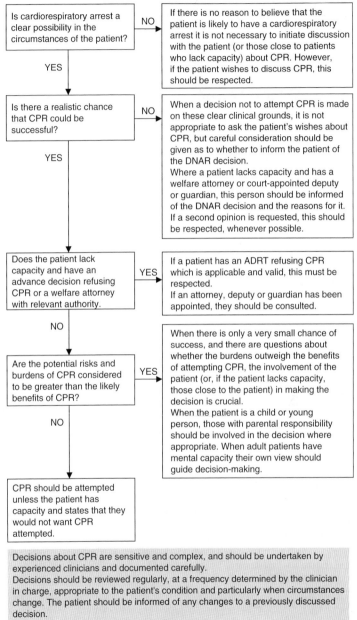

Figure 13.1 Decision-making framework in CPR, adapted from BMA guidelines.[11]

Box 13.E   Background information on CPR

CPR is undertaken in an attempt to restore breathing (sometimes with assisted ventilation) and spontaneous circulation in the patient after cardiorespiratory arrest. The benefits of possibly prolonging life must be weighed against the possible burdens.

It is an invasive medical intervention and generally includes chest compressions, attempted defibrillation with electric shocks, injection of drugs and ventilation of the lungs. In some cases spontaneous cardiac function may be restored with prompt use of an electric shock alone.

In hospital, the survival rate after cardiorespiratory arrest and CPR is low. The chances of surviving to discharge are at best 15–20%, and half that outside hospital.

The probability of success depends on factors including the cause of the arrest, how soon after the arrest CPR is started, and the equipment and staff available.

Undesirable effects of CPR include rib or sternal fractures, hepatic or splenic rupture, and possible treatment subsequently in a coronary care or intensive care unit. This may include artificial ventilation and other life support measures.

There is a risk of brain damage and resulting disability, particularly if there is delay between the arrest and the initiation of CPR.

A decision to attempt CPR does not automatically mean that all other intensive treatments and procedures will also be appropriate. Even if the heart has been restarted, prolonged support for multi-organ failure with artificial ventilation or renal dialysis in an intensive care unit may be clinically inappropriate if the patient already had a very poor prognosis.

CPR may be seen as 'traumatic', with death occurring in a manner which the patient, family and friends would not have wished.

However, even for patients with a DNAR decision, it could still be appropriate to provide CPR for situations that are easily reversible, e.g. choking, blocked tracheostomy tube. If the patient is at high risk of such events, their management should be discussed with the patient and their wishes ascertained.

Prolonging life is not always beneficial. Even when there is a slight chance that CPR may be successful, it is lawful to withhold CPR on the basis that it would not be in the patient's best interests, because the burdens outweigh the benefits. This should be done only after discussion with the patient, or those close to patients who lack capacity, and careful consideration of relevant factors including:
- the likely clinical outcome, including the likelihood of successfully restarting the patient's heart and breathing for a sustained period, and the level of recovery that can realistically be expected after successful CPR
- the patient's known or likely wishes, based on previously expressed views
- feelings, beliefs and values
- the patient's human rights, including the right to life and the right to be free from degrading treatment
- the likelihood of the patient experiencing severe unmanageable pain or suffering
- the level of awareness the patient has of their existence and surroundings.

Communicating DNAR decisions to patients

When a DNAR decision has been made because CPR will not be successful, it is *not* necessary or appropriate to initiate discussion with the patient to explore their wishes regarding CPR, unless the patient expresses a wish to discuss CPR.

The guidelines add that for patients approaching the end of their life, information about interventions which would not be clinically successful is unnecessarily burdensome and of little or no value. In other situations, it is necessary to decide how much information the patient wants to know (or, if the patient lacks capacity, those close to them). If it is decided not to inform the patient, the reason for this should be written in the medical records.

When a patient is informed of a DNAR decision, clinicians should:

- offer as much information as they want in a manner and format which they can understand
- answer questions as honestly as possible
- explain the aims of treatment
- assure them that a DNAR decision applies only to CPR and that all other appropriate treatment and care will continue.

To avoid confusion, it is recommended that DNAR decisions should specify 'do not attempt *cardiopulmonary* resuscitation'.

If a patient without capacity has a welfare attorney whose authority extends to making these clinical decisions, or if there is a court-appointed deputy or guardian with similar authority, this person should be informed of the decision and the reason for it. If a second opinion is requested, this should be arranged, if possible.

Requests for CPR in situations where it would not be successful

Patients, those close to them, a welfare attorney or court-appointed deputy cannot demand a treatment which is clinically inappropriate. The reasons for a DNAR decision should be sensitively explained by a senior clinician. If the decision is still not accepted, a second opinion should be offered. If this fails to resolve a disagreement between the clinical team and a welfare attorney or court-appointed guardian, the Court of Protection can be asked to make a declaration.

Decisions about CPR based on benefits and burdens

When CPR may be successful in restarting the patient's heart and maintaining breathing for a sustained period, the benefits of prolonging life must be weighed against the potential burdens to the patient. This must involve consideration of the patient's broader best interests, including their known or likely wishes. In these circumstances, discussion with the patient about whether CPR should be attempted is an essential part of the decision-making process.

A patient should be informed sensitively of the facts, including the risks and possible undesirable effects, to enable them to make an informed decision (see Box 13.E, p.416). When the patient lacks capacity, the clinical team and those close to the patient must decide what are the patient's best interests (see Box 13.D, p.413). If feasible, it should be explained to the patient that they are informing the decision-making process but that they have no legal authority to make the final decision, which rests with the senior clinician. If the patient has nobody to speak on their behalf, an IMCA should be consulted.

Refusal of CPR

A patient with capacity has the right to refuse any medical treatment, even if that refusal will result in their death. The decision must be respected, but it is necessary to ensure that the patient's decision is based on accurate information and not on any misunderstanding.

Communicating the decision

The clinician making the decision must document it clearly in the medical records. They (or a designated deputy) must also communicate the decision to other relevant health professionals in both primary and secondary care, particularly when the patient is transferred within or between establishments. National guidance to ambulance crews advise that CPR should be attempted, unless:

- there is a formal DNAR decision, or a valid and applicable ADRT
- the patient is known to be terminally ill and is being transferred to a palliative care facility (unless specific instructions to attempt CPR have been received).

Ambulance transfers will thus require the provision of appropriate information/ documentation.

Allow Natural Death

It has been suggested that, in palliative care, the DNAR status should be substituted by 'Allow Natural Death' (AND) because:[12,13]

- it is a positive rather than a negative statement
- there is a clear acknowledgement by all concerned that the patient is imminently dying
- it implies that everything being done for the patient is solely with the aim of making dying as comfortable as possible, but not prolonging it
- it means that artificial nutrition is likely to be discontinued, IV hydration scaled down (or not started), antibacterials strictly limited to symptom relief, and ventilators not considered.

One way of achieving this is to introduce the Liverpool Pathway for Care of the Dying (see p.424).

CONTINUITY OF CARE

Although a health professional may feel powerless in the face of rapidly approaching death, patients are generally more realistic. They know you cannot perform a miracle and time is limited. However, once the patient is faced with the fact that death is inevitable and imminent, support and companionship are of paramount importance.[14] Thus, despite possibly having nothing new to offer, it is important to:

- continue to visit
- quietly indicate that 'At this stage the important thing is to keep you as comfortable as possible'
- simplify medication: 'Now that your husband is not so well, he can probably manage without some of his tablets'
- anticipate a time when the patient will not be able to swallow, and supply drug formulations which can be given SL, PR or SC

- continue to inform the family of the changing situation:
  - ▷ 'He's very weak now, but could still live for several days'
  - ▷ 'Although he seems better today, he's still very weak. He could quickly deteriorate and die within a few days'
- control agitation even if it results in sedation
- listen to the nurses.

Remember: existing symptoms may worsen or new symptoms arise (see p.424). These will necessitate further changes in management, including new measures to ensure the comfort of the patient. Given professional diligence, a peaceful death is generally possible.[15]

WITHHOLDING AND WITHDRAWING LIFE-PROLONGING MEDICAL TREATMENT

In addition to CPR (see p.414), other medical interventions prolong life and, in some circumstances, allow time for recovery when organ or system failure would otherwise result in death, e.g. renal dialysis, artificial nutrition, hydration and ventilation. However, none can reverse a chronic progressive disease process.

In the UK, guidance is available from professional organizations on how to reach a decision about withholding or withdrawing a life-prolonging treatment.[16,17] Guidance from the GMC is currently being revised and updated. As with CPR, similar principles and factors must be taken into account when making a decision.

Those of particular relevance to palliative care include:
- the primary goal of medical treatment is to benefit the patient by restoring or maintaining the patient's health as far as is possible, maximizing benefit and minimizing harm; in the dying patient symptom management and comfort are paramount
- there is no obligation to provide a treatment that cannot achieve this goal and the treatment should, ethically and legally, be withheld or withdrawn
- good quality care and relief of symptoms should continue
- an act where the doctor's intention is to bring about a patient's death is unlawful.

Effective and sensitive communication with all concerned is vital to ensure understanding that:
- it is the underlying disease which is bringing about the death of the patient, not the withholding or withdrawing of a particular treatment
- all care which will enhance the comfort of the patient will continue.

ARTIFICIAL NUTRITION AND HYDRATION

The provision of artificial nutrition or hydration is regarded as a medical treatment and is not part of basic care.[18,19] In the terminal stage, food and fluid intake generally diminish. It is at this time that a relative may ask about the possibility of nutrition or hydration by artificial means.[18]

Artificial nutrition has known risks, and there is no evidence of net benefit to dying patients.[20] This should be explained sensitively to those concerned. Generally, in

UK palliative care practice, this view also extends to artificial hydration. Further, fluid depletion in the dying patient may be beneficial as a result of:

- reduced pulmonary, salivary and GI secretions with a consequent reduction in cough, 'death rattle', and vomiting, and less need for interventions such as oropharyngeal suctioning
- reduced urinary output, and thus less incontinence and less need for an indwelling urinary catheter
- less oedema and ascites with fewer associated symptoms.

Several studies suggest that thirst correlates poorly with fluid intake,[21–25] and dry mouth can generally be relieved by conscientious mouth care and small amounts of fluid, e.g. 1–2mL of water delivered by pipette or syringe into the dependent side of the mouth every 30–60min. Small ice chips can also be used.[26]

IV hydration may have negative psychosocial effects in that the infusion acts as a barrier between the patient and the family. It is more difficult to embrace a spouse who is attached to a plastic tube, and doctors and nurses tend to become diverted from the more human aspects of care to the control of fluid balance and electrolytes.[27]

Opinions differ about fluid administration.[28–33] This reflects the heterogeneity of attitudes of clinicians, ethicists, patients, those close to them and local practice. Proponents of fluid therapy argue hydration decreases the risk of symptoms such as:

- delirium, or opioid toxicity, especially if renal failure develops
- sedation and myoclonus
- constipation, pressure sores and dry mouth.[34–37]

However, in two RCTs, hydration did not reduce the incidence of delirium.[22,36] Further, dry mouth is a common problem in cancer patients, and is related to several factors other than dehydration, e.g. drugs, oxygen therapy, and mouth breathing.[25,38–40] In most patients, artificial hydration alone is unlikely to resolve dry mouth.[23]

A systematic review of the literature on fluid status in the dying concluded that there was insufficient evidence to draw firm conclusions about either the beneficial or harmful effects of fluid administration in dying patients.[41] Such conflicting data emphasize the need for individual evaluation and review in keeping with professional guidance. When there is uncertainty about the potential benefit of artificial hydration, a time-limited trial with specific goals could be undertaken, for example, give parenteral fluid for 48h, and see if the patient's delirium improves.[11,17]

VOLUNTARY REFUSAL OF FOOD AND FLUID

Most patients with advanced life-limiting disease sooner or later become anorexic (see p.77). Food intake becomes less, often the result of cachexia, or simply associated with extreme weakness and disinterest. Particularly when a patient is deteriorating on a daily basis, it is important to prevent 'forced feeding' by the family or other carers.

However, sometimes a patient voluntarily and deliberately stops taking both food and fluid with the primary intention of hastening death.[42–44] Generally, patients pursue this option for one or more of the following closely-related reasons:

- feel ready to die
- consider continued existence pointless
- quality of life poor
- a desire to be in control.

It is necessary to explore with a patient the reasons for their decision. Occasionally it is because of misunderstandings which, if resolved, results in a change of mind. However, if a patient with capacity confirms their intention, it is a legal obligation to respect this decision.[45]

Discussion between both doctor and nurse on the one hand and the family on the other is clearly also important. If not already discussed between themselves, the family is likely to need time to work through their immediate distressed reaction before they are willing to 'come on side'. Thus, for example, suggest that everybody thinks about it for 2 days and then discusses the matter again. This may prevent a lot of distress within the family and reduce the possibility of the family putting pressure on the patient not to go ahead.

In one report of >100 patients who stuck with their decision to refuse food and fluid, 85% died within 2 weeks. Almost all died peacefully (60% had cancer; the rest mainly neurological or cardiorespiratory disease).[44]

The patient should be 'given permission' to change their mind at any time, and to start taking fluid and/or food again without loss of face. In practice, only a few do this. Reasons for a change of mind include:

- family pressure
- hunger discomfort
- lifting of depression
- alleviation of concerns.[44]

'GIVE DEATH A CHANCE'

In patients who are close to death it is often appropriate to 'give death a chance'. All patients must die eventually; ultimately nature will take its course. In this respect, the skill is to decide when the burdens of any life-sustaining treatments are likely to outweigh any benefits, and thus when to allow death to occur without further impediment. Treatments which provide comfort and symptom relief should be continued.

For example, antibacterials are generally appropriate for the patient with advanced cancer who develops a chest infection while still relatively active and independent. However, in those who have become bedbound as a result of general progressive deterioration, and seem close to death, pneumonia should still be allowed to be 'the old person's friend'. In such circumstances it is generally appropriate *not* to prescribe antibacterials (see p.4).

If it is difficult to make a decision, the '2-day rule' should be invoked, namely, if after 2–3 days of straightforward symptom management the patient is clearly holding his own, prescribe an antibacterial but, if the patient is clearly much worse, do not.

If feasible, such decisions should be taken with the patient. If the patient lacks capacity, seek the patient's views from an ADRT, welfare attorney with appropriate powers, or those close to the patient.

On the other hand, not all terminally ill patients who develop a chest infection die from it. Some patients progress only to a 'grumbling pneumonia' but no further. A continuing wet cough may cause much distress and, possibly, loss of sleep. In circumstances when the patient is neither better nor worse after 3–4 days, an antibacterial may well be indicated for symptom relief.

DYING AT HOME

Dying in comfort at home is possible, but generally requires:
- family or community support for the patient
- someone to be present to care for the patient
- empowerment of the family or community member, e.g. by providing information, support and access to help
- ready availability of professional support, e.g. visits from the primary healthcare or palliative care team, telephone advice
- access to appropriate medications
- access to appropriate practical aids, e.g. wheelchair, commode, pressure relieving mattress
- access to inpatient care if needed, e.g. for a period of time to manage symptoms.

Advance planning is vital. In the UK the Gold Standards Framework is a nationally recommended tool to support high quality palliative and terminal care in primary care.[46–48] This facilitates:
- identification of patients approaching the end of life in need of palliative care
- evaluation of their care needs and preferences
- planning of their care
- communication across all relevant agencies throughout.

The Framework focuses on optimizing continuity of care, teamwork, advanced planning (including 'out of hours'), symptom management and patient carer and staff support. It can be used for any life-limiting disease and in care homes.

Planning for the last days will require an understanding by the patient and the family of what might happen and of available resources. Open and honest communication and regular support are vital. Ideally, this will include routine home visits from the primary health $\pm$ palliative care teams as well as being available for any emergency. If possible, indicate when the next home visit will be:

'I'll call in again next Wednesday, possibly between 12noon and 3pm. If I can't, I'll phone and let you know.'

Generally, the patient and family will feel better supported by this approach compared with one where the professional offers a visit at any time 'if you have any problems'.

Most situations are manageable in the home, although even carefully made plans may turn out to be inadequate. Particularly towards the end, the situation can change rapidly. Common problems, notably delirium (see p.207) and death rattle (see p.427), should be discussed with the relatives so as to prepare them psychologically and practically.

Generally, a point is reached when the patient will no longer be able to swallow reliably. The continuing administration of essential medicines needs to be anticipated and alternatives put in place. These include:

- intermittent SC bolus or by CSCI (this is the norm in the UK)
- sublingual or buccal administration, e.g. depositing a liquid concentrate into the dependent cheek of the moribund patient
- the rectal route, in patients not troubled by diarrhoea.

Ideally, a supply of drugs in injectable or suppository form should be prescribed and made available in the home in case they are needed, either for terminal symptoms or in the event of an emergency such as a seizure or massive haemorrhage.[49] Some services/associations promote the use of kits containing small quantities of a range of drugs for emergency use, e.g. 'Just in case' kit, MND 'breathing space kit'.[50,51] Care of the dying pathways, e.g. Liverpool Care Pathway (LCP), also prompt anticipatory prescribing.[52]

Despite earlier expressing a wish to be cared for at home, many patients and families change their minds as the disease progresses. In a group of patients receiving palliative care at home in the UK, preference for home care eventually fell to about 1/2.[53] Ultimately:

- about 1/3 died at home
- about 1/3 were admitted 1–3 days before death
- about 1/3 were inpatients for longer periods.

It remains to be seen if advance care plans, e.g. Preferred Place of Care, will successfully focus professional efforts and resources to allow more patients to die at home.

DIAGNOSING IMMINENT DEATH

Estimating prognosis is difficult, even when death may be fairly imminent.[54–57] A number of variables have been associated with decreased survival in patients with cancer (Box 13.F).[56,58–60]

Box 13.F Factors associated with decreased survival in cancer patients[58]

Clinical features	Biological factors	Other
Anorexia	Anaemia	Co-morbidity
Ascites	Raised CRP	Single status
Breathlessness	Hypo-albuminaemia	Older age
Delirium	Raised LDH	Poor performance status
Dry mouth	Leucocytosis	Metastatic disease
Dysphagia	Lymphocytopenia	Primary site of cancer, e.g.
Fever	Proteinuria	SCLC, ovary, pancreas,
Nausea	Hypercalcaemia	glioblastoma
Oedema	Hyponatraemia	
Pain		
Tachycardia		
Tiredness		
Weight loss		

Using such variables, attempts have been made to produce a reliable prognostic index. However, even the best of the currently available scales, the PaP score, provides only general guidance based on probability. Thus, patients are categorized as having a probability of >70%, 30–70% or <30% of surviving 30 days.[58]

Fortunately, in practice, the following 'rule' is generally an accurate enough guide to prognosis in advanced cancer. If a patient is deteriorating (without an obvious reversible cause):

- month by month, they probably have several months to live
- week by week, they probably have only weeks to live
- day by day, they probably have only days to live.

Further, in the absence of a reversible cause for the deterioration, the following features collectively indicate that a patient almost certainly has only days to live:

- physically wasted and profoundly weak → bedbound
- drowsy for much of the day → coma
- very limited attention span → disoriented (→ delirium)
- unable to take tablets or has great difficulty swallowing them
- little or no oral intake of food and fluid.[23,61]

LIVERPOOL CARE PATHWAY FOR THE DYING PATIENT

The Liverpool Care Pathway (LCP) for the dying patient is a nationally recommended tool to support high-quality terminal care.[46] Although initially for patients dying from cancer in hospital, it is increasingly used in other settings, and for patients dying from other life-limiting diseases.[52]

At the most basic level, the LCP is a way of acknowledging that death is almost certainly imminent, and that it is now necessary and appropriate to focus primarily (but not necessarily exclusively) on comfort measures.[62–64] A standard protocol is used, which becomes a part of the patient's clinical records. This includes a checklist of things to be considered, e.g.:

- *simplifying medication*: particularly stopping long-term prophylactic medication, e.g. statins, warfarin, antihypertensives, oral hypoglycaemics
- *anticipatory prescribing*: using the guidelines supplied to prescribe p.r.n. medication should the patient develop symptoms such as pain, breathlessness, vomiting, delirium, and ensuring that generally drugs are prescribed both PO and SC/IV
- *IV hydration*: is it still appropriate? Can it be stopped?
- *communication*: discuss the changing situation with the patient's family.

Similar care pathways have been used elsewhere, e.g. in the USA.[65–67]

SYMPTOM RELIEF

Symptom relief in the last days of a patient's life is generally a continuation of what is already being done. However, previously well-managed symptoms can recur or new symptoms develop.[15,68–71] The same principles of management apply as before (see p.6). However, because time is short, there is a greater need for urgency on the part of the caring team.

General considerations

When death is close, medication should be simplified. Those providing no symptomatic benefit can be discontinued. In the last few days it is often appropriate to discontinue laxatives and antidepressants.

In patients with insulin-dependent diabetes mellitus, the dose of insulin should be reduced as oral intake diminishes and the regimen simplified. However, a decision to stop insulin completely should normally be taken only after discussion with the patient (if still has capacity) and the family. It is generally appropriate to stop insulin injections completely when the patient has become irreversibly unconscious as part of the dying process, and not because of hypoglycaemia or diabetic keto-acidosis, and when all other life-prolonging treatments have been stopped.[72]

If it is felt strongly that the insulin should be continued, a simple regimen of once daily long-acting, or b.d. intermediate-acting insulin can be used, with the minimum of routine monitoring, i.e. once daily.[73]

Similarly, in the last days, some nursing procedures which are normally regarded as essential may be discontinued. For example, care of pressure areas may cause a moribund patient to become distressed. If so, such care should be reduced or stopped.

Incontinence and retention of urine

In patients close to death, incontinence is generally best managed by an indwelling urinary catheter.[74] This provides maximum comfort with minimum ongoing disturbance.

A loaded rectum may well be the cause of retention in dying patients. This may necessitate treatment with a laxative suppository, an enema, or digital evacuation of the rectum.

Stopping dexamethasone in patients with intracranial malignancy
See p.285.

Pain
Also see Chapter 2.

About 90% of patients dying from cancer require a strong opioid. Data from several specialist palliative care centres, expressed in oral morphine equivalents, indicate that:
- the median dose in the last 24h of life is 50–150mg
- individual dose requirements vary widely, e.g. 20mg–2g/24h.[75–77]

At one centre, over the course of an admission until death, the dose was increased in about 2/3, decreased in about 1/3 and unchanged in a few. The overall median increase in daily dose was about 20mg (a median increase of 50%).[77] Generally, a single increase in the dose of the strong opioid is all that is necessary.[71]

However, patients in specialist palliative care units often have more challenging symptoms, and may have received opioids for some time. In non-specialist settings, the proportion of patients and the dose required are likely to be correspondingly less. Thus, in a hospital survey:
- only 2/3 of patients dying from all causes required a strong opioid
- the median dose in the last 24h of life, expressed in oral morphine equivalents, was 30mg, ranging from 7.5–90mg.[77,78]

Generally, pain will not be troublesome at the very end if relief has previously been good. However, even when the patient is close to death, careful evaluation is still necessary. Dying patients may call out to check whether someone is with them or when they are aware that they are unattended. These cries may be misinterpreted as pain, and be a source of concern to family and carers.

Some patients show signs of discomfort when being turned in bed, even when apparently deeply unconscious, and may moan or cry out. Although this may be pain caused by joint stiffness for example, it could instead be an 'alarm response' to an unexpected disturbance. Disturbance distress is likely to be reduced by warning a patient (even when unconscious) of any intended interventions by describing the procedure to be undertaken, and by gentle slow handling.

Even so, new pains are relatively common in the last days.[71] Causes include:
- painful bedsore (consider the local application of a local anaesthetic gel $\pm$ topical morphine)
- distended bladder (relieve by catheterization)
- NSAID withdrawal (restart by a non-oral route).

Most patients experience difficulty in swallowing PO medication in the last days of life. Continuation of a regular strong opioid by an alternative route is the norm in this circumstance. Abrupt discontinuation risks a return of pain $\pm$ withdrawal symptoms. e.g. restlessness, diarrhoea.

Patients who have been taking an NSAID for metastatic bone pain may suffer a recurrence of pain after 12–24h if the NSAID is discontinued when swallowing tablets is no longer possible. Some NSAIDs are available in liquid, suppository or injection formulations, allowing them to be administered in this circumstance.

Severe breathlessness in the last days of life
Also see Chapter 4.

Patients often fear suffocating to death and a positive approach to the patient, their family and colleagues about the relief of terminal breathlessness is important:
- no patient should die with distressing breathlessness
- failure to relieve terminal breathlessness is a failure to utilize drug treatment correctly.

Because of the distress, inability to sleep and exhaustion, patients and their carers generally accept that drug-related drowsiness may need to be the price paid for greater comfort. However, unless there is overwhelming distress, deep sedation (reduced awareness/consciousness) is not the initial step. Some patients become mentally brighter when anxiety is reduced by light sedation, and there is an associated improvement in their breathlessness.

Even so, because increasing drowsiness also generally reflects a deteriorating clinical condition, it is important to stress the gravity of the situation and the aim of treatment to the relatives.

Drug treatment typically comprises:[79]
- parenteral administration of an opioid and a sedative-anxiolytic, e.g. morphine and midazolam or lorazepam by CSCI and p.r.n.
- haloperidol if the patient develops an agitated delirium (may be aggravated by a benzodiazepine (see Box 13.H, p.433).

Death rattle

Death rattle is a term used to describe noisy rattling breathing which occurs in about 50% of patients near the end of life.[80] It is caused by fluid pooling in the hypopharynx, and arises from one or more sources:
- saliva (most common)
- respiratory tract infection
- pulmonary oedema
- gastric reflux.

Rattling breathing can also occur in patients with a tracheostomy and infection. Because the patient is generally semiconscious or unconscious, drug treatment for death rattle is mainly for the benefit of relatives, other patients and staff.

Non-drug treatment

- ease the family's distress by explaining that the semiconscious/unconscious patient is not distressed by the rattle[80,81]
- position the patient semiprone to encourage postural drainage; but upright or semirecumbent if the cause is pulmonary oedema or gastric reflux
- oropharyngeal suction but, because it is distressing to many moribund patients, generally reserve for unconscious patients.

Drug treatment

For more information, see PCF3.

Saliva

An antimuscarinic is the drug of choice. This needs to be given promptly because it does not affect existing pharyngeal secretions. Such drugs are probably most effective for rattle associated with the pooling of saliva in the pharynx and least effective for rattle caused by bronchial secretions (as a result of infection or oedema) or related to the reflux of gastric contents.

In the UK, in this circumstance, antimuscarinics are generally given SC (Table 13.1). However, in some countries, the SL route is preferred. For example, glycopyrronium 0.01% oral solution prepared locally from glycopyrronium powder, 1mL (100microgram) SL q6h p.r.n.

Table 13.1 Antimuscarinic antisecretory drugs for death rattle: typical SC doses

Drug	Stat SC dose	CSCI dose/24h
Glycopyrronium	200microgram	600–1,200microgram
Hyoscine *hydrobromide*	400microgram	1,200–2,400microgram
Hyoscine *butylbromide*	20mg	20–120mg

Note:
- by injection, the efficacy of the different drugs is broadly similar; the rattle is reduced in 1/2–2/3 of patients[80]
- the onset of action of glycopyrronium is slower compared with hyoscine *hydrobromide*[82]

- hyoscine *hydrobromide* crosses the blood-brain barrier and possesses anti-emetic and sedative properties,[82] but there is also a risk of developing or exacerbating delirium
- atropine also dries secretions and, like hyoscine, it crosses the blood-brain barrier but it tends to stimulate rather than sedate, and could increase the need for midazolam or haloperidol.

Respiratory tract infection
Occasionally it is appropriate to prescribe an antibacterial in an imminently dying patient if death rattle is caused by profuse purulent sputum associated with an underlying chest infection:

- e.g. ceftriaxone, mix 1g ampoule with 2.1mL lidocaine 1% (total volume 2.6–2.8mL), and give 250mg–1g SC/IM once daily
- some centres use larger volumes of lidocaine 1% (up to 4mL) and administer a divided dose at separate SC/IM sites once daily or b.d.

Pulmonary oedema
Consider furosemide 20–40mg SC/IM/IV q2h p.r.n. Beware precipitating urinary retention.

Gastric reflux
Consider metoclopramide 20mg SC/IV q3h p.r.n., but do not use with an antimuscarinic because the latter blocks the prokinetic effect of the former.

Rattling breathing causing distress to a patient
In a semiconscious patient, if rattling breathing is associated with breathlessness, supplement the above with an opioid (e.g. morphine) ± an anxiolytic sedative (e.g. midazolam).

Noisy tachypnoea in the moribund
Noisy tachypnoea in the moribund is distressing for the family and other patients, even though the patient is not aware. It represents a desperate last attempt by a patient's body to respond to irreversible terminal respiratory failure ± airway obstruction.

Consider alleviating the noise by reducing the depth and rate of respiration to 10–15/min with diamorphine/morphine, best initially titrated IV to identify an effective dose. This may be double, or even treble, the previously satisfactory analgesic dose.

When there is associated heaving of the shoulders and chest, midazolam should be given as well, e.g. 5–10mg IV. The diamorphine/morphine ± midazolam can be repeated IV/SC hourly as needed.

Severe acute stridor as a terminal event
This may be caused by haemorrhage into a tumour pressing on the trachea. Administer diazepam/midazolam IV until the patient is asleep (5–20mg). If IV administration is not possible, alternatives include midazolam 10mg IM or diazepam solution 10mg PR.

Myoclonus
Multifocal myoclonus is a central pre-epileptiform phenomenon (see p.279). It is exacerbated by hypoglycaemia and, in the moribund, may be caused or exacerbated by dopamine antagonists (antipsychotics, metoclopramide) and opioids (particularly

at higher doses) or as a result of drug withdrawal (benzodiazepines, barbiturates, anti-epileptics, alcohol).

It is seen in cancer patients dying with encephalopathy associated with organ failure, e.g. renal failure, hepatic failure. It occurs with cerebral oedema and hypoxia, and also with hyponatraemia. Treat with a benzodiazepine (see p.279).

Generalized convulsive seizures
See p.279.

Delirium
Delirium develops in 80–90% of dying cancer patients at some stage during the last week of life.[83,84] Delirium is generally best treated with haloperidol ± midazolam given p.r.n. or by CSCI in an individually optimized dose. If delirium is not controlled on haloperidol 10–15mg/24h, a more sedating antipsychotic should be given instead, e.g. SC levomepromazine (see Box 13.H, p.433).

INTOLERABLE SUFFERING

'A realistic goal in palliative care is not to eliminate suffering but rather to alleviate it.'[85]

Palliative care professionals have to cope with the fact that it is not always possible to achieve 'a good death' for our patients (Box 13.G). Consider the patient with an eroded malodorous face or perineum.[86] There are times when a person's distress (or that of their family) seems unbearable.

Box 13.G   Where was God?[a]

Where was God when Brian shat from his mouth?
Where was God when Elsie's belly eroded
And liquid faeces rolled over her loins, soiled her sacred pubis
And soaked the sheets of her bed?
Where was God when spinster Jill couldn't fart or crap,
Blew up like the expectant mum we believe she never was
And cursed us all, supposedly behind our backs,
Hurling insults and expletives through the side-room door
On our departures, destroying our All
And filling other patients with fear?
I simply don't know where God was.
All I know is that God was there.

---

a. by John Chambers, Specialist in Palliative Medicine.

Indeed, a doctor who has never been tempted to deliberately kill a distressed dying patient probably has had limited clinical experience or is not able to empathize with those who suffer. Further, it could be claimed that a doctor who leaves a

---

patient to suffer intolerably is morally more reprehensible than the doctor who performs euthanasia. This does not necessarily mean that euthanasia (intentional drug-induced death) should be a legally enshrined 'human right' for dying patients.[87,88] However, it does mean that we must heed the emancipation principle of palliative care:

'No efforts should be spared to free dying persons from intolerable suffering which invades and dominates their consciousness, and leaves no space for other things'.[89]

This principle stems from society's general commission to health professionals to relieve suffering. And occasionally the only possible way of easing the person's intractable and overwhelming distress is to decrease a patient's awareness deliberately, even to the point of drug-induced coma (see below).[90-92]

PALLIATIVE SEDATION

Palliative sedation is a term used to describe the intentional drug-induced reduction of awareness/consciousness in a patient who is imminently and irreversibly dying in order to relieve an otherwise intolerable refractory symptom.[20,93,94] The term implies the use of appropriate sedative drugs titrated carefully to the cessation of symptoms, not the cessation of life (Table 13.2).

Table 13.2   Comparison of palliative sedation and euthanasia[a]

	Palliative sedation	Euthanasia
Intention	Relief by reducing awareness	Relief by killing the patient
Method	Dose titration	Standard doses
Drugs	Sedative	Lethal cocktail
Proportionate	Yes	No
Criterion of success	Relief of distress	Immediate death

a. but if not imminently dying, continuous deep sedation = *slow euthanasia* unless time-limited + hydration. On the other hand, if death is imminent, artificial hydration is irrelevant, and is best discouraged.

Palliative sedation is an extreme treatment, for 'when all else has failed'. Although the incidence appears to vary widely, particularly from country to country,[90,95] some of the variation relates to imprecise definition.[20,96] In the Netherlands, a recent national study suggested that 7% of all deaths in 2005 were preceded by palliative sedation.[97] In contrast, in a palliative care centre in Belgium, the incidence fell from 7% in 1999 to 2.5% in 2005.[94] The decrease was attributed to an improved standard of palliative care and a team approach to decision-making.

Regrettably, sometimes palliative sedation is implemented with insufficient justification.[98] However, local guidelines should help to minimize this.[20,99]

Indications for palliative sedation

The commonest indications for palliative sedation are:

- agitated delirium
- breathlessness
- pain.[20,90]

In Japan, 1% of palliative care patients are deeply sedated primarily or solely because of persistent intolerable existential distress (see p.432).[100]

Prevent the preventable

As always, prevention is better than cure. Because of present psychological turmoil, or past repressed bad experiences, the following are possibly at higher risk of developing a severe agitated delirium:

- adolescents and young adults
- parents with young children
- Armed Forces veterans
- concentration camp survivors
- victims of abuse or torture
- those who continue to deny that they are dying despite unremitting deterioration.

Ideally, patients in these categories (and anyone else manifesting severe emotional/existential distress) should be evaluated by a clinical psychologist, psychotherapist, or liaison psychiatrist, and continuing support provided if possible.

Further, the early recognition and prompt treatment of delirium may prevent matters from escalating out of control (see p.207).

Relieve physical symptoms

Palliative sedation is not an alternative to the provision of high quality palliative care. All feasible efforts must be made to relieve physical symptoms, e.g. pain or breathlessness, with appropriate non-drug and drug treatments, and advice sought from colleagues before concluding that a symptom is 'refractory'.

Choice of sedative drugs in the imminently dying

Note:
- mild delirium is not always easy to detect
- an antipsychotic is essential if a patient manifests features suggestive of delirium
- the use of a benzodiazepine alone may precipitate or exacerbate delirium[101]
- if in doubt, treat an agitated imminently dying patient with both an antipsychotic and midazolam.

Good practice dictates a step-by-step approach (Figure 13.2 and Box 13.H). Thus, sedation is not 'all or none' but a continuum, with p.r.n. sedation at one end and continuous deep sedation at the other.

Abrupt deep sedation is rarely necessary, e.g. sudden massive arterial haemorrhage. Particularly for existential distress, respite deep sedation for a few hours (up to 1–2 days in some centres) is an important intermediate step.

In the imminently dying, it is uncommon to lighten the depth of the sedation once the patient is settled. However, at one centre, after the patient's distress has been

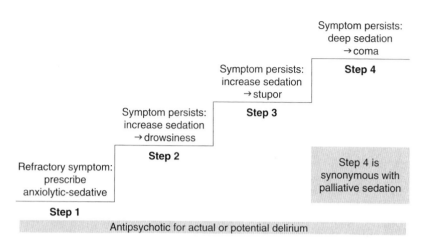

Figure 13.2 Progressive and proportionate treatment for an intolerable refractory symptom in the imminently dying.

relieved, medication is scaled down so that the patient is physically and mentally comfortable (albeit drowsy/sleeping for most/all of the time) but can be roused for short periods to permit meaningful communication: 'our target in sedation is calming and comfort without lowering the level of consciousness deep enough to lose communication.'[92]

REFRACTORY EXISTENTIAL DISTRESS

Suffering has been defined as a state of severe distress caused by events which threaten a person's sense of integrity or intactness.[103] When defined in this way, it becomes self-evident that suffering can occur in the absence of any physical symptoms whatsoever. Bystanders may also suffer when obliged to witness helplessly someone else's pain, particularly that of a loved one. Indeed, helplessness in itself is a potent source of suffering.[104]

There are occasions when a dying patient may be physically comfortable but mentally severely distressed. The question then arises: is it legitimate to escalate to continuous deep sedation in someone who is experiencing intolerable existential suffering?

Logically the answer is 'yes', but following through the logic can be profoundly disturbing to health professionals. This is particularly so when, although 'terminally ill', the person does not completely fit the pen portrait of an imminently dying patient (see p.427):

• what if the patient's prognosis is 2–3 weeks/months, rather than 2–3 days?
• can we be sure that the existential suffering is refractory?
• should artificial hydration and nutrition be provided?

Box 13.H   Drugs for sedation in the imminently dying

For more information, see *PCF3*.

First-line drugs
Midazolam
- start with 5–10mg stat and q1h p.r.n.
- if necessary, increase progressively to 20mg SC/IV stat
- maintain with CSCI/CIVI 10–60mg/24h.

Although some centres, if necessary, titrate the dose of midazolam up to 200mg/24h,[92] it is probably better to add in an antipsychotic if midazolam 30–40mg/24h is inadequate to settle the patient.

Haloperidol
- start with 5–10mg q1h p.r.n. (2.5–5mg q4h in the elderly)
- if necessary, increase progressively to 10mg IV stat
- maintain with CSCI/CIVI 10–20mg/24h.

Second-line drugs
Levomepromazine
Generally given only if it is intended to reduce the patient's level of consciousness:
- start with 25mg SC stat and q1h p.r.n. (12.5mg in the elderly)
- if necessary, titrate dose according to response
- maintain with 50–300mg/24h CSCI.

Although high-dose levomepromazine (⩾100mg/24h) is generally best given by CSCI, smaller doses can be conveniently given as an SC bolus at bedtime or b.d., and p.r.n.

If levomepromazine is not available, use chlorpromazine; doses generally need to be higher, e.g. double those of levomepromazine.

Third-line drugs
Phenobarbital
Because of the irritant nature of the injection, stat doses are generally given IM/IV, but can be followed by CSCI:
- start with 100–200mg IM/IV stat and q1h–q2h p.r.n.
- maintain with 600–1,200mg/24h CSCI (dilute with WFI, e.g. 10mL per 200mg ampoule; if necessary, changing the syringe every 8–12h)
- if necessary, increase the dose to 2,400mg/24h.

Propofol
Some centres use propofol instead of phenobarbital. This is a specialist only treatment, and necessitates an IVI and appropriate variable-rate syringe driver.[102]

Experienced professional palliative carers will all have had patients seemingly trapped in refractory existential suffering but who over time (2–3 months, or even longer) have worked through to either a neutral acquiescence in, or a more positive acceptance of, their predicament.[105,106]

In a report from palliative care services throughout Japan, 1% of patients (about 90/9,000) were treated by continuous deep sedation for refractory existential distress.[100] The reasons given were:
• meaninglessness/worthlessness
• burden on others/dependency
• death anxiety
• the patient's need to remain in control
• lack of social support/isolation.

Prerequisites for continuous deep sedation for existential distress
Although continuous deep sedation for refractory existential distress is disturbing to most health professionals, there will be occasions when doctors and/or nurses will find themselves being inexorably drawn towards it.[107] Thus clear criteria for its application should be established:
• the designation of symptoms as refractory must be done only after repeated skilled psychological evaluation
• the decision must be made by the team because individual feelings or burn-out can bias decision-making
• sedate initially on a respite (intermittent) basis.[108]

Respite deep sedation should also be approached on a step-by-step basis. For example, initially offer the patient an afternoon sleep for several hours, in addition to 7–8h at night, by prescribing an after-lunch 'night' sedative:

'Because of the effort needed to cope with an ongoing illness, I can see that both your physical and psychological stamina are at a low point. And that 16 continuous hours awake each day is too much for your present resources. What I suggest we do is to give you a night sedative after lunch each day, so that you can sleep for at least 2–3 hours in the afternoons. This will break up the long 16-hour stretch, and that will be helpful...'.

This may be enough. But sometimes, as a further step, a more prolonged period of deep sedation for, say, 48h becomes necessary. In the report from Japan, >90% progressed to continuous deep sedation only after periods of respite deep sedation.[100] The following data are also noteworthy:
• >50% were stated to be depressed (not all of whom were prescribed antidepressants)
• only 35% had specialist psychological evaluation
• <60% received specialist psychiatric, psychological or religious support.[100]

Survival after the initiation of continuous deep sedation for refractory existential distress varied widely:
• about 2/3 = <1 week
• about 1/3 = >1 week, <1 month
• only 1 patient > 1 month.[100]

Although not stated, some, if not all, patients would have received IV hydration throughout this time.

It is important that health professionals continue to feel uncomfortable about continuous deep sedation for refractory existential distress.[94,109] The following words from the 1950s are still relevant:

'Patients tend to be sedated when the carers have reached the limit of their resources and are no longer able to stand the patient's problems without anxiety, impatience, guilt, anger or despair. Perhaps many of the desperate treatments in medicine can be justified by expediency, but history has an awkward habit of judging some as fashions, more helpful to the therapist than to the patient.'[110]

WHEN ALL HAS BEEN SAID AND DONE

Palliative care developed as a reaction to the attitude, spoken or unspoken, that 'There's nothing more we can do for you', with the inevitable consequence for the patient and family of a sense of abandonment, hopelessness and despair. It was stressed that this is never true; there is always something which can be done. Even so, there are times when the doctor or nurse feels that they have nothing more to offer. In this circumstance one is thrown back on who one is as an individual:

'Slowly, I learn about the importance of powerlessness.
I experience it in my own life and I live with it in my work.
The secret is not to be afraid of it – not to run away.
The dying know we are not God.
All they ask is that we do not desert them.'[111]

When there is nothing to offer except ourselves, a belief that life has meaning and purpose helps to sustain the carer. However, to speak glibly of this to a patient who is in despair is cruel. At such times, actions speak louder than words. The essential message is conveyed by the words of Cicely Saunders:

You matter because you are you.
You matter to the last moment of your life,
and we will do all we can,
not only to help you die peacefully,
but to live until you die.

1 Agency for Healthcare Research and Quality (2007) Advance care planning. Preferences for care at the end of life. Available from: www.ahrq.gov/populations/eolix.htm
2 Austin Health (2007) Respecting Patient Choice: An advance care planning program. Available from: www.respectingpatientchoices.org.au
3 Royal College of Physicians of London (2009) Concise guidance to good practice number 12: National guidelines advance care planning. Available from: www.rcplondon.ac.uk
4 Lancashire and South Cumbria Cancer Network Preferred Place of Care Plan. NHS. Available from: www.cancerlancashire.org.uk/ppc.html
5 NICE (2004) Improving supportive and palliative care for adults with cancer. In: London. National Institute for Clinical Excellence. Available from: www.nice.org.uk
6 Univesity of Nottingham (2007) Advance Care Planning: A Guide for Health and Social Care Staff. NHS. Available from: www.endoflifecare.nhs.uk
7 ADRT (2007) Advance Decisions to Refuse Treatment. NHS. Available from: www.adrtnhs.co.uk
8 National Council for Palliative Care/National End of Life Care Programme (2008) Advance Decisions to Refuse Treatment. A Guide for Health and Social Care Professionals. Available from: http://www.endoflifecareforadults.nhs.uk/eolc/files/NHS_NEoLC_ADRT_082008.pdf

9 Anonymous (2000) Adults with Incapacity (Scotland) Act. Available from: www.scotland-legislation.hmso. gov.uk/legislation/scotland/acts2000

10 Anonymous (2005) Mental Capacity Act 2005: Elizabeth II. Chapter 9 Reprinted May and December 2006; May 2007. Available from: www.opsi.gov.uk/acts/acts2005/20050009.htm

11 BMA (2007) Decisions relating to cardiopulmonary resuscitation. British Medical Association, The Resuscitation Council (UK) and the Royal College of Nursing. Available from: www.bma.org.uk/ap.nsf/ Content/CPRDecisions07

12 Venneman SS et al. (2008) "Allow natural death" versus "do not resuscitate": three words that can change a life. Journal of Medical Ethics. 34: 2–6.

13 Meyer C A new designation for allowing natural death (AND). Hospice Patients Alliance. Available from: www.hospicepatients.org/and.html

14 Murray SA et al. (2007) Patterns of social, psychological, and spiritual decline toward the end of life in lung cancer and heart failure. Journal of Pain and Symptom Management. 34: 393–402.

15 Fainsinger R et al. (1991) Symptom control during the last week of life on a palliative care unit. Journal of Palliative Care. 7 (1): 5–11.

16 British medical Association (2007) Withholding and Withdrawing Life-prolonging Medical Treatment. Guidance for decision making (3e). Blackwell Publishing, Oxford, UK.

17 General Medical Council (2002) Withholding and Withdrawing Life-prolonging Treatments: Good Practice in Decision Making. Available from: www.gmc-uk.org

18 Campbell C and Partridge R (2007) Artificial nutrition and hydration – guidance in end of life care for adults. National Council for Palliative Care. Available from: http://www.ncpc.org.uk/publications/ pubs_list2.html (subscription only)

19 Morita T et al. (2007) Development of a national clinical guideline for artificial hydration therapy for terminally ill patients with cancer. Journal of Palliative Medicine. 10: 770–780.

20 de Graeff A and Dean M (2007) Palliative sedation therapy in the last weeks of life: a literature review and recommendations for standards. Journal of Palliative Medicine. 10: 67–85.

21 Burge F (1993) Dehydration symptoms of palliative care cancer patients. Journal of Pain and Symptom Management. 8: 454–464.

22 Cerchietti L et al. (2000) Hypodermoclysis for control of dehydration in terminal-stage cancer. International Journal of Palliative Nursing. 6: 370–374.

23 Ellershaw JE et al. (1995) Dehydration and the dying patient. Journal of Pain and Symptom Management. 10: 192–197.

24 McCann RM et al. (1994) A comfort care for terminally ill patients: the appropriate use of nutrition and hydration. Journal of the American Medical Association. 272: 179–181.

25 Musgrave CF et al. (1995) The sensation of thirst in dying patients receiving i.v. hydration. Journal of Palliative Care. 11: 17–21.

26 Billings J (1985) Comfort measures for the terminally ill: is dehydration painful? Journal of the American Geriatrics Society. 808–810.

27 Editorial (1986) Terminal dehydration. Lancet. 1: 306–306.

28 Craig GM (1994) On withholding nutrition and hydration in the terminally ill: has palliative medicine gone too far? Journal of Medical Ethics. 20: 139–143; discussion 144–135.

29 Gillon R (1994) Palliative care ethics: non-provision of artificial nutrition and hydration to terminally ill sedated patients. Journal of Medical Ethics. 20: 131–132, 187.

30 Ashby M and Stoffell B (1995) Artificial hydration and alimentation at the end of life: a reply to Craig. Journal of Medical Ethics. 21: 135–140.

31 Dunlop RJ et al. (1995) On withholding nutrition and hydration in the terminally ill: has palliative medicine gone too far? A reply. Journal of Medical Ethics. 21: 141–143.

32 Dunphy K et al. (1995) Rehydration in palliative and terminal care: if not - why not? Palliative Medicine. 9: 221–228.

33 Craig GM (1996) On withholding artificial hydration and nutrition from terminally ill sedated patients: the debate continues. Journal of Medical Ethics. 22: 147–153.

34 Fainsinger R and Bruera E (1994) The management of dehydration in terminally ill patients. Journal of Palliative Care. 10 (3): 55–59.

35 Bruera E et al. (1995) Changing pattern of agitated impaired mental status in patients with advanced cancer: association with cognitive monitoring, hydration, and opioid rotation. Journal of Pain and Symptom Management. 10: 287–291.

36 Bruera E et al. (2005) Effects of parenteral hydration in terminally ill cancer patients: a preliminary study. Journal of Clinical Oncology. 23: 2366–2371.

37 Lawlor PG et al. (2000) Occurrence, causes, and outcome of delirium in patients with advanced cancer: a prospective study. Archives of Internal Medicine. 160: 786–794.

38 Hanks GW (1983) Management of symptoms in advanced cancer. Update. 26: 1961.

39 Holmes S (1991) The oral complications of specific anticancer therapy. International Journal of Nursing Studies. 28: 343–360.

40 Morita T et al. (2001) Proposed definitions for terminal sedation. Lancet. 358: 335–336.

41 Viola RA et al. (1997) The effects of fluid status and fluid therapy on the dying: a systematic review. Journal of Palliative Care. **13**: 41–52.

42 Quill T et al. (1997) Palliative options of last resort: a comparison of voluntarily stopping eating and drinking, terminal sedation, physician-assisted suicide and voluntary active euthanasia. Journal of the American Medical Association. **278**: 2099–2104.

43 Quill T and Byock I (2000) Responding to intractable terminal suffering: the role of terminal sedation and voluntary refusal of food and fluids. Annals of internal medicine. **132**: 408–414.

44 Ganzini L et al. (2003) Nurses' experiences with hospice patients who refuse food and fluids to hasten death. The New England Journal of Medicine. **349**: 359–365.

45 Sandra J (2003) Death by voluntary dehydration – what the caregivers say. The New England Journal of Medicine. **349**: 325.

46 NICE (2004) Improving supportive and palliative care for adults with cancer. National Institute for Clinical Excellence, London, UK. Available from: www.nice.org.uk

47 Gold Standards Framework A programme for Community Palliative Care. NHS End of Life Care Programme. Available from: www.goldstandardsframework.nhs.uk/

48 Thomas K (2003) Caring for the Dying at Home: Companions on the Journey. Radcliffe Publishing, Oxford.

49 LeGrand S et al. (2001) Dying at home: emergency medications for terminal symptoms. American Journal of Hospice and Palliative Care. **18**: 421–423.

50 Palliativedrugs.com (2007) Research and Guidance Panel. Available from: www.palliativedrugs.com

51 MNDA (2008) Motor Neurone Desease Association. Available from: www.mndassociation.org

52 Liverpool Care Pathway and Marie Curie Cancer Care (2006) The Liverpool Care Pathway for the dying patient. Available from: http://www.mcpcil.org.uk/liverpool_care_pathway

53 Hinton J (1994) Can home care maintain an acceptable quality of life for patients with terminal cancer and their relatives? Palliative Medicine. **8**: 183–196.

54 Glare P et al. (2003) A systematic review of physicians' survival predictions in terminally ill cancer patients. British Medical Journal. **327**: 195–198.

55 Christakis N and Lamont E (2000) Extent and determinants of error in doctors' prognoses in terminally ill patients: prospective cohort study. British Medical Journal. **320**: 469–473.

56 Vigano A et al. (2000) Survival prediction in terminal cancer patients: a systematic review of the medical literature. Palliative Medicine. **14**: 363–374.

57 Ellershaw J and Ward C (2003) Care of the dying patient: the last hours or days of life. British Medical Journal. **326**: 30–34.

58 Stone PC and Lund S (2007) Predicting prognosis in patients with advanced cancer. Annals of Oncology. **18**: 971–976.

59 Maltoni M et al. (2005) Prognostic factors in advanced cancer patients: evidence-based clinical recommendations – a study by the Steering Committee of the European Association for Palliative Care. Journal of Clinical Oncology. **23**: 6240–6248.

60 Chuang RB et al. (2004) Prediction of survival in terminal cancer patients in Taiwan: constructing a prognostic scale. Journal of Pain and Symptom Management. **28**: 115–122.

61 Higgs R (1999) The diagnosis of dying. Journal of the Royal College of Physicians of London. **33**: 110–112.

62 Ellershaw JE and Wilkinson S (eds) (2003) Care of the Dying: A Pathway to Excellence. Oxford University Press, Oxford.

63 Jack BA et al. (2003) Nurses' perceptions of the Liverpool Care Pathway for the dying patient in the acute hospital setting. International Journal of Palliative Nursing. **9**: 375–381.

64 Swart S et al. (2006) Dutch experiences with the Liverpool Care Pathway. European Journal of Palliative Care. **13(4)**: 156–159.

65 Bookbinder M et al. (2005) Improving end-of-life care: development and pilot-test of a clinical pathway. Journal of Pain and Symptom Management. **29**: 529–543.

66 Luhrs CA et al. (2007) Pilot of a pathway to improve the care of imminently dying oncology Inpatients in a Veterans Affairs Medical Center. Journal of Pain and Symptom Management. **29**: 544–551.

67 Ellershaw J (2002) Clinical pathways for care of the dying: an innovation to disseminate clinical excellence. Journal of Palliative Medicine. **5**: 617–621.

68 Exton-Smith AN (1961) Terminal illness in the aged. Lancet **2**: 305–308.

69 Wilkes E (1984) Dying now. Lancet. **1**: 950–952.

70 Ventafridda V et al. (1990) symptom prevalence and control during cancer patients' last days of life. Journal of Palliative Care. **6 (3)**: 7–11.

71 Lichter I and Hunt E (1990) The last 48 hours of life. Journal of Palliative Care. **6(4)**: 7–15.

72 Poulson J (1997) The management of diabetes in patients with advanced cancer. Journal of Pain and Symptom Management. **13**: 339–346.

73 McCann M-A et al. (2006) Practical management of diabetes mellitus. European Journal of Palliative Care. **13**: 226–229.

74 Fainsinger RL et al. (1992) The use of urinary catheters in terminally ill cancer patients. Journal of Pain and Symptom Management. **7**: 333–338.

75 Good PD et al. (2005) Effects of opioids and sedatives on survival in an Australian inpatient palliative care population. Internal Medicine Journal. 35: 512–517.

76 Thorns A and Sykes N (2000) Opioid use in last week of life and implications for end-of-life decision-making. Lancet. 356: 398–399.

77 Wilcock A and Chauhan A (2007) Benchmarking the use of opioids in the last days of life. Journal of Pain and Symptom Management. 34: 1–3.

78 Wilcock A and Chauhan A (2008) Re: Benchmarking the use of opioids in the last days of life. Journal of Pain and Symptom Management. 35: 456–457.

79 Navigante AH et al. (2006) Midazolam as adjunct therapy to morphine in the alleviation of severe dyspnea perception in patients with advanced cancer. Journal of Pain and Symptom Management. 31: 38–47.

80 Hughes A et al. (2000) Audit of three antimuscarinic drugs for managing retained secretions. Palliative Medicine. 14: 221–222.

81 Hughes A et al. (1997) Management of 'death rattle'. Palliative Medicine. 11: 80–81.

82 Back I et al. (2001) A study comparing hyoscine hydrobromide and glycopyrrolate in the treatment of death rattle. Palliative Medicine. 15: 329–336.

83 Massie MJ et al. (1983) Delirium in terminally ill cancer patients. Amercian Journal of Psychiatry. 140: 1048–1050.

84 Bruera E et al. (1987) Delirium and severe sedation in patients with terminal cancer. Cancer Treatment Reports. 71: 787–788.

85 Daneault s et al. (2004) The nature of suffering and its relief in the terminally ill: a qualitative study. Journal of Palliative Care. 20 (1): 7–11.

86 Lawton J (1998) Contemporary hospice care: the sequestration of the unbounded body and 'dirty dying'. Sociology of Health and Illness. 20: 121–143.

87 Twycross RG (1990) Assisted death: a reply. Lancet. 336: 796–798.

88 Twycross RG et al. (2008) Introducing Palliative Care (5e). palliativedrugs.com, Nottingham.

89 Roy DJ (1990) Need they sleep before they die? Journal of Palliative Care. 6: 3–4.

90 Fainsinger RL et al. (2000) A multicentre international study of sedation for uncontrolled symptoms in terminally ill patients. Palliative Medicine. 14: 257–265.

91 Rousseau P (2002) Existential suffering and palliative sedation in terminal illness. Progress in Palliative Care. 10: 222–224.

92 Muller-Busch HC et al. (2003) Sedation in palliative care – a critical analysis of 7 years experience. BMC Palliative Care. 2: 2.

93 Rietjens J et al. (2004) Physician reports of terminal sedation without hydration or nutrition. Annals of internal medicine. 141: 178–185.

94 Claessens P et al. (2007) Palliative sedation and nursing: The place of palliative sedation within palliative nursing care. Journal of Hospice and Palliative Nursing. 9: 100–106.

95 Claessens P et al. (2008) Palliative sedation: a review of the research literature. Journal of Pain and Symptom Management. 36: 310–333.

96 Murray SA et al. (2008) Continuous deep sedation in patients nearing death. British Medical Journal. 336: 781–782.

97 Rietjens J et al. (2008) Continuous deep sedation for patients nearing death in the Netherlands: descriptive study. British Medical Journal. 336: 810–813.

98 Harrison PJ (2008) Continuous deep sedation: Please, don't forget ethical responsibilities. British Medical Journal. 336: 1085.

99 Treloar AJ (2008) Continuous deep sedation: Dutch research reflects problems with the Liverpool Care Pathway. British Medical Journal. 336: 905.

100 Morita T (2004) Palliative sedation to relieve psycho-existential suffering of terminally ill cancer patients. Journal of Pain and Symptom Management. 28: 445–450.

101 Breitbart W et al. (1996) A double-blind trial of haloperidol, chlorpromazine, and lorazepam in the treatment of delirium in hospitalized AIDS patients. American Journal of Psychiatry. 153: 231–237.

102 Lundstrom S et al. (2005) When nothing helps: propofol as sedative and antiemetic in palliative cancer care. Journal of Pain and Symptom Management. 30: 570–577.

103 Cassell E (2003) The Nature of Suffering and the Goals of Medicine (2e). Oxford University Press, Oxford.

104 Cassell EJ (1983) The relief of suffering. Archives of Internal Medicine 143: 522–523.

105 Lichter I (1991) Some psychological causes of distress in the terminally ill. Palliative Medicine. 5: 138–146.

106 Weddington W (1950) Euthanasia. Clinical issues behind the request. Journal of the American Medical Association. 246: 1949–1950.

107 Rousseau P (2001) Existential suffering and palliative sedation: A brief commentary with a proposal for clinical guidelines. American Journal of Hospice and Palliative Care. 18 (3): 151–153.

108 Cherny NI (1998) Commentary: sedation in response to refractory existential distress: walking the fine line. Journal of Pain and Symptom Management. 16: 404–406.

109 Hunt R (2002) Existential suffering and palliative sedation in terminal illness: a comment. Progress in Palliative Care. 10: 225–226.

110 Main T (1957) The ailment. British Journal of Medical Psychology. 30: 129–145.

111 Cassidy S (1988) Sharing the Darkness. Darton, Longman and Todd, London, pp. 61–64.

Index